ZOLLINGER

OXFORD MEDICAL PUBLICATIONS

Geographical and environmental epidemiology

Geographical and Environmental Epidemiology
Methods for Small-Area Studies

Edited by

P. Elliott

Environmental Epidemiology Unit,
Department of Public Health and Policy,
London School of Hygiene and Tropical Medicine

J. Cuzick

Department of Mathematics, Statistics, and Epidemiology,
Imperial Cancer Research Fund,
61 Lincoln's Inn Fields, London

D. English

Department of Public Health,
Queen Elizabeth II Medical Centre,
University of Western Australia

and

R. Stern

World Health Organization,
European Centre for Environment and Health,
Bilthoven, The Netherlands

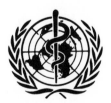

PUBLISHED ON BEHALF OF THE WORLD HEALTH
ORGANIZATION REGIONAL OFFICE FOR EUROPE BY
OXFORD UNIVERSITY PRESS
Oxford   New York   Tokyo
1992

Oxford University Press, Walton Street, Oxford OX2 6DP
Oxford New York Toronto
Delhi Bombay Calcutta Madras Karachi
Kuala Lumpur Singapore Hong Kong Tokyo
Nairobi Dar es Salaam Cape Town
Melbourne Auckland Madrid
and associated companies in
Berlin Ibadan

Oxford is a trade mark of Oxford University Press

Published in the United States
by Oxford University Press Inc., New York

A catalogue record for this book is available from the British Library

Library of Congress Cataloging in Publication Data
Geographical and environmental epidemiology : methods for small-area
studies / edited by P. Elliott . . . [et al.].
(Oxford medical publications)
Includes bibliographical references.
1. Medical geography. 2. Epidemiology. I. Elliott, P. (Paul)
II. Series.
[DNLM: 1. Environmental Exposure—congresses. 2. Environmental
Health—congresses. 3. Epidemiologic Methods—congresses. WA 950 G345]
RA791.G47   1992   614.4'2—dc20   92-13056
ISBN 0 19 262280 3

Typeset by Downdell, Oxford
Printed in Great Britain by
Bookcraft Ltd, Midsomer Norton, Avon

Foreword

Health for all by the year 2000 is the blueprint for change adopted by the Member States of the World Health Organization (WHO). In Europe, this blueprint is built upon 38 regional targets, many of which have the underlying theme of uncovering new knowledge and using existing knowledge more effectively. The targets for a healthy environment are to be achieved by safeguarding human health against environmental hazards, and enhancing the quality of life through the provision of clean and safe water, air, food, and working and living conditions.

These goals are also an integral part of the WHO-initiated European Charter on Environment and Health, adopted by 29 European countries and the Commission of the European Communities in December 1989. The Charter stresses that protecting the environment is the shared responsibility of everyone; it also stresses that everyone should be given adequate and accurate information, and be involved in decision-making. It outlines the principles for public policy as well as what needs to be done to transform them into action. In all this, strong information systems have a vital role to play by helping to monitor the trends analysed and the priorities set, as well as the effectiveness of measures taken and decisions made.

In keeping with the letter and spirit of the Charter, Member States need to develop multisectoral policies that effectively protect the environment from health hazards, ensure community awareness and involvement, and support international efforts to reduce hazards affecting more than one country. Similarly, the machinery for implementing such policies must be developed, especially through the monitoring, assessment, and control of a wide range of potential environmental hazards.

This book is the first to bring together the experience of environmental epidemiologists, statisticians, geographers, and map-makers in a single volume devoted to the study of adverse health outcomes in small areas. It is also one of the first results of the Regional Office's programme on environment and health information systems, which has been generously supported by the German Federal Ministry for the Environment, Nature Conservation and Nuclear Safety, the Italian Ministry of Environment, and the Department of Health in the United Kingdom. This programme is being carried out by a large number of institutions in Europe and coordinated by the WHO European Centre for Environment and Health, a recent extension of the WHO Regional Office for Europe, with operational units in Copenhagen, Bilthoven, and Rome.

The wide use of this book is expected to improve the ability of the European Region to identify environmental priorities and to improve public health planning policy.

J.E. Asvall
Regional Director
WHO Regional Office for Europe

Preface

This book represents a timely convergence of the dramatic growth of public concern about environmental health and the new possibilities for 'micro-epidemiology', resulting from developments in computing technology, statistics, and data.

Epidemiologists have always liked to see maps of the distribution of disease; but these have generally been on a broad scale, or based on inappropriate administrative areas, or displaying case numbers not rates. It is now, for the first time, becoming possible to produce small-area analyses with a quite new efficiency and speed. One result has been a proliferation of reports of disease clusters, which has stimulated advances in statistical methods designed to separate real from chance effects. New questions are also raised concerning the validity of the data themselves when applied to these new questions, the correlation of disease rates with environmental measures, confounding, and many other issues.

Here is an exciting, important, and rapidly developing field, and this book presents experience at its forefront.

London   Geoffrey Rose
February 1991

Introductory remarks by the editors

There is a growing awareness of environmental pollution and its potential effects on health. In particular, concern about the possible adverse health effects of living near to certain industrial or nuclear plants has led to public anxiety and considerable media scrutiny. The apparent tendency for some diseases to 'cluster' has also raised questions about local exposure to environmental hazards. These issues have captured the attention of the public, the scientific community, and the media alike, and their resolution will involve collaboration among public health physicians, epidemiologists, statisticians, toxicologists, and environmentalists.

Epidemiology is crucial to the analysis of relationships between the environment and health. However, traditional epidemiological techniques are ill-suited to detect purely local effects, possibly related to low-level environmental pollution: new epidemiological and analytical methods are required. Small-area studies, in which health (and often environmental exposure) data are analysed with much finer geographical resolution than has hitherto been possible, represent an important new approach to this problem, and promise to enhance our knowledge of environmental hazards and their impact on the health of human populations.

As part of a WHO initiative on small-area health studies, a consultation on 'Data requirements and methods for the analysis of spatial patterns of disease in small areas' was held at the Istituto di Sanita Superiore, Rome, 22–24 October 1990. The scientific programme drew upon many of the leading researchers in this area. For this book, extended contributions were invited from a number of the meeting's participants and further chapters were sought from other experts to give a broad and comprehensive overview. To our knowledge this is the first book to be published summarizing the important new developments in data availability, methodology, and execution of small-area health studies.

The book is divided into five parts. Part I gives an introduction to geographical and small-area studies, and includes an assessment of the role of chemicals and radiation in the aetiology of disease. Part II summarizes data requirements for small-area health studies, including reviews on the use of mortality and morbidity data, denominator (population) data, and exposure data. Chapters are also included in this section on confidentiality, record linkage and data-base management techniques, mapping of disease and of exposure data, and on the problems of socio-economic confounding in ecological studies of small areas. Part III summarizes the currently available statistical methodology and identifies areas for future work in geographical correlation studies, mapping and map smoothing, the analysis of disease risk around a putative 'point source', and the assessment of clustering. Part IV gives an historical perspective of environmental epidemiology, and guidelines on the investigation and interpretation of disease clusters. Part V gives some examples of small-area and geographical correlation studies. These were chosen to demonstrate some of the methodological difficulties involved, as well as to illustrate the type of study that has been undertaken and the range and scope of the geographical approach, especially for small areas.

We have aimed for an up-to-date and authoritative account of recent developments in environmental and geographical epidemiology. Thus we hope that the book will be of interest to practising epidemiologists, geographers, environmentalists, statisticians, toxicologists, and public health physicians concerned with the impact of environmental exposures on the health of populations. We hope also that the book will interest students on undergraduate and postgraduate courses in environmental epidemiology and environmental science, and be a valuable source of reference for more general courses in epidemiology, medical statistics, environmental health, and medical geography. In addition, we anticipate that the book's scope and topicality will make it a useful source of reference for health policy makers, health economists, politicians in the fields of environment and health, and informed lay-persons.

The editors wish to thank Marie-Thérèse Barnes (Imperial Cancer Research Fund) and Alison Willmett (London School of Hygiene and Tropical Medicine) for their invaluable secretarial and administrative support in preparing this volume.

July 1991   P.E.
London   J.C.
                                                               D.E.
                                                               R.S.

Postscript

It was with deep sorrow that we learned of the death of Dr Ole Møller Jensen, as this book was going to press. Ole was a contributor and participant at the Rome meeting, where we greatly benefited from his wisdom, knowledge, and expertise. He would also have been a contributor to this volume but for his untimely illness. He will be greatly missed.

Contents

Contributors

A. Ahlbom Karolinska Institute, National Institute of Environmental Medicine, Department of Epidemiology, Box 60208, S-104 01 Stockholm, Sweden

F. E. Alexander University of Southampton, Department of Medical Oncology, Room G071/72, Royal South Hants Hospital, Southampton, UK

J. M. Antó Department of Epidemiology and Public Health, Institut Municipal de Investigació Medica, Passeig Maritim 25–29, 08003 Barcelona, Spain

J. E. Asvall World Health Organization, Regional Office for Europe, 8 Scherfigsvej, DK 2100 Copenhagen, Denmark

Y. I. Baris Department of Chest Diseases, Hacettepe School of Medicine, TIP Fakultesi, Gogus Hastaliklari Bilim Dali, TR-Sihhiye Ankara, Turkey

J. A. Beresford Environmental Epidemiology Unit, Department of Public Health and Policy, London School of Hygiene and Tropical Medicine, Keppel Street, London WC1E 7HT, UK

L. Bernardinelli Institute of Hygiene and Preventive Medicine, University of Sassari, Via P. Manzella 4, 07100 Sassari, Italy

P. A. Bertazzi Istituto di Medicina del Lavoro, Università di Milano, Via San Barnaba 8, 20121 Milano, Italy

J. F. Bithell Department of Statistics, Oxford University, South Parks Road, Oxford OX1 3TB, UK

J. Boreham ICRF Cancer Studies Unit, Nuffield Department of Medicine, University of Oxford, Oxford OX2 6HE, UK

D. J. Briggs Department of Geographical and Environmental Sciences, Polytechnic of Huddersfield, Queensgate, Huddersfield HD1 3DH, UK

T. C. Campbell Department of Nutritional Biochemistry, Cornell University, Ithaca, New York, USA

J. Chen Institute of Nutrition, Chinese Academy of Preventive Medicine, Beijing, People's Republic of China

D. Clayton MRC Biostatistics Unit, Institute of Public Health, University Forvie Site, Robinson Way, Cambridge CB2 2SR, UK

J. Cuzick Department of Mathematics, Statistics, and Epidemiology, Imperial Cancer Research Fund, 61 Lincoln's Inn Fields, London WC2A 3PX, UK

P. De Wals   Département des Sciences de la Santé Communautaire, Faculté de Médicine, Université de Sherbrooke, Sherbrooke, Quebec J1H 5NA, Canada

I. Diamond   Department of Social Statistics, University of Southampton, Southampton SO9 5NH, UK

H. Dolk   Department of Epidemiology, Catholic University of Louvain, School of Public Health EPID 30.34, Clos Chapelle aux Champs, B-1200 Brussels, Belgium

G. J. Draper   Childhood Cancer Research Group, Department of Paediatrics, University of Oxford, 57 Woodstock Road, Oxford OX2 6HJ, UK

P. Elliott   Environmental Epidemiology Unit, Department of Public Health and Policy, London School of Hygiene and Tropical Medicine, Keppel Street, London WC1E 7HT, UK

D. English   Department of Public Health, Queen Elizabeth II Medical Centre, University of Western Australia, Nedlands, WA 6009, Australia

J. Estève   Unit of Biostatistics, International Agency for Research on Cancer, 150 cours Albert-Thomas, 69372 Lyon, Cedex 08, France

Z. Feng   Institute of Nutrition, Chinese Academy of Preventive Medicine, Beijing, People's Republic of China

M. J. Gardner   MRC Environmental Epidemiology Unit, University of Southampton, Southampton General Hospital, Southampton SO9 4XY, UK

N. Hammar   Karolinska Institute, National Institute of Environmental Medicine, Department of Epidemiology, Doktorsringen 18, Box 60208, S-104 01 Stockholm, Sweden

M. Hills   Environmental Epidemiology Unit, Department of Public Health and Policy, London School of Hygiene and Tropical Medicine, Keppel Street, London WC1E 7HT, UK

B. Jarman   Department of General Practice, St Mary's Hospital Medical School, Lisson Grove Health Centre, Gateforth Street, London NW8 8EG, UK

D. J. Jolley   Environmental Epidemiology Unit, Department of Public Health and Policy, London School of Hygiene and Tropical Medicine, Keppel Street, London WC1E 7HT, UK

I. Kleinschmidt   Environmental Epidemiology Unit, Department of Public Health and Policy, London School of Hygiene and Tropical Medicine, Keppel Street, London WC1E 7HT, UK

J. Li   Cancer Institute, Chinese Academy of Medical Science, Beijing, People's Republic of China

A. D. Lopez   Global Health Situation Assessment and Projections Unit, World Health Organization, 20 Avenue Appia, 1211 Geneva 27, Switzerland

G. K. Matthew Flat 2, Pond House, 21 Craven Hill, London W2 3EN, UK

D. M. Parkin Unit of Descriptive Epidemiology, International Agency for Research on Cancer, 150 cours Albert-Thomas, 69372 Lyon, Cedex 08, France

S. H. Pattenden Environmental Epidemiology Unit, Department of Public Health and Policy, London School of Hygiene and Tropical Medicine, Keppel Street, London WC1E 7HT, UK

A. C. Pesatori Istituto di Medicina del Lavoro, Università di Milano, Via San Barnaba 8, 20122 Milano, Italy

R. Peto ICRF Cancer Studies Unit, Nuffield Department of Medicine, University of Oxford, Oxford OX2 6HE, UK

E. Pukkala Finnish Cancer Registry, The Institute for Statistical and Epidemiological Cancer Research, Liisankatu 21, SF-00170 Helsinki, Finland

M. J. Quinn Office of Population Censuses and Surveys, St. Catherine's House, 10 Kingsway, London WC2, UK

S. Richardson Unité de Recherches Epidémiologiques et Statistiques sur l'Environnement et la Santé, INSERM U.170, 16 Avenue Paul-Vaillant-Coutourier, 94807 Villejuif Cedex, France

G. Rose Department of Epidemiology and Population Sciences, London School of Hygiene and Tropical Medicine, Keppel Street, London WC1E 7HT, UK

R. B. Rothenberg National Center for Chronic Disease Prevention and Health Promotion, Centers for Disease Control, Atlanta GA 30333, USA

R. Saracci Unit of Analytical Epidemiology, International Agency for Research on Cancer, 150 cours Albert-Thomas, 69372 Lyon, Cedex 08, France

L. Simonato Registro Tumori del Veneto, Via Giustiniani 2, 35100 Padua, Italy

M. Smans Unit of Biostatistics Research and Informatics, International Agency for Research on Cancer, 150 cours Albert-Thomas, 69372 Lyon, Cedex 08, France

R. Stern World Health Organization, European Centre for Environment and Health, PO Box 1, 3720 BA Bilthoven, The Netherlands

J. Sunyer Department of Epidemiology and Public Health, Institut Municipal de Investigació Medica, Passeig Maritim 25–29, 08003 Barcelona, Spain

A. J. Swerdlow Epidemiological Monitoring Unit, Department of Epidemiology and Population Sciences, London School of Hygiene and Tropical Medicine, Keppel Street, London WC1E 7HT, UK

B. Terracini Dip. di Scienze Biomediche e Oncologia Umana, Università di Torino, Via Santena 7, 10126 Torino, Italy

S. B. Thacker Epidemiology Program Office, Centers for Disease Control, Atlanta GA 30333, USA

Contributors

J. Urquhart Information and Statistics Division, Scottish Health Service, Trinity Park House, South Trinity Road, Edinburgh EH5 3SQ, UK

A. J. Westlake Environmental Epidemiology Unit, Department of Public Health and Policy, London School of Hygiene and Tropical Medicine, Keppel Street, London WC1E 7HT, UK

R. Winkelmann Unit of Analytical Epidemiology, International Agency for Research on Cancer, 150 cours Albert-Thomas, 69372 Lyon, Cedex 08, France

L. Youngman ICRF Cancer Studies Unit, Nuffield Department of Medicine, University of Oxford, Oxford OX2 6HE, UK

G. A. Zapponi Laboratorio di Igiene Ambientale, Istituto Superiore di Sanita, Viale Regina Elena 299, 1-Roma 00161, Italy

C. Zocchetti Clinica del Lavoro, Istituto Clinici di Perfezionamento, Via San Barnaba 8, 20122 Milano, Italy

I Introduction

1. Geographical epidemiology and ecological studies

D. English

Geographical epidemiology

Geographical epidemiology can be defined as the description of spatial patterns of disease incidence and mortality. It is a part of descriptive epidemiology, which is more generally concerned with describing the occurrence of disease with respect to demographic characteristics (e.g. age, race, sex), place, and time.

Historically, geographical studies have provided important clues to the aetiology of disease. Snow (1854), for example, developed his hypothesis about the mode of transmission of cholera on the basis of his observations of variations in the mortality rate in London. Palm (1890) suspected that lack of sunshine was the major cause of rickets. He obtained data on the geographical variation in the prevalence of rickets in various countries, which confirmed his suspicions. The geographical distribution of mortality from malignant melanoma led Lancaster (1956) to conclude that, in contrast to rickets, its major cause was excessive sunlight. (This example is illustrated in detail later in this chapter.) A major resource for cancer epidemiologists seeking hypotheses to test has been the series *Cancer Incidence in Five Continents*, which is a compilation of cancer incidence data from registries in many countries and which is now in its fifth volume (Muir *et al.* 1987). Differences in rates among the registries up to a hundredfold have provided cancer epidemiologists with many hypotheses about the aetiology of cancer.

As the examples suggest, a major aim in studying geographical variation in disease rates is to formulate hypotheses about the aetiology of disease by taking into account spatial variation in environmental factors. Hypotheses developed from descriptive studies need to be tested by more rigorous methods, such as intervention, cohort, and case-control studies. It is generally not possible to test hypotheses about causes of disease in descriptive studies because exposure to a particular agent (e.g. water containing *Vibrio cholerae* or lack of sunlight) and outcome (e.g. cholera or rickets) are not measured in the same individuals.

Geographical studies at an international level have been successful in identifying possible risk factors for disease because they exploit large differences in both the frequency of disease and the prevalence of exposure. The relationship between lack of sunlight and rickets is an example; it was demonstrated by data from numerous countries where the amount of sunlight and the prevalence of rickets both showed substantial variation. Whether studies in small areas, where rates of disease and environmental exposures are likely to be relatively homogeneous, will be able to produce similar results, is as yet unknown. Small-area studies have other purposes, though, which will be discussed in the next chapter.

Types of geographical studies

Three major types of studies of geographical variation in disease frequency can be distinguished. The first category includes studies where the aim is simply to describe the distribution of disease with respect to place of occurrence. The results of these studies are often presented in maps. The second category includes ecological studies (sometimes known as geographical correlation studies) in which the aim is to describe the relationship between geographical variation in disease and concomitant variation in degree of exposure to a particular factor (usually an environmental agent or a life-style-related characteristic, such as diet). Estimates of the relative risk corresponding to different levels of exposure can be obtained from ecological studies, though, as will be discussed below, the estimates are rarely unbiased. A third category of geographical studies involves studies of migrants, in which the aim is to determine whether the risk of disease among migrants from a region of high (or low) risk to another region with low (or high) risk changes after migration. These can be considered as geographical studies because they exploit geographical variation in frequency of disease in an attempt to separate the effects of place (i.e. the environment) from the effects of person (i.e. genetic factors). Although migrant studies have been particularly useful in epidemiology (see, for example, Steinitz *et al.* 1989), they are not considered further in this book.

Potential problems in the interpretation of geographical studies

Studies of geographical variation need to be interpreted with caution since many factors apart from environmental exposures can contribute to such variation in the recorded frequency of disease. For example, the quality of diagnosis and classification of disease may vary from one place to another. There may also be substantial variation in the reporting of disease; in some areas underenumeration of cases may be substantial. In addition, population estimates may also vary in quality. Mortality data, while more generally available than morbidity data, may be affected by differential survival among regions. Genetic and ethnic factors may confound geographical variations. (Migrant studies have been used to help overcome this problem.) Migration patterns may also affect geographical comparisons if there are substantial inward or outward movements. Chance can also play a role in creating spatial variation in the distribution of disease, especially for rare diseases and in small or sparsely populated areas.

As will be seen in subsequent chapters of this book, some of these issues are of less concern for studies conducted in small areas than, for example, in international studies where the variation in many of these factors may be considerable. However, chance, migration, and errors in population estimates are likely to have greater effects in studies of small areas.

Presentation of geographical data

Maps provide the most succinct summary of descriptive geographical data since they display the spatial distribution of the characteristic of interest. On a map, the geographical distribution of disease is readily visible to the eye. The recent production of cancer maps for many countries (Boyle *et al.* 1989) testifies to the appeal of this approach. A well-known example is the Chinese atlas of cancer mortality (Chinese Academy of Medical Sciences 1981). The maps in that atlas show substantial regional variation in mortality for many cancer sites.

Statistical tables, while able to present more data than maps, cannot easily convey these spatial patterns and so are a less comprehensible or accessible means of presenting geographical data. Subtle patterns may be missed in tables which cannot take account of the spatial relationships between populations. On the other hand, it is difficult to present more than one variable on a single map so that important features of the data (e.g. the number of cases on which a rate is based) may not be portrayed. Ideally, supporting tabular data should be presented alongside maps. The question of which variable to map, and other technical issues related to map production, are considered in detail in Chapter 14.

When examining an atlas of mortality or incidence, it is easy to forget that the instant visual impression of regions of high and low risk and of spatial patterns of disease frequency is based upon descriptive data which are subject to the problems of interpretation mentioned previously. Furthermore, as was noted by Barker (1981): 'Maps of disease compel speculation about aetiology, but only rarely has such speculation by itself led directly to the discovery of causes.'

Ecological studies

The aim of ecological studies is to describe, in quantitative terms, the relationship between the frequency of a disease and the level of exposure to a particular agent. Ecological studies are used in conjunction with simple descriptive studies of geographical variation in an attempt to determine how much of the variation in rates among populations is associated with concomitant variation in level of exposure.

In an ecological study, place and time of residence are used to create surrogate measures of the real exposure of interest. This can be direct, as is the case where the exposure of interest is latitude or altitude. In most instances, though, the relationship between place and exposure is indirect. Thus, for example, in an ecological study of tobacco consumption, sales figures in various regions of a country are sometimes used to relate place of residence to exposure (Friedman 1967). Using place and time of residence as a surrogate for actual exposure generally means that large groups of people (e.g. whole countries) are assigned the same level of exposure. The levels of exposure assigned to the various populations of interest are then compared with the rate of disease in each of the populations.

An estimate of the relative risk associated with exposure, whether the exposure be quantitative (e.g. the amount of alcohol consumed), or dichotomous (e.g. ever-usage of the oral contraceptive pill), can be obtained from the slope of the regression line relating the frequency of disease to the population prevalence of exposure (Morgenstern 1982). (Statistical methods for the analysis of data from geographical correlation studies are given in Chapter 17.) In fact, in most ecological studies, only the correlation coefficient is calculated, hence the alternative name for the type of study. The correlation, though, is of less value than the regression slope, since it gives no indication of the size of the relationship between level of exposure and risk of disease apart from measuring how close the relationship is to a straight line. Furthermore, the value of the correlation coefficient is subject to bias induced by the study design. It can be arbitrarily increased by choosing populations to maximize the between-population difference in levels of exposure (Piantodosi *et al.* 1988).

Potential strengths and weaknesses of ecological studies

The advantages and disadvantages of ecological studies are best considered in relation to analytical studies, which are based on data in which the disease of interest and the exposure have been assessed in the same individuals. On the one hand, ecological studies may be less subject to the effects of random error in the measurement of exposure, while on the other hand, they are more prone to the problems of confounding. The validity of the ecological approach depends on how well the surrogate indicator of exposure (place of residence) for an individual who develops the disease of interest measures the actual exposure.

An attractive feature of ecological studies is that random errors in measuring exposure may be greater for individuals than for populations. It is well known that such random errors (non-differential misclassification) attenuate effects in analytical studies (Gardner and Heady 1973). This bias, which is sometimes referred to as the 'regression-dilution' bias, may be substantial.

Consider, as an example, the relationship between blood pressure and stroke. Single measurements from a number of individuals will provide a good estimate of the mean blood pressure for the group when the sample is sufficiently large, but a single measurement of an individual's blood pressure will not be a good estimate of his or her usual blood pressure because of intra-individual variability. As a result, studies in individuals in which blood pressure is measured only once will underestimate the effect of high blood pressure on the risk of stroke. An analysis of data from several cohort studies has shown that the regression-dilution bias resulting from single measurements of blood pressure reduced the strength of the association between blood pressure and relative risk of stroke by 60 per cent (MacMahon *et al.* 1990).

While ecological studies may be less prone to the effects of random errors, they may be more subject to bias induced by systematic errors in the measurement of exposure. If these systematic errors differ geographically, ecological studies may be subject to substantial bias. For example, the possibility of systematic differences in assessing national consumption of dietary fats in international ecological studies has been advanced as part of the explanation of the association between the incidence of breast cancer and the apparent consumption of dietary fat (Willett and Stampfer 1990).

Although systematic errors in assessing exposure are a problem, the major disadvantage of ecological studies is that the measure of exposure, place of residence, is only a surrogate and is based on an average level of exposure in the community. Within a population (or area) in which individuals are classified to have the same level of exposure, the range in exposure among individuals may actually be quite large. (As a matter of interest for this book, the smaller the area used for classifying individuals, the more likely it is that the grouped data will apply to the individuals.) As a result, associations in ecological studies apply to groups. The real interest, however, is in the relationship between exposure and risk of disease among individuals. To assume that the relationship between exposure and disease in groups is the same as that in individuals is to commit the 'ecological fallacy' (Selvin 1958). Associations that occur in aggregated data might be spurious and may be subject to considerable ecological confounding. This problem was first discussed by Robinson (1950), who cautioned against the use of ecological analyses as a means of predicting the behaviour of individuals.

An often-discussed example of the ecological fallacy is the analysis of suicide rates in regions of Prussia by Durkheim (1951). The rate of suicides was positively correlated with the proportion of Protestants in a region, suggesting that Protestants were more likely than Catholics to commit suicide. In the absence of information about the religious persuasion of those persons who actually committed suicide, however, an equally plausible explanation is that the correlation is due to high suicide rates among Catholics living in regions of Prussia which were predominantly Protestant. In this instance, therefore, knowledge of the religion of the majority of the population in a region may not be a good measure of the religion of an individual.

Ecological studies can lead to conclusions at odds with known epidemiological evidence. Hakama *et al.* (1982) compared the results of a municipality-based ecological analysis of the incidence of cancer and socio-economic status in Finland, with an analysis in which they used data on socio-economic status of individuals. The incidence of cancer of the cervix was highest in municipalities of high socio-economic status, whereas *individuals* of high socio-economic status had the *lowest* incidence of cancer of the cervix, which is the expected result.

A discussion of the conditions necessary for ecological bias to occur is given in Chapter 17, so only brief details are provided here for the simplest case of a dichotomous risk factor. If the rate of disease in people who are not exposed to a particular agent of interest is the same in all populations (i.e. there are no other determinants of disease distributed differently among populations), and the effect of exposure is the same in all populations (i.e. there are no effect modifiers distributed differently among populations), the ecological analysis will be unbiased. If either of these conditions is violated, the ecological analysis will be biased (Greenland and Morgenstern 1989). The bias may be substantial, even to the point of reversing the true exposure–disease relationship, as was seen above in the example on cancer of the cervix. Note that ecological confounding should not be confused with the usual notion of confounding at an individual level, since ecological bias can occur in the absence of such individual-level confounding (Greenland and Morgenstern 1989).

To illustrate these properties, consider a single dichotomous exposure, and one other variable, for example ethnic origin. First, assume that ethnic origin is a determinant of risk of disease and that it is distributed differently among populations. An ecological analysis of crude rates (i.e. not ethnic origin-specific) will be biased. Ethnic origin need not be associated with exposure within populations at the level of individuals for the ecological analysis to be biased. In the example on melanoma and latitude, which is discussed below, an analysis which was not restricted to white populations would be biased even if the level of exposure to sunlight was the same in all ethnic groups within populations. The results of such an analysis might show that latitude is inversely related to risk of melanoma because low-risk populations tend to live at low latitudes. Suppose now that ethnic origin modifies the effect of exposure. If it is distributed differently among populations, the ecological analysis will be biased, even in the absence of other extraneous variables which affect the rate of disease in the unexposed.

Analyses based on individuals are not subject to the same degree of confounding since the conditions for confounding at an individual level are more stringent. Furthermore, in analytical studies it is usually possible to take into account the effect of confounding variables. In an ecological analysis, even if the variable that causes the ecological bias is known, its effects cannot readily be removed (Greenland and Morgenstern 1989), because to do so requires satisfying stringent assumptions which are unlikely to be met in practice (Richardson and Hémon 1990).

Several techniques can be used, though, to reduce the possibility of ecological confounding. These include performing separate analyses within categories of determinants of risk (e.g. age, sex, ethnic origin), incorporation of time-lags to allow for latent periods, and statistical adjustment for potentially confounding variables. For example, in an analysis of sodium intake and blood pressure among populations, separate analyses were performed for economically developed and undeveloped communities (Law *et al.* 1991). The effect of sodium intake on blood pressure was weaker than in other geographical analyses which did not take level of development into account. The authors suggested that this difference was due to ecological confounding in the crude analysis, since economic development is related to a number of determinants of blood pressure (e.g. weight, potassium intake) which would confound the ecological analysis.

Despite the obvious problems with ecological studies, they do have a continued role. Information about individuals' exposure histories may be unavailable, or, within populations, exposure among individuals may be so homogeneous as to be considered to occur only at a group level. For example, the International Agency for Research on Cancer is co-ordinating an ecological study of childhood leukaemia in Europe in relation to exposure to radiation from the Chernobyl accident. The incidence of childhood leukaemia generally shows little geographical variation, and there are few known risk factors apart from ionizing radiation, so ecological analyses are unlikely to be seriously biased, particularly if rates prior to the accident can be incorporated into the analysis. Estimates of radiation doses for populations in relatively large areas have been calculated by the United Nations Scientific Committee on the Effects of Atomic Radiation. Uniformly calculated estimates are not available for small areas.

Example

As an example of an ecological study, consider the relationship between the frequency of occurrence of malignant melanoma and latitude. This example demonstrates both the strengths and weaknesses of correlation studies.

In 1956, Lancaster noted that mortality from malignant melanoma was higher in Australia and South Africa than in the parts of Europe from which these populations originated; that mortality in Australia, New Zealand, and the United States increased with proximity to the equator; but that within Europe it was higher in Norway and Sweden in the north than in France and Italy in the south. These patterns are also evident in recent incidence data for melanoma among white populations (Muir *et al.* 1987), as is illustrated for

white males in Fig. 1.1. The results of a regression analysis between latitude
and the age-adjusted incidence rate of melanoma, weighted by numbers of
cases, predict that the incidence decreases by 0.33 per 100 000 person-years for
each degree of latitude. The correlation is − 0.67. A similar relationship holds
for females.

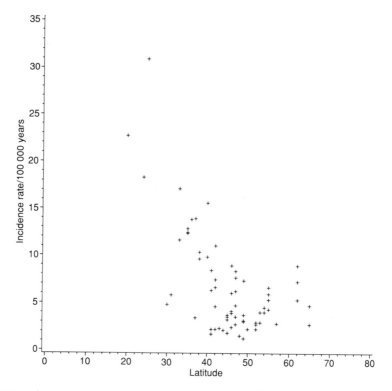

Fig. 1.1 The incidence rate of melanoma among white males by latitude of the
reporting cancer registry, approximate years 1978–82. Incidence rates are
directly standardized to the world population. The data are for white males in
Europe, North America, Australia, and New Zealand. (Data from Muir et al. 1987.)

After observing these patterns, Lancaster hypothesized that sunlight was a
major cause of melanoma. Prior to 1956, sunlight was not considered to be a
major factor in the aetiology of melanoma because of the anatomical site
distribution (melanomas occur frequently on body sites which are not usually
exposed) and the relatively high frequency in indoor workers (Blum 1948).

Lancaster's analysis illustrates all the potential strengths of the ecological
approach. It exploited large differences in exposure among populations,
avoided the difficulty and uncertainty of measuring exposure in individuals,
and was simple and cheap.

People living at widely varying latitudes are likely to be exposed to a wide range of ultraviolet B radiation, which is believed to play a major role in melanoma, since it varies markedly with latitude. Within populations, the range of exposure to ultraviolet B radiation is much more limited, and measurement of sun exposure among individuals in analytical studies has proved to be a major problem leading to substantial attenuation of effects (Armstrong 1988).

The example also illustrates the potential problems with the ecological approach, namely the inability to determine the behaviour of individuals within populations and the difficulty of taking into account potential confounding factors. At high latitudes (i.e. in northern Europe and the Nordic countries), the relationship between latitude and incidence of melanoma is reversed. At first glance, this reversal appears to contradict Lancaster's hypothesis, but does it? The use of latitude as a proxy for exposure means that, for example, every individual living in Norway is considered to have less exposure than is every individual living in Italy, where melanoma is less common. It is possible, though, that some individuals in Norway have more relevant exposure than do individuals living in more southerly parts of Europe.

A further problem with these data relates to the form of the relationship between exposure and disease. From Fig. 1.1 a simple linear relationship seems appropriate (at least at lower latitudes). However, the relationship between exposure to sunlight and risk of melanoma is complex (Armstrong 1988). Intermittent bursts of intense exposure may be more important than total accumulated exposure to the sun, and constant exposure may actually be protective. This complex pattern is obscured in an analysis in which the level of exposure is based on average levels within populations.

The analysis also fails to take into account other variables that influence the risk of melanoma. Among European populations, degree of skin pigmentation is strongly related to risk of melanoma, and the populations of southern Europe may be protected, to some extent, from melanoma by virtue of their generally darker pigmentation than the populations of the Nordic countries.

Conclusion

Ecological studies have a number of strengths and are useful as a first step in identifying possible associations between risk of disease and environmental exposures. However, because of the potential for bias, they should never be considered anything other than initial steps in investigating associations between environmental agents and occurrence of disease.

Lancaster and Palm succeeded in formulating correct hypotheses about aetiology on the basis of geographical and ecological studies of disease frequency. As it happened, in each case, the relative effect of the exposure was strong, and the proportion of cases that could be attributed to the exposure was also high. In the presence of strong determinants of risk which are distributed unevenly in space, this approach is unlikely to have success. Maps of lung cancer mortality, for example, are likely to give an accurate representation of the prevalence of smoking at some time in the past but may be of little value in helping to identify other causes of lung cancer, such as air pollution, unless the prevalence of smoking is low.

In contrast to ecological studies, analytical studies have generally been conducted in single populations. Random errors in the measurement of exposure, relatively small variation in exposure within populations, and small sample sizes have all contributed to the difficulties that these studies have had in detecting weak to moderate effects of exposure. (See Prentice and Sheppard (1990) for a review of these issues with respect to dietary fat.) Recently, however, there have been a number of international studies of individuals, which have been conducted in populations with widely varying levels of exposure and frequency of disease. One such study is the INTERSALT study of electrolyte excretion and blood pressure (Intersalt Cooperative Research Group 1988). It had a large sample, 5045 men and 5034 women randomly selected, and was conducted in 52 centres around the world, with a large range in mean blood pressure and sodium intake. In addition, duplicate measurements were taken for a number of the participants to enable the investigators to adjust for the regression-dilution bias. Studies such as the INTERSALT study, which incorporate the best features of analytical and ecological studies, offer much promise in epidemiology.

References

Armstrong, B. K. (1988). Epidemiology of malignant melanoma: intermittent or total accumulated exposure to the sun? *Journal of Dermatologic Surgery and Oncology*, **14**, 835–49.

Barker, D. J. P. (1981). Geographical variations in disease in Britain. *British Medical Journal*, **283**, 398–400.

Blum, H. F. (1948). Sunlight as a causal factor in cancer of the skin of man. *Journal of the National Cancer Institute*, **9**, 247–58.

Boyle, P., Muir, C. S., and Grundman, E. (ed.) (1989). Cancer Mapping. *Recent Results in Cancer Research*, **114**.

Chinese Academy of Medical Sciences (1981). *Atlas of cancer mortality in the People's Republic of China*. China Press, Beijing.

Durkheim, E. (1951). *Suicide: A study in sociology*. Free Press, New York.

Friedman, G. D. (1967). Cigarette smoking and geographic variation in coronary heart disease mortality in the United States. *Journal of Chronic Diseases*, **20**, 769–79.

Gardner, M. J. and Heady, J. A. (1973). Some effects of within-person variability in epidemiologic studies. *Journal of Chronic Diseases*, **26**, 781–93.

Greenland, S. and Morgenstern, H. (1989). Ecological bias, confounding and effect modification. *International Journal of Epidemiology*, **18**, 269–74.

Hakama, M., Hakulinen, T., Pukkala, E., Saxén, E., and Teppo, L. (1982). Risk indicators of breast and cervical cancer on ecologic and individual levels. *American Journal of Epidemiology*, **116**, 990–1000.

Intersalt Cooperative Research Group (1988). Intersalt: an international study of electrolyte excretion and blood pressure. Results for 24 hour urinary sodium and potassium excretion. *British Medical Journal*, **297**, 319–28.

Lancaster, H. O. (1956). Some geographical aspects of the mortality from melanoma in Europeans. *Medical Journal of Australia*, **1**, 1082–7.

Law, M. R., Frost, C. D., and Wald, N. J. (1991). By how much does dietary salt reduction lower blood pressure? I-Analysis of observational data among populations. *British Medical Journal*, **302**, 811–15.

MacMahon, S., *et al.* (1990). Blood pressure, stroke and coronary heart disease. Part 1, prolonged differences in blood pressure: prospective observational studies corrected for the regression dilution bias. *Lancet*, **335**, 765–74.

Morgenstern, H. (1982). Uses of ecologic analysis in epidemiologic research. *American Journal of Public Health*, **72**, 1336–44.

Muir, C., Waterhouse, J., Mack, T., Powell, J., and Whelan, S. (ed.) (1987). *Cancer incidence in five continents*, Vol. V. International Agency for Research on Cancer, Scientific Publication 88, Lyon.

Palm, T. A. (1890). The geographical distribution and aetiology of rickets. *Practitioner*, **45**, 270–9.

Piantodosi, S., Byar, D. P., and Green, S. B. (1988). The ecological fallacy. *American Journal of Epidemiology*, **127**, 893–904.

Prentice, R. L. and Sheppard, L. (1990). Dietary fat and cancer: consistency of the epidemiologic data, and disease prevention that may follow from a practical reduction in fat consumption. *Cancer Causes and Control*, **1**, 81–97.

Richardson, S. and Hémon, D. (1990). Ecological bias and confounding (letter). *International Journal of Epidemiology*, **19**, 764–6.

Robinson, W. S. (1950). Ecological correlations and the behavior of individuals. *American Sociological Review*, **15**, 351–7.

Selvin, H. C. (1958). Durkheim's 'Suicide' and problems of empirical research. *American Journal of Sociology*, **63**, 607–19.

Snow, J. (1854). *On the mode of communication of cholera*, (2nd edn). Churchill Livingstone, London.

Steinitz, R., Parkin, D. M., Young, J. L., Bieber, C. A., and Katz, L. (1989). *Cancer incidence in Jewish migrants to Israel 1961–1981*. International Agency for Research on Cancer, Scientific Publication 98, Lyon.

Willett, W. C. and Stampfer, M. J. (1990). Dietary fat and cancer: another view. *Cancer Causes and Control*, **1**, 103–9.

2. Small-area studies: purpose and methods

J. Cuzick and P. Elliott

As outlined in the previous chapter, large-scale geographical and correlation studies are useful epidemiological techniques, especially suited to forming and refining hypotheses about aetiology. More rigorous tests of these hypotheses can then be carried out at the individual level, usually by means of case-control methodology. The very scale on which these geographical surveys take place limits their value to the study of risk factors that are widely distributed and vary gradually over geographical regions, and implies that they are unable to detect risks associated with environmental factors that are spatially localized. Thus diseases affected by proximity to industrial plants that emit potentially dangerous chemicals or radiation into the surrounding air, water, or soil, and diseases with a possible contagious aetiology cannot be studied in this way.

At the same time, in our increasingly health-conscious and environmentally aware society, members of the public are much more likely to notice unusual aggregations of disease in a small neighbourhood and to attribute them to some nearby industrial source of pollution. To investigate these claims quickly it is essential to have ready access to all cases of disease in a given area and relate the number of cases to the number expected for a typical population of the same size and age structure as the neighbourhood in question. With this information, the local population can be reassured if, in fact, no excess is observed, or further studies can be initiated when significant excess disease is found.

Thus there is a need for high-quality, routinely collected morbidity and mortality data on a scale fine enough to enable the study of these questions. Fortunately, advances in computer technology, geographical data systems, and statistical methodology have meant that a variety of small-area studies are now feasible using routine data. However, the type of study undertaken and the methods required depend on the question to be answered. Whereas for some kinds of enquiry, the geographical, statistical, and epidemiological methodologies are firmly embedded within a standard and accepted framework (for example, examining the hypothesis that a particular industrial process is associated with adverse health outcomes in the vicinity of industrial plants), for others an established theoretical framework does not exist (e.g. searching through a data set to detect disease 'clusters'). The level of evidence

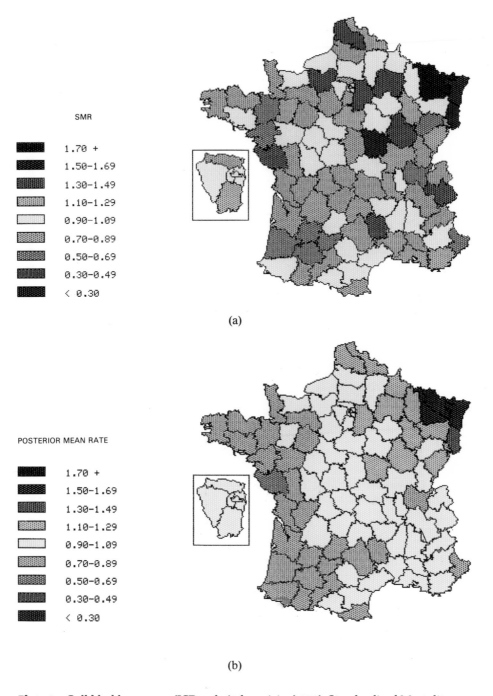

Plate 1 Gall bladder cancer (ICD code (8th revision) 156), Standardized Mortality Ratio (SMR) France males, 1971–78 (a) unsmoothed (b) smoothed using Gibbs sampler (from Mollié 1990, with permission).

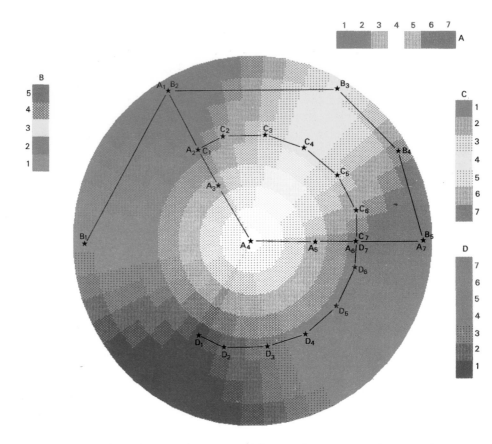

Plate 2 Colour disc showing the range of hue and saturation. See text for explanation of colour pathways.

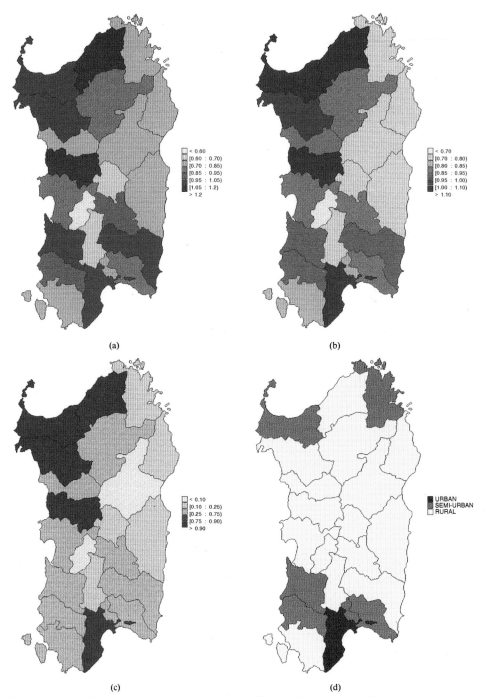

Plate 3 (a–c) Breast cancer mortality in Sardinia 1983–7, for 22 larger areas
(Unitá Sanitarie Locali)

    a) unsmoothed SMRs;

    b) smoothed SMRs;

    c) smoothed map based on exceedance probabilities

(d) Urban/rural status

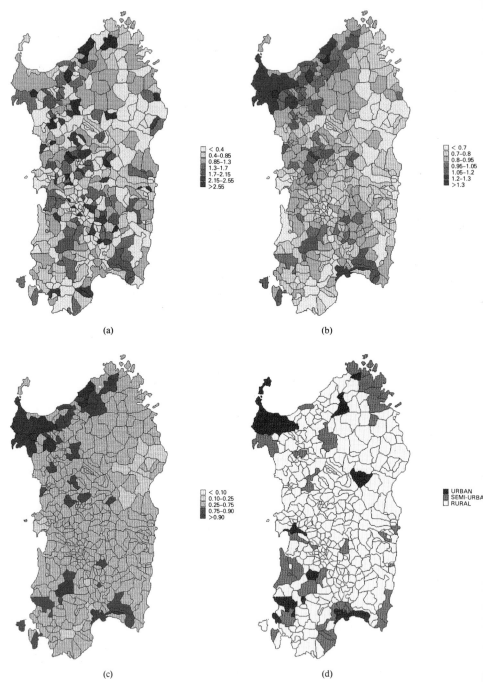

Plate 4 (a–c) Breast cancer mortality in Sardinia 1983–7, for 366 smaller areas
(communes)

　　a) unsmoothed SMRs;

　　b) smoothed SMRs;

　　c) smoothed map based on exceedance probabilities

d) Urban/rural status

required and the interpretation of such studies need to reflect this spectrum of uncertainty.

Types of study

Several types of small-area study can be identified, as follows:

(1) studies of reports of disease excess ('clusters') in specific localities without a putative source;
(2) studies of point sources of industrial pollution;
(3) studies of clustering as a general phenomenon;
(4) ecological-correlation studies;
(5) descriptive studies of the distribution of disease in small areas;
(6) geographical surveillance to detect areas with high disease incidence;
(7) studies following acute chemical or nuclear accidents.

Each type of study is introduced briefly below and some of the problems of interpretation are discussed. Several examples of geographical and small-area studies can be found in the remainder of this book.

Clusters without a putative source

Here the problems of interpretation are severe as many apparent clusters are certain to arise by chance. Efforts to document carefully the extent of a cluster and to investigate to what extent the cases in question share a common aetiology are important. Two examples are the cluster of multiple myeloma at Thief River, Minnesota (Kyle *et al.* 1970) and the cancer cluster in Randolph, Massachusetts (Day *et al.* 1988), for which a likely potential source was not identified. Often clusters surviving this initial screening process are subsequently linked with at least one putative source, for example the excess of childhood leukaemias observed in Woburn, Massachusetts which was linked to contaminated well water (Lagakos *et al.* 1986).

Point sources

A major difficulty here is how to deal with *post hoc* reports of disease excesses in the vicinity of a particular source of pollution. Often the suspicion of an excess in a local community leads to evaluation by the local public health physician, and in these circumstances, strictly speaking, the use of statistical hypothesis testing is invalid. The steps to be undertaken in the validation and investigation of such reports are discussed in Chapter 23.

Ideally, a decision to evaluate the effects of a point source of pollution should be undertaken without prior knowledge of the disease incidence in the locality, as in the investigation of a zinc smelter by Brown *et al.* (1984).

However, this is not usually possible in practice unless prior suspicion has been raised at another similar site. The problem is highlighted by the studies of excess leukaemia around the nuclear reprocessing plant at Sellafield, reviewed in detail in Chapter 25. An example of a *post hoc* enquiry around one site leading to replication around other similar sites, is given in Chapter 29.

Clustering as a general phenomenon

Another, somewhat more abstract and less tangible purpose is to be able to study the tendency for certain diseases to show a pattern of clustering over a large area without particular regard to any one cluster or putative source of clustering. A number of studies have shown this to be the case for Hodgkin's disease (Alexander *et al.* 1989; Glaser 1990), and there is some evidence that it may be true for childhood leukaemia, especially at very young ages (Alexander 1991; Black *et al.* 1991). This has important implications for aetiology and should serve to intensify the search for a virus related to these cancers, although other explanations are possible, including localized variations in environmental exposures, and artefacts relating to local diagnostic, coding, and registration practices, to population mobility, and to variations in birth-rates.

Ecological-correlation studies

When health, environmental exposure, and population data are available for areas at comparable high levels of geographical resolution, there is the potential to carry out ecological studies correlating health and the environment at a much finer scale than considered in the previous chapter. Unfortunately, for most environmental exposures, only low-level resolution data are routinely collected (e.g. a few monitoring sites across a whole country) so that only crude ecological-correlation studies could be considered. Because of the problems of unmeasured ecological confounding, including variations in the underlying socio-demography of areas leading to variations in disease incidence, these studies should be regarded at best as providing data for 'hypothesis generation', at worst as giving a misleading and confusing picture, possibly leading to the 'ecological fallacy' (Piantodosi *et al.* 1988).

With the advent of disaggregated, high-resolution, health and population data, and the availability of schemes to classify areas by measures of their socio-economic characteristics, some of the problems associated with ecological studies may be overcome, provided that high-quality environmental data at similar levels of aggregation are forthcoming. Here, the level of analysis (for example, the enumeration district) is closer to individuals and hence confounding and interpretation may (under certain circumstances) be less problematic.

A good example of ecological-correlation studies for which exposure data exist at a localized level is in the field of radiation, where studies of leukaemia with respect to background radiation and household radon exposure are now being pursued. An example of an ecological-correlation study at a higher level of aggregation, conducted in China, is given in Chapter 30.

Descriptive studies

Although variations in disease rates have been studied in detail in large geographical areas, e.g. regions in England and Wales (Britton 1990), municipalities in Finland (Teppo *et al.* 1980), counties in the USA (Mason and McKay 1973), little is known about the variations in rates over small areas. This is particularly relevant to the interpretation of studies around point sources, or to the investigation of disease 'clusters', where studies at higher levels of aggregation can miss important local excesses. An example is childhood leukaemia in Britain which shows regional and subregional variation in incidence rates such that, at district level, known local areas of high incidence (e.g. around Sellafield) fall well within the observed distribution of incidence rates for Britain as a whole (Stiller *et al.* 1991). Additionally, local anomalies need to be referred to the appropriate reference distribution, which should ideally take account of socio-economic factors as well as age and sex. This point is pursued further in Chapters 11 and 29.

Geographical surveillance

Systems for carrying out small-area analyses using routine data offer the possibility of surveillance to detect areas of high disease incidence. This is a potentially dangerous activity because, if used naively, many spuriously positive results will arise solely by chance. Such investigation needs to be conducted with great care, and before any results are announced publicly they should be replicated (e.g. in at least two independent time intervals) or confirmed at a separate location where the previously hypothesized causal agent is also present.

Acute accidents

Studies of acute chemical or nuclear accidents have much in common with studies of point sources of pollution. The major new factor here is time. The exposure occurs at a well-defined instant in time and is generally, but not always, short lived. Examples of acute accidents include the explosions at a factory in Seveso, described in Chapter 28, and of a nuclear reactor at Chernobyl (for which the exposure was neither short lived nor localized), and the poisoning of the water supply with aluminium sulphate at Camelford, Cornwall in England (Clayton 1989).

Methods for small-area studies

We now consider what data and methods are available to address the various types of studies outlined above. First, what is meant by a small area? This will depend on the context, as it relates to the number of cases of disease that are observed. As a rough guide, any region containing fewer than about 20 cases of disease can be considered a small area. The geographical area that this relates to will depend upon the time period over which the data have been collected, the incidence rate of disease, and the population density. Many cancers have annual incidence rates of around 5 per 100 000, so for a collective period of 5 years a small area constitutes a population of around 100 000 or fewer. In some instances, such as a cluster of disease in a remote area or small village, it could be much less, but usually populations of at least 10 000 are needed to form an aggregation of minimal size.

The simplest method of anlaysis is to choose a particular area and to compare the observed number of cases with the number that would be expected if the area had a similar incidence as some larger reference area, such as a region, state, *département*, or the entire country. A naive analysis assumes that the observed count differs from the expected value only because of Poisson sampling variation. However, many problems can occur, including:

(1) how to choose the area;
(2) *post hoc* nature of the analysis;
(3) non-Poisson sampling variation;
(4) assessment of trends of decreasing risk with distance from a source.

These problems are elaborated in Chapters 19, 20, 21, and 24.

A modification of this approach is to assume that each case of disease defines the centre of a cluster, and then to compare the number of other cases observed in circles of different radii around each point to the expected number. If used naively, this method will necessarily generate many false clusters. However, when appropriate account is taken of the number of false clusters likely to be generated, this idea can be useful and forms the basis of a number of tests for clustering in general. Additionally, the points that make the largest contribution to the overall test are prime candidates for being within aetiologically significant clusters. Again, these methods are discussed more fully in Chapter 21.

This strategy is not particularly powerful for detecting isolated clusters for a disease that does not have a general tendency to cluster, unless the cluster is of overwhelming magnitude. In this situation, the identification of a putative source is essential before any further progress can be made. This will generally be a *post hoc* association in the first instance, and replication is necessary before it can be put on a firm footing.

One attractive approach is to have a catalogue of all the major sources of a large number of potentially hazardous emissions and then to test a hypothesis generated around one such source by carrying out small-area studies around the remaining sources. To do this requires a large initial expenditure of resources, first to create the catalogue of sources (although it may already be known to the appropriate government departments, or regulatory authorities), and, secondly, to set up a system with the population and disease data available at a sufficiently fine level of resolution to be able to compute the necessary observed and expected numbers. The development of such a system for the UK (in the Small Area Health Statistics Unit at the London School of Hygiene and Tropical Medicine) is discussed in Chapter 10.

Many problems also arise when this approach is pursued. First, factories and other potential sources of pollution are likely to produce emissions of more than one substance, and each source will produce pollutants in different proportions, with different dispersion patterns, etc., so that even approximate replication of sites may be difficult. Secondly, it may not be possible to isolate one source of pollution from among many potential candidates in an industrial complex (the range of industry along the Humber estuary is a case in point when considering the alleged cluster of central nervous system malignancies near Capper Pass; Alexander *et al.* 1991).

Even for a single exposure agent, the level of exposure will differ from site to site, often by orders of magnitude. This is well illustrated by studies of leukaemia around nuclear installations, since the emissions from the nuclear reprocessing plant at Sellafield are much larger than for a nuclear power generating station, and other installations, such as research centres and weapons centres, have intermediate levels (Gardner 1989). At least, for (many of) these sources of radiation regular measurements of environmental contamination are available. When considering other pollutants, estimates of population exposure may be absent or are likely to be far less numerous and reliable.

Discussion

When faced with a report of a cluster of disease, a multi-stage screening strategy needs to be employed. Guidelines of how to proceed are presented in Chapter 23 in which epidemiological, statistical, legal, social, and psychological issues are addressed. Here we outline briefly the statistical and epidemiological problems of a typical cluster investigation. First, one needs to discover whether the number of cases are truly in excess of the number expected. To do this one must first pick a geographical sampling frame and a time period. Although these are likely to be highly data-dependent, in many instances, even with this bias, the ratio of observed to expected numbers of cases may not be much above unity. The ability to establish this quickly can be a valuable activity for helping to eliminate concern over a cluster and to reassure the public that disease rates are not elevated. When an elevated rate is found, a number of potential confounding and biasing factors need to be considered. Socio-economic factors are one source of confounding and may be an explanation of disease rates higher than the national average in some small areas (see Chapter 11).

Possible biases relating to choice of area and time have been discussed above, and an examination of the extent by which the degree of disease excess depends on the choice of time period, geographical boundaries, age-group, etc. is usually the next step.

Clusters that pass this hurdle can then be examined further by replication in different areas, by detailed case studies, and by (more formal) case-control studies in the same area. The choice between these options depends on whether there is a strong candidate for a putative source, as this is necessary before replication can be attempted, and on which approach is most easily carried out. For example, the choice may depend on the existence of an automated system to carry out replicate studies. In the absence of confirmatory evidence, a formal case-control study may still be needed to alleviate public anxiety. Case-control studies require epidemiological expertise and detailed planning, and are expensive and time-consuming to carry out. They may also raise unachievable expectations (particularly if small numbers are involved) and should only be undertaken after careful and thoughtful evaluation of the evidence. Sometimes a preliminary case study can give some idea of what the relevant factor might be before embarking on a full-scale study.

When the provision exists for replication at other sites, this is often a much more sensible next step. If the appropriate data systems are in place, replication can be done without embarking on field work and offers the chance to strengthen the hypothesis before carrying out a detailed study, or, alternatively, it may fail to reproduce the initial findings, making the hypothesized association less likely.

In conclusion, many new techniques exist to study the incidence of disease in small areas, including those in the vicinity of point sources of environmental pollution. Interpretation of any study needs to be cautious, and much confirmatory evidence is required (usually including local field studies) before a causal association can be accepted. These themes are developed further throughout this book.

References

Alexander, F. E. (1991). Investigations of localised spatial clustering, and extra-Poisson variation. In *Geographical epidemiology of childhood leukaemia and non-Hodgkin's lymphoma in Great Britain, 1966–83*, (ed. G. Draper), pp. 69–76. Studies on Medical and Population Subjects No. 53. HMSO, London.

Alexander, F. E., Williams, J., McKinney, P. A., Cartwright, R. A., and Ricketts, T. J. (1989). A specialist leukaemia/lymphoma registry in the UK. Part 2: clustering of Hodgkin's disease. *British Journal of Cancer*, **60**, 948–52.

Alexander, F. E., McKinney, P. A., and Cartwright, R. A. (1991). The pattern of childhood and related adult malignancies near Kingston-upon-Hull. *Journal of Public Health Medicine*, **13**, 96–100.

Black, J., Sharp, L., and Urquhart, J. D. (1991). An analysis of the geographical distribution of childhood leukaemia and non-Hodgkin lymphomas in Great Britain using areas of approximately equal population size. In *Geographical epidemiology of childhood leukaemia and non-Hodgkin's lymphoma in Great Britain, 1966–83*, (ed. G. Draper), pp. 61–7. Studies on Medical and Population Subjects No. 53. HMSO, London.

Britton, M. (ed.) (1990). *Mortality and geography: A review in the mid-1980s England and Wales*. HMSO, London.

Brown, L. M., Pottern, L. M., and Blot, W. J. (1984). Lung cancer in relation to environmental pollutants emitted from industrial sources. *Environmental Research*, **34**, 250–61.

Clayton, B. (chairman) (1989). *Water Pollution at Lowermoor, North Cornwall*. Report of the Lowermoor Incident Health Advisory Group. Cornwall and Isles of Scilly District Health Authority, Truro.

Day, R., Ware, J. H., Wartenberg, D., and Zelen, M. (1988). An investigation of a reported cancer cluster in Randolph, Massachusetts. *Journal of Clinical Epidemiology*, **42**, 137–50.

Gardner, M. J. (1989). Review of reported increases of childhood cancer rates in the vicinity of nuclear installations in the UK. *Journal of the Royal Statistical Society, Series A*, **152**, 307–25.

Glaser, S. L. (1990). Spatial clustering of Hodgkin's disease in the San Francisco bay area. *American Journal of Epidemiology*, **132**, (1), S167–S177.

Kyle, R. A., Herber, L., Evatt, B. L., and Heath, C. W. (1970). Multiple myeloma: a community cluster. *Journal of the American Medical Association*, **213**, (8), 1339–41.

Lagakos, S. W., Wesser, B. J., and Zelen, M. (1986). An analysis of contaminated well water and health effects in Woburn, Massachusetts (with discussion). *Journal of the American Statistical Association*, **81**, 583–614.

Mason, T. J. and McKay, F. W. (1973). *U.S. cancer mortality by county: 1950–1969*. DHEW Publication No. (NIH) 74–615. US Government Printing Office, Washington, DC.

Piantodosi, S., Byar, D. P., and Green, S. B. (1988). The ecological fallacy. *American Journal of Epidemiology*, **127**, 893–904.

Stiller, G. A., Draper, G. J., Vincent, T. J., and O'Connor, C. M. (1991). Incidence rates nationally and in administratively defined areas. In *Geographical epidemiology of childhood leukaemia and non-Hodgkin's lymphoma in Great Britain, 1966–83*, (ed. G. Draper), pp. 25–35. Studies on Medical and Population Subjects No. 53. HMSO, London.

Teppo, L., Pukkala, E., Hakema, M., Hakulinen, T., Herva, A., and Saxen, E. (1980). Way of life and cancer incidence in Finland. A municipality-based ecological analysis. *Scandinavian Journal of Social Medicine, Supplement*, **19**, 5–84.

3. Health and the environment: the significance of chemicals and radiation

*G. K. Matthew**

How great is the damage to the health of people living in prosperous indus-trialized countries, and to the environment, from chemicals or radiation? What are we to make of the widespread use of chemicals at work, on farms, and in the home? How significant for health is long-range transport of pollutants in food, air, or water? What about indirect harm to people, secondary to effects on the environment, including climate? Finally, do discharges, or waste from factories, power plants, and other sources of local-ized pollution ('point' sources) ever harm members of the general public living near to them? Despite all that is done to prevent harm, there are many un-certainties in the answers that can, so far, be given to these questions. The methods discussed in this book are most relevant to the last of these questions. They are, of course, only a part of the scientific armoury required for chemical and radiation risk assessment and risk management, but they promise sub-stantial help in reducing the uncertainties that face us.

Any public discussion on health and the environment should take account of all that we already know about risks from hazardous chemicals and radiation and the measures that are taken to prevent or limit harm. The remaining risks should be seen in just perspective with other threats to public health and well-being, so that further action in the fields of chemical safety and public health has the greatest effect. This chapter aims to set the book's specific, technical subject matter in these wider contexts. It reviews accepted knowledge of the main present-day burdens of environmental chemicals and radiation on the health of the general population in industrialized countries, and indicates how advances in environmental and geographical epidemiology, as applied to the study of health in small areas and of disease clusters, fit into the broad context.

* The author would like to thank his former colleagues in the Toxicology Division of the Department of Health for their helpful comments in the development of the views expressed in this chapter, but its contents represent his personal views and are not necessarily those of the Department of Health.

The current health burden of contamination in prosperous countries

The following pages review the current main chemical and radiation hazards to the health of the general public in prosperous industrialized countries, which are associated with contamination of food, drinking water, or the public and domestic environments. The review is restricted mainly to effects where there is a strong scientific consensus that harm is certain or probable, and to exposures that leave a troublesomely small safety margin. However, it also considers examples of geographical associations between contamination and disease, for which a causal interpretation is not, at least yet, adequately backed by other types of evidence. It deals with the direct consequences for health of contamination by chemicals at ground level and by radiation, but discussion of the indirect effects of contamination on a global scale is beyond the scope of this book. There are theoretical considerations suggesting that the total burden of contamination on health could be greater than is demonstrable directly from current evidence on exposures or effects in populations, but it is surely right to base any discussion of the place of chemicals in society primarily on a recital of what is known with fair certainty.

Contamination of food or the public and domestic environments is far from the main way by which chemicals and radiation do harm. Routine and accidental exposures are far higher in occupational environments, and some jobs still involve the acceptance of a considerable risk of occupational disease. Poisoning in the home, following the gross misuse of medicines or household and garden chemicals, is the cause of considerable mortality and morbidity, particularly amongst small children who gain access to carelessly stored chemical products. Serious incidents of poisoning of populations due to the deliberate gross adulteration of food and wine, or the misuse of material known to be contaminated, is most characteristically a problem of impoverished communities but incidents in western Europe involving the use of ethylene glycol to sweeten wine, or the sale of contaminated oil leading to the toxic oil syndrome, demonstrate that no country should assume that it is free from the possibility of criminal adulteration. The side-effects of medical treatment provide another category of harm, which is sometimes deliberately risked on the basis of a rational risk–benefit analysis, but which is too often incurred unnecessarily. All these problems pose a challenge to preventive medicine and chemical safety regulation, and they illustrate the care required in the use of chemicals and radiation. But they are not the problems of environmental pollution on which we focus here.

Chemical contamination: ground level

Serious health effects probable or certain

Carbon monoxide

Deaths continue to occur from carbon monoxide produced by badly maintained and inadequately regulated fires and heaters. Vehicle emissions can produce dangerous levels in garages and tunnels. Carbon monoxide is a postulated cardiovascular disease risk factor at lower levels.

Lead

Environmental pollution by lead is now largely the legacy of past practices and body burdens are falling. Recent evidence on the relationship between body lead burden and intelligence testing is consistent with a small negative effect on intellectual performance (MRC-LAG 1989). A small harmful effect due to current levels of exposure, particularly to some tap waters, is thought to be more probable than not, and action is being taken widely to reduce environmental lead further. Acute toxicity with occasional deaths still occurs, due in particular to the ingestion of old lead paint by children.

Environmental tobacco smoke

There is now a strong consensus that inhalation of side-stream smoke is a risk factor for acute and chronic respiratory disease in small children and of lung cancer in significantly exposed persons.

Other mixtures of substances each at trace level

All environmental media contain an ill-specified mixture of organic chemicals at trace levels, including many that are animal carcinogens and/or mutagens in high-dose experiments. Some (certain polycyclic aromatic hydrocarbons or chlorinated solvents) are of particular concern because of their toxicology, and/or because of environmental levels. Additive effects or other interactions may occur. These micro-pollutants probably make a contribution to cancer incidence, but it is likely to be small. It is impossible to assess which substances are active in humans at the levels found. It is suggested that the micro-pollutants contribute only a minor part of the total burden of avoidable death and disease. However, there are profound uncertainties behind this assessment, which can only be resolved, if at all, by extensive long-term research.

Safety margins small

The classical air pollutants: SO_2 and NO_x

Sulphur dioxide and associated smoke are more closely monitored and regulated than any other forms of air pollution. Hazardous levels occur in certain industrialized regions of the world, particularly where brown coal is used widely. Even in countries with strict controls there may be local and transient problems when smoke from high stacks is blown to ground level. Such exposures cause discomfort and may produce a short-term effect on respiratory function. The highest environmental levels of the oxides of nitrogen occur indoors in association with the combustion of gas. Short-term peaks occur. Despite extensive studies, there is no sound evidence of persistent effects on lung function or the incidence of chronic respiratory disease from current environmental levels in prosperous industrialized countries but research continues, the safety margin can be small and there is concern that the risk may be greater for vulnerable groups, such as those with asthma.

Ozone and photochemical smog

Photochemical smogs, due to complex chemical interactions involving hydrocarbons, oxides of nitrogen, ozone, and sunlight, are a serious problem in certain metropolitan areas characterized by long hours of sunlight and entrapment of air. On occasion they develop to a less grave extent elsewhere. A severe photochemical smog is extremely unpleasant, but the clearly demonstrated effects are only of small reductions in lung function, within the range of normal variability; however, there is concern lest there may be longer-term effects, especially in vulnerable people.

Mercury

Discharges of mercury directly or indirectly into coastal waters result in the formation of the organic form, methyl mercury, and to the contamination of fish, particularly predatory species up the food chain. The effects of methyl mercury are known from direct observations in people as a result of incidents of gross poisoning, for example an incident in Iraq when seed corn deliberately treated with methyl mercury as a fungicide was improperly used for human consumption (IPCS 1990). It causes widespread damage to the nervous sytem, often of delayed onset. The effects in the milder cases include paraesthesia, blurred vision, and malaise, and are reversible, but irreversible damage and even death can occur. The fetus is particularly sensitive. Levels of mercury intake by extreme fish consumers can approach dangerous levels, in rare instances, and equivocal evidence of marginal effects has been published. A main source of contamination of coastal waters by mercury was the traditional practice in the chloralkali industry of using liquid mercury as an electrode and estuary water as the electrolytic medium, a prime example of a grossly polluting industrial technology dating from the nineteenth century. It has been replaced largely by a cleaner process but has left a residue of long-lasting environmental contamination which is difficult to ameliorate and impossible to clear up entirely.

Cadmium

Cadmium has very many industrial uses and there is concern that unacceptable levels of contamination will be reached eventually in many environmental media unless usage is severely restricted. There is particular concern about cadmium in sewage sludge as a result of small-scale discharges to the sewers, affecting sludge-treated farm land and crops grown on it. There are also natural sources and historical residues in the form of old mine tippings. Cadmium in sufficient amount can damage many organs of the body, but the first effect, as the cumulative body burden increases, is on the kidneys, with the asymptomatic presence of low molecular weight protein in the urine. Extreme exposure in a famous Japanese incident led to severe illness and many deaths, with multiple symptoms; the population affected was poorly nourished and the illness, known as Itai-Itai, was thought to result from the interaction of these factors (JECFA 1989). Studies in a healthy British population exposed to intakes far above those normally possible, as a result of consuming home-grown vegetables from land contaminated by ancient mine spoil, showed no ill health attributable to cadmium (Morgan 1988). However, in this case, the usual safety margin was seriously eroded and there have been other instances where this has occurred.

The dioxins, PCBs, organochlorine pesticides, etc., in food and breast milk

The 'dioxins', polychlorinated biphenyls (PCBs) and triphenyls, organochlorine pesticides, and certain other complex organohalogens are not readily biodegradable and tend to accumulate in the food chain and in human fat. The best studied, dioxin (2,3,7,8-TCDD), is toxic in experimental animals at remarkably low dose, and it and the large class of related halogenated dioxins and furans are produced as unintended by-products in many combustion and manufacturing processes. Although levels in food and the environment are also low (too low to have been measurable until recently), there is concern that the apparent safety margin is relatively modest, given the imprecision of our knowledge of the toxicity of the dioxins in humans (Interdepartmental Working Group on Dioxins 1989). It is of particular concern that human breast milk contains relatively high levels. Polychlorinated biphenyls were manufactured and used widely; their use is now banned but they continue to contaminate the environment and the food chain. The organochlorine pesticides had an extremely destructive effect on wildlife until they were replaced by less persistent alternatives, at least in developed countries. There is concern about them and, indeed, about a whole class of persistent complex organohalogen compounds that can accumulate in the food chain and reach relatively high levels in human body fat and breast milk. This concern is, however, based in large part on evidence of liver toxicity and carcinogenicity in laboratory animals. These chemicals are prime examples of compounds where the validity of extrapolation from laboratory evidence to human beings is particularly open to question. Incidents of poisoning due to gross misuse have been reported from several countries, but there is no direct evidence of harm to people at environmental levels.

Nitrate contamination resulting from agricultural practice

Nitrate contamination illustrates a number of important problems in risk assessment and management. The nitrate ion is a simple substance, an essential nutrient for plants, and an inevitable constituent of them and of the soil; it has, however, no biological function in humans. It is a potential health problem due to the use of manure or artificial nitrate-containing fertilizer to increase crop yields. Since contaminated water in soil may take decades to percolate through rock to reach ground waters used for drinking, nitrate contamination is a prime example of an environmental problem which is not easy to correct once it has been allowed to develop. In many areas an early reduction of exposure could only be achieved by denitrification of the source water, and the question raised is whether there is sufficient assurance that the processes of denitrification are themselves entirely safe. Nitrate also poses peculiarly difficult problems in toxicological assessment:

1. The clear-cut risk is of methaemoglobinaemia in infants, a condition that is detectable medically before it is harmful and can be reversed easily. The threshold of this effect is not determined exactly and there is reason for uncertainty about how stringent the regulation of levels in supply should be.
2. There is a theoretical risk, without sound supporting epidemiological evidence, that nitrate may contribute to cancer incidence, but indirectly, by complex chemical processes within the body. There are differences of opinion on how much weight should be given to this possibility.

Asbestos and other mineral fibres

Asbestos provides an example of a substance for which a cancer risk has been clearly demonstrated in human populations, but in relation to former high levels of exposure in industry. There is now also suggestive epidemiological evidence of a lung cancer risk associated with past occupational exposure to man-made mineral fibres at high levels which no longer occur with modern industrial practice. Because of the particular physical and chemical nature of these fibrous substances, there is greater than usual uncertainty on whether a threshold to the carcinogenic effect exists. There is particular difficulty in deciding whether asbestos-based materials installed in buildings in the past, and widely used insulation based on man-made mineral fibres, represent any degree of health hazard. It is likely that, if there are risks, they are small. The extremely stringent policies adopted in relation to public exposure to asbestos proved an awkward precedent when, later, suspicion also fell, unforeseen, on the substitute materials.

Aflatoxin and other natural food toxicants

Aflatoxin is the prime example of a class of natural toxicants. It is derived from food moulds, is characterized by liver toxicity, and is an unusually potent carcinogen in experimental animals. The recent detection of a previously unsuspected source, namely figs grown and prepared in a Mediterranean country, illustrates the ceaseless vigilance required to minimize the likelihood of undetected contamination of foods and unacceptable levels of exposure.

Geographical associations not confirmed by other evidence

Marked differences from place to place in the incidence of many diseases, particularly urban/rural differences, raise the suspicion of an environmental aetiology but, generally, no convincing hypotheses concerning specific substances have emerged to explain these geographical associations. Recently, in a few instances, hypotheses based in whole or in part on such geographical associations have been under active examination.

Aluminium in food and drinking water

Aluminium is widely and naturally present in food and the environment, with a number of approved uses in food manufacture, water treatment, and pharmaceutical practice. Water contaminated by aluminium and used in renal dialysis is established as the cause of the encephalopathy and bone disease formerly seen in dialysis patients but now prevented by the use of appropriate water. However, the low bioavailability of many forms of aluminium, and the normally ready excretion of aluminium by the healthy kidney, have long led to the view that aluminium taken by mouth is essentially non-toxic except in individuals with gross renal failure, although there has been some concern of toxicity at the extremes of life. A recent episode of gross contamination of a water supply by the acid salt, aluminium sulphate, which caused secondary contamination by other metals, led to immediate effects on the gastrointestinal tract in individuals who managed to swallow the foul-tasting water (Clayton 1989). However, a more fundamental concern is the hypothesis of an association between exposure to aluminium and Alzheimer's disease. The hypothesis is based on post-mortem findings in individuals with this condition, although recent epidemiological research in two European countries has suggested a geographical association between levels of aluminium in drinking water and the incidence of the disease (Flaten 1986; Martyn *et al.* 1989). The association is surprising, given that drinking water provides only a few per cent of the daily intake of aluminium. More research on the bioavailability of different forms of aluminium, and further epidemiological studies, are under way as part of the wider effort to establish the causes of Alzheimer's disease. The aluminium/Alzheimer's disease story is a prime example of the difficult decisions on policy that arise, when the public is aware of a hypothesis of a major toxic effect relating to an important and frightening disease, but where scientific consensus is lacking and the research required to investigate the truth of the matter is likely to take some years to complete.

Water supply management and cancer

Drinking water taken from rivers downstream of major towns and industrial areas contains many trace pollutants. Chlorination, particularly of peaty upland waters, produces increased quantities of various halogenated organic chemicals, some of them potential carcinogens. Epidemiological research has found some evidence, from particular areas, suggestive of an increased cancer risk associated with so-called indirect reuse of water, with the use of upland water rich in humic acids, and with chlorinated surface water. However, the evidence has been inconsistent and is insufficiently strong to have led to recommendations for any radical change of present water industry practices. This experience provides a prime example of the limitations of observational epidemiology in testing hypotheses of weak effects.

Water mineral content and cardiovascular disease

Perhaps the most compelling finding of environmental epidemiology is a strong negative association between the hardness of water in supply and cardiovascular disease incidence. This has been noted internationally and the finding stands up both in well-controlled studies based on routine statistics and in prospective studies based on the records of individuals (Pocock *et al.* 1980; Shaper *et al.* 1981). However, a plausible mechanism for the effect, consistent with the range of evidence, has never been suggested. Evidence from populations whose drinking water has changed is not helpful. It might have been hoped that here was a clue that would lead to the prevention of a large proportion of premature deaths from cardiovascular disease but, in the event, the evidence has not been judged sufficiently clear-cut to justify action. This is a prime example of the very different criteria employed when judging whether to add a potentially beneficial substance to food or water from those employed when judging when to eliminate a potentially hazardous contaminant.

Environmental radiation

Environmental radiation is the current environment health issue of greatest public and political concern. Only in the case of radiation is there direct evidence for the absence of a threshold to a carcinogenic effect in human populations; in addition, exposure to significant levels of certain forms of radiation are ubiquitous and inevitable, and there are important limitations in our knowledge of the toxicokinetics and biological effects of specific radionuclides. The nuclear energy industry is widely seen as presenting the greatest risk of catastrophic major accidents. There is also, no doubt, a psychological reaction to an agent that is potent but imperceptible. There are three major current issues: radon, nuclear installations handling or discharging alpha-emitting radionuclides, and electromagnetic fields.

Radon

Evidence from occupational exposure to the decay products of radon gas suggests that exposure to radon in the home could be an important contribution to lung cancer incidence. Concentrations of radon in houses varies considerably, depending on the nature and degree of influx from the underlying rock. This, together with the dominance of the effect of smoking, makes the extent of the risk difficult to determine. Nevertheless, radon, which is of natural origin, may be the major current cause of ill health from any form of environmental contamination (chemical or radiobiological).

Nuclear installations handling or discharging alpha-emitting radionuclides

Childhood leukaemia is a relatively rare condition, which tends to cluster geographically to an extent explicable as a normal statistical phenomenon. It is therefore difficult to determine whether the occurrence of a childhood leukaemia cluster close to an installation handling and/or discharging potentially leukaemogenic substances has occurred in that locality by coincidence or as the direct or indirect effect of the relevant exposure. A substantially above-average incidence of childhood leukaemia has now been reported from the neighbourhood of the only two nuclear fuel reprocessing plants in the UK (Black 1984; COMARE 1988); lesser excesses have been reported from the neighbourhood of some, but by no means all, other nuclear installations in the UK. A close examination of the evidence has failed to discover a mechanism whereby a perceptible excess risk could have been engendered by these operations, although there is recent evidence from the Sellafield site of an association with occupational exposure of fathers (see Chapter 25). The findings are sufficiently striking to suggest the need for further research and for all rigour in the limitation of exposures of neighbouring populations and workers alike. This is the prime example of the need for the most powerful available means for studying disease incidence in small areas close to point sources of environmental contamination, if environmental epidemiology is to make a contribution to our understanding of the links between environmental factors and health.

Electromagnetic fields

Powerful electromagnetic fields can induce biological effects such as body heating. Subtle, but not necessarily harmful, effects are observed at lower intensities. Recent epidemiological evidence is suggestive of a cancer risk associated with such fields and thus with the electricity supply. The evidence is inconsistent but warrants further work. At the same time, electromagnetic fields are proving a fruitful field for speculation amongst the practitioners of alternative medicine; various effects, including sudden infant death syndrome, have been suggested, although without the support of sound evidence, and allegedly protective devices are sold widely. This example suggests that any environmental factors that have been traditionally regarded as harmless are liable to come under scrutiny in the present wave of concern and speculation about the relationships between environment and health.

Discussion

There is little unequivocal, direct evidence that harm is being done to the health of the general population of prosperous countries at the present time, as a result of environmental contamination by chemicals or radiation. Even if one includes harm for which the evidence is controversial but which is judged likely by a consensus of scientific opinion, the total burden would seem to be modest amongst the full range of avoidable disease. There is, at least as yet, no sound evidence of any 'epidemic' of disease related to the greatly increased production and use of chemicals since the Second World War. On the face of it, accidents and deficiencies in food hygiene are far more important as environmentally related public health problems, while the misuse or dangerous storage of chemicals in the home and the chemical aspects of occupational health appear to be more important concerns of chemical safety than the effects of pollution on the physical health of the public.

There are, however, many reasons why the lack of clear evidence of harm should not be allowed to lead to complacency or to any slackening of effort to secure higher standards of chemical safety. First, of course, the control of pollution is required to protect ecosystems and other species, and controls required to meet that objective sometimes need to be tighter than those that would have been sufficient for the protection of human health. Secondly, some forms of current pollution threaten human health in the future, either by toxicological mechanisms following the continued accumulation of non-biodegradable substances, or indirectly, as with the immensely important phenomena of effects on the atmosphere and stratosphere. Thirdly, the infrequency of demonstrable effects due to agents in the immediate environment of individuals is due, in large part, to control actions taken in the past, as problems came to light; it is unlikely that all the contributions of chemicals to disease have yet been identified and, in particular, small contributions to the risk of common diseases from multiple low-level exposures, and various 'subtle' adverse effects on health cannot be excluded. It is worth noting that some of the forms of harm from chemicals which are now accepted as at least likely, such as the influence of lead on intellectual development, not to speak of the trend to global warming, were at first dismissed as implausible by many expert scientists.

The goal is to be able to use chemicals and radiation confidently for the benefit of the human race, and to eliminate, as far as is reasonably possible, avoidable harm and environmental damage, while responding to public concern about the safety of current practice. This means that the development of programmes of testing, assessment, and monitoring, in toxicology and radiation science, and of the underlying research required for their advance, should be pursued energetically. At the same time, our response to the potential risks of chemicals and radiation should be in just proportion to our response to other threats to the public health and the environment, and care should be taken not to waste scarce resources by the wrong response to sometimes exaggerated or unjustified fears.

Amongst the investigative disciplines that deal with chemical safety, and in which advances are required, epidemiology and medical geography, since they seek the information that we need directly, stand pre-eminent. In particular, advances are required in the methods available to detect increases in the incidence of disease in small populations, which may result, by whatever mechanism, from an industrial operation or a localized source of pollution in the neighbourhood. Since an important part of the requirement is to respond promptly to fears that are widely felt, but probably rarely justified, about local industry, waste disposal sites, etc., cost-effective techniques are needed for the rapid initial assessment of health in small areas, and to decide whether more extensive investigation is justified. In that connection, the expensively collected routine health statistics call out for fuller exploitation. The main challenges are: first, to focus analyses of those statistics far more closely on the populations that are most likely to be exposed to the consequences of a particular activity; and, secondly, to strengthen techniques for distinguishing circumstances where a much higher than expected incidence of disease might well be the result of a local hazardous exposure, from those that are very probably 'due to chance'.

In recent years a number of groups in universities and statistical agencies, particularly in the UK, have become interested in these questions. The Black Report on the incidence of childhood leukaemia near the Sellafield nuclear fuel reprocessing plant (see Chapter 25) recommended that means be established in the UK to co-ordinate work done with the available statistics. The Small Area Health Statistics Unit was subsequently established at the London School of Hygiene and Tropical Medicine by the British government departments responsible for health and for the environment (see Chapters 10 and 29). It was founded in order to further the development of the necessary techniques, to undertake studies for government, and to provide a focus for the collaboration of the groups active in the UK. Since then, major advances have been made in the technical and conceptual aspects of the subject, and a powerful network of collaboration amongst geographers, epidemiologists, and statisticians established, not only in the UK but internationally. The fruits of that collaboration are described in the remainder of this book.

References

Black, D. (chairman) (1984). *Investigation of the possible increased incidence of cancer in West Cumbria*. Report of the Independent Advisory Group. HMSO, London.

Clayton, B. (chairman) (1989). *Water pollution at Lowermoor North Cornwall*. Report of the Lowermoor Incident Advisory Group. Cornwall and Isles of Scilly District Health Authority, Truro.

COMARE (Committee on Medical Aspects of Radiation in the Environment) (1988). *Second Report: Investigation of the possible incidence of leukaemia in young people near the Dounreay Nuclear Establishment, Caithness, Scotland*. HMSO, London.

Flaten, T. P. (1986). An investigation of the chemical composition of Norwegian drinking water and its possible relationships with the epidemiology of some diseases. Unpublished Ph.D. thesis. Institutt for Uorganisk Kjemi, Universitetet I Trondheim.

Interdepartmental Working Group on Dioxins, Polychlorinated dibenzo-para-dioxins (PCDDs) and Polychlorinated dibenzofurans (PCDFS) (1989). *Dioxins in the environment*. Department of the Environment Pollution Paper No. 27. HMSO, London.

IPCS (International Programme on Chemical Safety) (1990). *Methylmercury*. Environmental Health Criteria 101. World Health Organisation, Geneva.

JECFA (Joint FAO/WHO Expert Committee on Food Additives) (1989). Cadmium. In *Toxicological evaluation of certain food additives and contaminants*, WHO Food Additive Series No. 24, pp. 163–219. Cambridge University Press, Cambridge.

Martyn, C. N., Barker, D. J. P., Osmond, H., Harris, E. C., Edwardson, J. A., and Lacey, R. F. (1989). Geographical relationship between Alzheimer's disease and aluminium in drinking water. *Lancet*, **i**, 59–62.

Morgan, H. (ed.) (1988). The Shipham Report. An investigation into cadmium contamination and its implications for human health. *Science of the Total Environment*, **75**, (1),

MRC-LAG (Medical Research Council Advisory Group on Lead and Neuropsychological Effects in Children) (1989). *The neuropsychological effects of lead in children. A review of the research 1984–1988*. Medical Research Council, London.

Pocock, S. J., *et al.* (1980). British regional heart study: geographic variations in cardiovascular mortality and the role of water quality. *British Medical Journal*, **280**, 1243–9.

Shaper, A. G., Pocock, S. J., Walker, M., Cohen, N. M., Wale, C. J., and Thompson, A. G. (1981). British regional heart study: cardiovascular mortality in middle-aged men in 24 towns. *British Medical Journal*, **283**, 179–86.

II Data, computational methods, and mapping

4. Mortality data

A. D. Lopez

Undoubtedly, the single, most comprehensive source of small-area health statistics is that concerned with mortality. Basic information on the number, age, and sex of deceased persons has been routinely collected in Europe for several hundred years. Information on the cause of death, albeit according to relatively imprecise nosological standards, was available from the records of the London parishes in the seventeenth century and formed the basis for John Graunt's foundation work on the *Bills of Mortality* (Graunt 1662). No comparable information base has been developed for other indicators of health status (e.g. morbidity) or for other aspects of the health system (e.g. health care delivery, health personnel). This is not to deny the importance of such data. However, no long, standard, and comparable time-series is available for most countries. This, to some extent, reflects definitional problems about what to measure (relevance) and how to obtain valid data on these indicators.

In Europe, virtually all deaths are registered and, with very few exceptions, the cause of death is medically certified according to the rules and procedures of the International Classification of Diseases (ICD). Mortality statistics are thus available for the entire population of Europe, including the former USSR, which are, in principle at least, valid and comparable. National-level statistics are then compiled from individual records and the annual national statistics are forwarded to WHO, where a mortality data-base, containing data as far back as 1950, is maintained.

Despite the ready availability of mortality data for Europe, the accuracy and relevance of these statistics for epidemiological research needs to be carefully examined. Thus, whereas the aggregation of national-level data according to broad categories of cause of death may yield a reasonably complete picture of the current epidemiological environment for Europe as a whole, or for particular subregions, the utility of these data for small-area studies requires a much more careful evaluation. This chapter will review some of the issues in the use of routine mortality data for small-area epidemiological research.

Data collection systems

Before looking into the quality of mortality data, it is perhaps worthwhile to review briefly how the data are generated. The basic medical record is the

International Form of Medical Certificate of Cause of Death, which is completed by the attending physician, after investigation by a medicolegal authority. On the basis of the information reported on the death certificate, a single, *underlying* cause of death is coded according to the rules and procedures of the ICD Revision in force at the time. Coding of death certificates may be done centrally or may be carried out locally, with or without a mechanism for ensuring consistency among coders. Most countries in Europe have instituted data quality checks and follow-up procedures in case of doubt about the cause of death, although the principles and practices obviously vary from country to country. In some cases, an autopsy is required before the death certificate can be issued. On the basis of these completed records, mortality statistics are compiled, first, for administrative subdivisions of a country, and then progressively aggregated to the national level. For subsequent tabulations, data may then be disaggregated according to administrative areas.

Table 4.1 provides a summary of some of the principal aspects of the cause of death information system in European countries and, where available, gives data on the extent of autopsy. It should be pointed out, however, that autopsy data are not always used to determine the underlying cause of death mentioned on the death certificate and, hence, the reliability of the cause-of-death is probably less than that suggested by the table.

Issues in the use of mortality data

The major advantages of routine mortality data (availability, coverage, medical certification, application of a common standard) have already been mentioned. The relative merits of a particular data system must, of course, be viewed within the context of its intended use, and for first-level health monitoring or for regional health situation assessment, these advantages are apparent. There are a number of issues affecting the quality and relevance of these data for other, more specific purposes, however, and these are discussed below according to the two principal phases in the process of reporting and ordering causes of death on the death certificate, namely:

(1) diagnosis (determination of pathologies present at or around the time of death); and
(2) certification and coding (ordering and coding of diseases and injuries on the death certificate according to the ICD).

Diagnosis of cause of death

Diagnostic accuracy is clearly of fundamental importance in the determination of the cause of death. Conditions present in the deceased which were not diagnosed or, for other reasons, were not entered on the death certificate will not be considered as one of the potential causes of death. It is, thus, extremely important that *all* major diseases or injuries be diagnosed. The medical practitioner's ability to do this depends on a wide variety of factors, which ultimately influence the quality of cause of death statistics.

Changes in the pattern of diseases with epidemiological transition has probably had a very significant impact on diagnostic accuracy. The progressive postponement of death to higher and higher ages has been accompanied by a dramatic rise in the average number of chronic conditions potentially contributing to death, a situation that was much less common under the regime of infectious diseases. Correctly identifying these conditions, particularly in the absence of diagnostic aids, is often very difficult, leading to ill-defined diagnoses, such as heart failure, senility, and the like. This effect is particularly evident for females in view of their longer life expectancy. Based on the experience of some (predominantly northern) European countries, the mean expectation of life at birth for females is now around 80 years, with more than 50 per cent of deaths occurring at ages 80 years or over. Of these, almost one-fifth occur at ages 90 or more. The likelihood of multiple pathologies at these ages is very high.

The increasing availability of diagnostic aids, such as electrocardiograms for heart disease, electroencephalograms for brain tumours, and haematological services for blood diseases such as leukaemia have undoubtedly improved the completeness and accuracy of diagnostic information entered on the death certificate. Another major factor in diagnostic ascertainment is the use of autopsy and histological diagnoses. However, as Table 4.1 indicates, typically only about one-quarter to one-third of deaths are the subject of autopsy, with the proportion as low as 7 per cent in Ireland. Moreover, there is a distinct tendency for the autopsy rate to decrease with age, with the result that comparatively few autopsies are carried out at the older ages where the vast majority of deaths occur. Under extensive pathological investigation, the underlying morbid process leading ultimately to death can usually be determined with a high degree of accuracy. Clinical opinions, on the other hand, are often based on presumptive evidence and may be quite inaccurate, particularly if the certifying physician was not well acquainted with the morbid history of the deceased.

Independent clinical and pathological evaluations of the cause of death may thus be expected to provide some insight into the accuracy of diagnosis offered by medical practitioners. Overall, the findings of these dual certification studies suggest that tabulations of the underlying cause of death be viewed with some caution. The classical study of Heasman and Lipworth (1966), based on almost 10 000 autopsies performed in a number of teaching hospitals in England and Wales, indicated that hospital clinicians and pathologists chose the same underlying cause of death for only about 45 per cent of deaths. Of the disagreements between the two, about one-half were cases where 'either the clinician's underlying cause of death was not mentioned in the pathologist's report or vice versa' (Heasman and Lipworth 1966). Physicians in England

Table 4.1 Background information (around 1985) on mortality statistics for the WHO European Region

Country	% of deaths medically certified	% of deaths occurring in a hospital or other medical establishment	% of deaths for which an autopsy was performed	Follow-up enquiries in case of doubt about the cause of death	Deaths recorded by date of	Coding procedure	Remarks on coverage of mortality statistics
Austria	100	60	_Age_ % 0 89 1–14 49 15–44 49 45–64 46 65+ 30 All ages 34	By Central Statistical Office in case of doubt (3–4% of all deaths)	Occurrence	Centrally coded except for deaths occurring in Vienna for which cause is coded by Municipal Council; centrally supervised	Foreigners with usual residence in Austria are included; Austrian citizens with usual residence abroad are excluded
Belgium	100	59	No information	Yes, in cases where the underlying cause of death is improbable or ill-defined	Occurrence	Decentralized	Since 1986, non-residents who die in Belgium are not included; nationals who die abroad (approx. 1000 each year) are not included either
Bulgaria	100	25	25	Yes	Occurrence	Decentralized since 1980, but under supervision of Ministry of Health	Statistics refer to permanent residents only
Czechoslovakia	100	60	_Age_ % 0 96 1–14 75 15+ 28 All ages 29	Yes, only rarely	Occurrence	Centrally coded in Prague and Bratislava	Czechoslovakia proper; statistics also cover nationals living abroad

Country			Age / %				
Denmark	100	56	*Age* % 0 — 65 1–19 — 27 20–34 — 43 35–54 — 30 55–74 — 27 75+ — 17 All ages — 32	Yes, for about 8% of deaths	Occurrence	Centrally coded	Statistics refer to Danish residents only; Danes dying abroad are excluded but deaths of foreign residents (about 0.6% of the total) are included; data do not include deaths occurring in Greenland and Faeroe Islands
Finland	100	75	*Age* % 0 — 93 1–14 — 84 15–44 — 82 45–64 — 52 65+ — 27 All ages — 36	Yes, 2% of death certificates were queried in 1985 (mainly those with improbable cause-of-death sequences and with ill-defined cause as the only cause mentioned)	Occurrence	Centrally coded	Finland, including Åland Islands; statistics refer to permanent residents only
France	100	50	No information	Yes	Occurrence	Centrally coded	Includes France proper, plus overseas departments
(former) German Democratic Republic	100	50	*Age* % 0 — 100 1–14 — 100 15–44 — 48 45–64 — 34 65+ — 14 All ages — 25	Yes	Occurrence	Coded by the certifying physician	German Democratic Republic
(former) German Federal Republic	100	53	8	For some cases, but not systematically	Occurrence	Decentralized but under guidance of Federal Statistical Office	Federal Republic of Germany, including Berlin (West); German nationals who died abroad are included

Table 4.1 *(cont.)*

Country	% of deaths medically certified	% of deaths occurring in a hospital or other medical establishment	% of deaths for which an autopsy was performed	Follow-up enquiries in case of doubt about the cause of death	Deaths recorded by date of	Coding procedure	Remarks on coverage of mortality statistics
Greece	99	46	Not available; autopsies are performed for deaths from accidents and for sudden deaths	Yes, if cause sequence is improbable or illegible	Occurrence	Centrally coded	Statistics include deaths of permanent residents as well as deaths of foreigners which occur in Greece
Hungary	100	55	49	Yes, at regional level	Occurrence	Centrally coded	Statistics do not include nationals who die abroad but include foreigners who die in Hungary irrespective of whether they are permanent residents or not (except for diplomatic and military personnel)
Iceland	100	80	38	Yes; all codes are systematically checked by the Dept of Public Health with additional enquiries of coders, if necessary	Occurrence	Centrally coded	Iceland proper; statistics include deaths abroad of residents, but exclude deaths of non-residents (e.g. tourists, foreign diplomatic personnel) who die in Iceland

Country							
Ireland	100	62	Age % 0 22 1–14 11 15–44 13 45–64 13 65+ 4 All ages 7	Yes, certifying doctor or coroner is queried for further information	Occurrence since 1970; prior to 1970 by date of registration	Centrally coded	Statistics do not include nationals who die abroad but include deaths of foreigners, whether they are permanent residents or not
Israel	100	68	No information	Since 1971 all death certificates with doubtful cause sequences are queried and corrected accordingly	Occurrence	Centrally coded	Statistics include deaths in Israel, plus those of Jews living in Judea, Samaria and Gaza Area
Italy	100	37	No information	Yes; in 1984, roughly 3500 death certificates were queried as to the cause of death	Occurrence	Centrally coded	Statistics include all deaths occurring in Italy but not those of Italians residing abroad
Luxembourg	100	69	No information (except for perinatal deaths for which the % of autopsies varies between 30% and 40%)	Yes, if cause stated on the death certificate is imprecise or illegible	Occurrence	Centrally coded	Statistics include all deaths occurring in Luxembourg irrespective of country of usual residence; however, deaths of residents which occur abroad are excluded
Malta	100	67	Age % 0 49 1–14 24 15–44 39 45–64 9 65+ 2 All ages 6	Yes, directly with certifying physician	Occurrence	Centrally coded	Nationals who die abroad are not included in the statistics; foreigners who die in Malta are also excluded unless they are permanent residents

Table 4.1 (*cont.*)

Country	% of deaths medically certified	% of deaths occurring in a hospital or other medical establishment	% of deaths for which an autopsy was performed	Follow-up enquiries in case of doubt about the cause of death	Deaths recorded by date of	Coding procedure	Remarks on coverage of mortality statistics
Netherlands	100	46	*Age* % 0 58 1–14 21 15–44 17 45–64 13 65 + 8 All ages 10	Yes, further information sought from certifying physician if necessary	Occurrence	Centrally coded	Nationals who die abroad are included if they are registered as residents in the Netherlands; statistics also include deaths of foreigners who were permanent residents of the Netherlands
Norway	100	62 (+ 11% in other institutions such as old-age homes)	*Age* % <50 30 50–69 18 70–79 13 80 + 6 All ages 16	Yes, particularly for deaths from cancer, external causes, sudden deaths, or deaths for which the stated sequence is incomplete or improbable	Occurrence	Centrally coded	Statistics include all deaths among the resident population, irrespective of where the death occurred
Poland	96	47	9	Yes	Occurrence	Decentralized (codes verified by district physician)	Statistics include deaths of all nationals irrespective of where the death occurred
Portugal	99	39	No information	Yes	Occurrence	Centrally coded	Statistics include deaths of Portuguese citizens with usual residence abroad

Country						
Spain	100	30	No information	Yes, in some regions	Occurrence	Decentralized but reviewed by National Institute of Statistics	Statistics do not include Spaniards who die abroad; however, deaths of foreigners in Spain are included
Sweden	100	79	*Age* % 0 74 1–14 66 15–44 76 45–64 56 65+ 36 All ages 37	About 3% of death certificates are queried, primarily deaths at ages 0–74 years	Occurrence	Centrally coded	Statistics include permanent residents who die abroad, irrespective of nationality, but exclude deaths of Swedes registered as living abroad
Switzerland	100	54	*Age* % 0 72 1–14 35 15–44 35 45–64 27 65+ 16 All ages 19	Yes, for about 10–15% of deaths to permit more precise coding	Occurrence	Centrally coded	Statistics refer to permanent residents only, including those who die abroad
(former) USSR	94% by physicians, 6% by 'feldschers' (medical auxiliaries) working primarily in rural areas	24	31	Yes	Occurrence	Regional level	No information

Table 4.1 (*cont.*)

Country	% of deaths medically certified	% of deaths occurring in a hospital or other medical establishment	% of deaths for which an autopsy was performed	Follow-up enquiries in case of doubt about the cause of death	Deaths recorded by date of	Coding procedure	Remarks on coverage of mortality statistics
United Kingdom: England and Wales	100	63	*Age* % 0–14 60 15–44 62 45–64 37 65+ 23 All ages 27	Yes; each year, 2–3% of death certificates are followed up, typically those with unspecified or poorly specified codes	Registration	Centrally coded	Statistics refer to deaths occurring in England and Wales only and include non-residents
United Kingdom: Northern Ireland	100	61	*Age* % <1 32 1–14 37 15–44 56 45–64 17 65+ 5 All ages 11	Yes; in case of doubt a query is sent to the coroner	Registration	Centrally coded	Statistics include non-nationals who die in N. Ireland irrespective of whether they are permanent residents or not; they do not include nationals who die abroad
United Kingdom: Scotland	100	65	*Age* % 0 67 1–14 58 15–44 57 45–64 24 65+ 11 All ages 15	Yes; medical enquiry forms are sent out when further information is required	Registration	Centrally coded	Statistics include all persons who die in Scotland, including non-nationals, irrespective of whether they are permanent residents or not; they do not include nationals who die abroad
(former) Yugoslavia	96	36	No information	No	Occurrence	Decentralized, but according to uniform criteria	Statistics refer to Yugoslav citizens dying in Yugoslavia

and Wales had a tendency to overdiagnose cerebrovascular diseases, while lung cancer and peptic ulcers were understated as causes of death. On the other hand, ischaemic heart disease and pneumonia and bronchitis displayed a 'good agreement' in the number of deaths assigned to these conditions by the two sources.

Among the many other factors that influence diagnostic quality and, particularly, the *comparability* of diagnostic information between countries, or even within a country, are diagnostic 'fads', medical training, and cultural norms. There is some suggestion that the comparatively high mortality from chronic obstructive lung diseases in Britain may be due to the greater tendency to diagnose these conditions which elsewhere may have been ascribed to cardiovascular disease, although this interpretation has been called into question (Preston *et al.* 1972). Obviously, any propensity for medical practitioners to prefer a 'fashionable' diagnosis on the basis of its prominence in the medical literature would lead to an overstatement of the true incidence of that disease. Coronary heart disease appears to be one condition that has been affected in this way, mostly at the expense of other cardiac disorders. A study of mortality trends in Australia between 1950 and 1967, reported that the rapid increase in ischaemic heart disease was substantially diminished when deaths from degenerative heart disease were included (McDonald 1972). Even though there was no direct evidence, the author concluded that the transfer of diagnosis from degenerative to ischaemic heart disease during this time was 'virtually certain'.

In other instances, a physician might refrain from making a specific diagnosis if it was thought that such information might be harmful to the memory of the deceased and/or cause some embarrassment to the survivors. Deaths from syphilis and other sexually transmitted diseases, suicide, tuberculosis, cancer, and causes related to alcoholism have probably been under-reported as a result of this practice. There is a direct corollary of this 'diagnostic reluctance' in relation to geographically specific data, where there may be particular concerns about a given locality and, hence, a reluctance to diagnose illnesses connected with it.

Variations in the experience, quality, and type of training of physicians could be expected to influence their diagnostic skills. Thus, better opportunities for postgraduate training in disciplines such as cardiology have undoubtedly led to a greater refinement of diagnosis for many chronic conditions. Further, it would appear unlikely that medical practitioners trained 20 or more years apart would share congruent views about the pathology of such diseases.

Certification and coding of diseases and injuries

Numerous studies have been conducted to assess the accuracy and comparability of coding and certification of conditions appearing on the death certificate

(Gittelsohn and Royston 1982; Kelson and Farebrother 1987; Mackenbach *et al.* 1987). For the most part, these studies have been based on a recoding of a sample of case histories (real or hypothetical), followed by comparison with some standard coding or certification source (e.g. by a WHO Collaborating Centre). Although the World Health Organization (1977) has issued standard rules and procedures for classifying underlying causes of death, the problem of selecting a single underlying cause, as has been the traditional practice in vital statistics, is often complicated by the sequence and combination of illnesses mentioned on the death certificate. This has been repeatedly demonstrated by comparative studies of coding and certification practices, which have identified significant differences between countries. A very good example is the recent study by Percy and Muir (1989) to assess the international comparability of the coding of death certificates mentioning cancer. Some of the principal factors affecting comparability and accuracy were the ordering of multiple sites of cancer on the death certificate, the co-existence of heart disease and cancer, and the interpretation of coding rules in different countries. As a result, the 'corrected' death rate from cancer was significantly altered in some countries, notably France, where there would appear to be an overstatement of cancer deaths of the order of 10 per cent compared with the USA. Similar comparative studies of coding and certification practices have been carried out in Europe for respiratory and occupation-related diseases, which have confirmed differences in certification and coding practices of the order of 10–20 per cent (Kelson and Farebrother 1987; Mackenbach *et al.* 1987).

Even though the above evidence would appear to indicate that the underlying causes of death may frequently be incorrect for chronic disorders, the overall situation is far from discouraging. An investigation of the diagnostic accuracy for deaths assigned to the cardiovascular–renal diseases in the USA, for example, revealed that although the underlying cause of death was incorrectly stated in 15 per cent of cases, the preferred diagnosis for 95 per cent of these deaths was another cardiovascular–renal disease (Moriyama *et al.* 1966). There is also some evidence to suggest that errors in certification, for the chronic diseases at least, may be largely compensatory (James *et al.* 1955; Heasman and Lipworth 1966) and, hence the final description of the underlying cause-of-death structure may, after all, be not too far removed from reality.

Clearly, traditional approaches to the selection of one single cause may have to be altered radically in the future, even if this will lead to discontinuity with adverse effects on trend analysis. The obvious strategy is to utilize all the information recorded on the death certificate rather than to select a single 'underlying' cause only. This approach is based on the premise that where multiple pathology is provided on the certificate, it does not seem appropriate to strive to derive a single underlying cause by the application of arbitrary rules, such as choosing the first-mentioned condition.

Interest in multiple cause-of-death statistics has been sporadic. In short, two opposing views can be identified. On the one hand, it has been argued that as death is more and more deferred to older ages, analysis of one single cause is becoming increasingly irrelevant and that the full potential offered by the medical certificate of death should be exploited. On the other hand, where there is limited appreciation by physicians of the purposes and the scientific potential of cause of death statistics, it is questionable whether certifiers who look at their task as a medicolegal commitment can provide meaningful epidemiological information. Using multiple cause tabulations requires, first and foremost, that the complex pathological processes involved are identified and accurately recorded on the death certificate. Unfortunately, experiments with multiple cause-of-death coding carried out so far have not been too encouraging. It would appear that to improve their utility one would need to make direct enquiries about the existence of certain diseases or conditions to the certifying physician, or else through more explicit questions on the death certificate itself. There is also the analytical problem of how the data should be interpreted. For multiple-cause analyses, it might be more appropriate to tabulate counts and rates of *mentions* per thousand deaths (i.e. proportionate mortality) than the conventional denominator of population exposed to risk.

Other analytical issues

In addition to the reliability issues identified above, what are some of the other considerations in the use of mortality data for small-area studies? Clearly, it is desirable to define population clusters/areas which are relatively homogeneous with respect to socio-behavioural factors likely to affect mortality. Against this, small areas (e.g. populations of 300 000 to 500 000 or so) will have relatively few deaths (3000–5000 in this example) each year, and when further disaggregated by sex, age, and cause, the robustness of mortality indices is clearly of concern, all the more so when the underlying reliability/comparability of the cause of death assignment is questionable. This is less likely to be of concern in large (e.g. national) populations where 'compensating errors' in the cause-of-death statistics are more likely to be 'self-correcting'.

Populations-at-risk (denominators) are another major concern. Small-area studies may be used to evaluate the effects of a specific exposure, or of the efficacy of health services, etc., which require that the population-at-risk be relatively uncontaminated by population movements. Inter-regional migration clearly violates this requirement and, hence, areal populations subject to comparatively high migration (in or out) are unsuitable for such studies. Again, this is not likely to be a problem at the national level due to compensatory flows and larger denominators.

Timeliness of data is also likely to vary among areas due to differences in procedures, follow-up, and administrative efficiency. Comparable calendar-year data for reporting units may thus be difficult to obtain for some countries, although this is unlikely to hinder comparisons seriously since the level and pattern of mortality by cause are relatively invariant over short intervals.

Finally, there is the issue of preserving confidentiality. Small-area analyses are often carried out on relatively small cell sizes, with the result that the cause of death or other potentially sensitive information on the deceased can be identified from other tabulated data, such as age, sex, and place of residence. Confidentiality is clearly fundamental to the integrity of small-area analyses and the research community must continue to ensure that it is respected (see Chapter 13).

References

Gittelsohn, A. M. and Royston, P. N. (1982). *Annotated bibliography of cause-of-death validation studies: 1958–1980*, Vital and health statistics, series 2, No. 89. US Government Printing Office, Washington, DC.

Graunt, J. (1662). *Natural and political observations mentioned in a following index and made upon the Bills of Mortality*, (ed. Walter F. Willcox). Reprinted in 1939 by the Johns Hopkins University Press, Baltimore.

Heasman, M. A. and Lipworth, M. B. (1966). *Accuracy of certification of cause of death*, Studies on Medical and Population Subjects, No. 20. General Registrar Office, London.

James, G., Patton, R. E., and Heslin, A. S. (1955). Accuracy of cause-of-death statements on death certificates. *Public Health Reports*, **70**, 39–51.

Kelson, M. and Farebrother, M. (1987). The effect of inaccuracies in death certification and coding practices in the European Economic Community (EEC) on international cancer mortality statistics. *International Journal of Epidemiology*, **16**, 411–14.

McDonald, P. F. (1972). Recent trends in mortality in Australia. *Journal of Biosocial Sciences*, **4**, 25–36.

Mackenbach, J. P., van Duyne, W. M. J., and Kelson, M. C. (1987). Certification and coding of two underlying causes of death in the Netherlands and other countries of the European Community. *Journal of Epidemiology and Community Health*, **41**, 156–60.

Moriyama, I. M., Dawber, T. R., and Kannel, W. B. (1966). Evaluation of diagnostic information supporting medical certification of deaths from cardiovascular disease. In *Epidemiological approaches to the study of cancer and other chronic diseases*, (ed. W. Haenszel), National Cancer Institute Monograph, No. 19, pp. 405–19. Government Printing Office, Washington, DC.

Percy, C. and Muir, C. (1989). The international comparability of cancer mortality data. *American Journal of Epidemiology*, **129**, 934–46.

Preston, S. H., Keyfitz, N., and Schoen, R. (1972). *Causes of death: life tables for national populations*. Seminar Press, New York.

World Health Organization (1977). *International classification of diseases. Manual of the international statistical classification of diseases, injuries and cause of death* Vol. 1, (9th revision). WHO, Geneva.

5. Cancer incidence data for adults

A. J. Swerdlow

This chapter describes the sources of cancer incidence data for small-area analyses, the data requirements for such analyses, and issues that need to be considered in interpreting the results. The limitations of small-area analyses using cancer registry data are discussed, and ways in which investigation can go beyond calculation of geographical rates from the registry data are outlined with examples. Since long-established, high-quality cancer registration and population data on computer are not available in many countries, illustrations are given of classic small-area analyses of cancer incidence which have provided important results without these facilities.

Collection of cancer incidence data

Cancer incidence data for small-area analyses are usually obtained either from cancer registration or, less conveniently, from *ad hoc* data collection by processes similar to those of registration. Cancer registration has been defined as 'the process of continuing systematic collection of data on the occurrence and characteristics of reportable neoplasms' (MacLennan *et al*. 1978). It may be population-based, attempting to collect information on all cases of cancer occurring in a defined population, or hospital-based, collecting information on all patients attending particular hospital(s). The former is preferable for epidemiological purposes; the latter is often used for clinical studies.

Registries may also be divided into specialist registries, which cover only particular sites of cancer or cancers at particular ages (for instance children), and general registries, which try to register all malignancies at all ages. Even within the latter, however, the exact scope varies. For instance, many general registries do not attempt to register non-melanoma skin cancers, even though these are classified as malignant in the International Classification of Diseases (ICD) (WHO 1977). Conversely, many registries try to register, in addition to malignant neoplasms, selected tumours from outside the malignant neoplasm section of the ICD. For instance, data collected by the England and Wales registry include: neoplasms of uncertain behaviour; carcinomas *in situ*; benign neoplasms and neoplasms of unspecified nature of the bladder and brain, including the pineal and pituitary glands; and hydatidiform mole.

Cancer registration is well established in many countries. The oldest population-based registry, in Connecticut, holds data on cancers incident since 1935 in residents of the state. The first national population-based registry was established in Denmark in 1942. Subsequently, all of the other Scandinavian countries, New Zealand, Australia, Canada, Israel, England and Wales, Scotland, and several other countries have founded national registries. In large countries, national registration is often achieved by a network of regional registries, which pool registrations to give national data. Thus in England and Wales, a national registry was established in 1945, and in 1950 there were 74 centres in the country contributing registrations to it. In 1962 full national geographical coverage was achieved, and now 12 independent registries covering populations of from 2 million to 14 million, contribute to the national data set. In many other Western countries, for instance the USA, France, and Italy, registration is conducted in certain areas but not others. In much of Asia, Africa, and South America there is little registration.

The duration for which data are available varies considerably between registries. This is of particular importance to small-area analyses, because they are often based on small populations with few cases of cancer per year, and therefore need several years of data to give stability to the risk estimation. Cancer registration data in Scandinavia, Britain, New Zealand, and some other countries, cover the entire population for 25 or more years, but many registries in continental Europe are of far more recent origin, and often registries in Africa have operated for some years and then closed. The volume of data accumulated by registries can be very large—in the national files for England and Wales about 5 million registrations since 1954 are held.

Data collection methods vary considerably between registries, and knowledge of these is of importance to users of the data. Possible methods include notifications by doctors, examination by registry staff of hospital notes and pathology records, use of computerized hospital in-patient listings, scanning of death certificates for mention of cancer, and use of several other sources. It is usual to utilize multiple sources to improve completeness. The methods used by many registries can be found in Muir *et al.* (1987). Registration in some countries is legally compulsory, and in others is voluntary, but, in general, the distinction does not appear to be critical to the completeness or accuracy of the data.

Registration data from many different areas of the world can be found in *Cancer incidence in five continents*, Volumes I–V, covering data from the 1950s through to around 1982 (Muir *et al.* 1987). The sixth volume of this publication is now in preparation, adding a further quinquennium of data.

Data needed for small-area studies of cancer incidence

For small-area analyses it is desirable that *population-based* cancer incidence data be available. Desirable, but not always essential. For instance, Burkitt's

(1962) important findings on the geographical distribution of Burkitt's lymphoma in East and Central Africa were made by a 'tumour safari': he visited 56 hospitals and contacted the staff of many others, to enquire about the frequency of the tumour in their area (without calculation of population-based rates). As he comments: 'This form of investigation, touring the African bush in a Ford station wagon that had already seen eight years of service in the Congo, is foreign to accepted concepts of cancer research, but has nevertheless proved fruitful.'

Many other intriguing variations in cancer risk by geography were shown in Africa by Cook and Burkitt (1971), analysing proportions of suspected tumours (irrespective of method of diagnosis) seen at different medical centres. These analyses, although not population-based, showed, for instance, great variations in risk over relatively short distances for oesophageal cancer and penile cancer. Similarly, hospital registry data on cancer incidence in many developing countries (Parkin 1986) have given valuable insight into high- and low-incidence areas in parts of the world where no population-based data exist. Nevertheless, population-based data are desirable if more precise estimates of risk, with less risk of bias, are to be attained, and are needed particularly if lesser differences in risk by geography are to be investigated satisfactorily. It is desirable also that the data be *complete, not duplicated, and accurate*. These issues are discussed further below.

For analyses based on registration (incidence) rates in small areas, it is necessary that *population denominators* be available for the same geographical boundaries as for the cancer data to be analysed. This will limit the detail of geography that can be analysed to the smallest units that are coded, or can be formed by aggregation of coded units, in both the cancer and population data, with age- and sex-specific information available for both. Although this limitation applies to calculation of geographical rates based on registration data, it should be noted that it does not apply to several other types of small-area analysis. Thus Knox (1964) showed space–time clustering of childhood leukaemia incidence in Northumberland and Durham by analysing whether more cases were incident close together in both time and space than would be expected from their distributions in these dimensions separately—a method not requiring population denominators. Case-control or proportional analyses, too, do not need small-area population denominators, and cohort studies of geographical risk will not be limited by availability of small-area population data from outside the study, since the person-years at risk in the cohort will form the denominators. (Such studies may use population denominators to calculate rates in the general population of the country or region, for comparison with the study cohort rates, but this is a different requirement, on a larger geographical scale.)

It is desirable that sufficient *years of cancer incidence data* are available to give reasonable stability of risk estimation in small areas. If the analysis is in relation to an exposure that occurred at a particular time, it is necessary that data be available for the relevant years after the exposure (with allowance for an induction period, if known).

Storage of *data on a magnetic medium*, and hence the potential for computer processing, will facilitate large-scale retrieval of data, although it is not essential to small-area analyses. For analyses based on small numbers, clerical processing may be easy and, even on a large scale, computer processing is not a necessity. Stocks (1936, 1937, 1939), for example, mapped the distribution of mortality from several cancer sites across England and Wales for 1921–30 entirely by clerical processes, and also mapped cancer mortality in small areas of London (Stocks 1947) well before computers were available.

It is necessary that the cancer data set includes the *variables required for the analysis*. At a minimum this would normally be, for each case, the site of cancer, age, sex, and geographical location. The latter is usually the place of residence at incidence of the cancer (the date taken to represent 'incidence' varies between registries; commonly used dates are the date of first treatment, or that of first diagnosis). However, as discussed below, it is often desirable, if possible, to analyse risks in relation to geographical location at other times in life. The geographical data will be easier to use if they are coded, but if so, it is important that the coding system is fully understood, and that it is compatible between different years of data. Often, administrative areas are convenient for anlaysis. Thus, Teppo *et al.* (1980) analysed cancer incidence in Finland by municipality in relation to the distribution of various socio-economic factors, and atlases of cancer incidence have been prepared by county in Scandinavia (Jensen *et al.* 1988) and England and Wales (Swerdlow and dos Santos Silva 1992), and by local government district in Scotland (Kemp *et al.* 1985).

A frequent difficulty in geographical analyses over long periods of time is that administrative boundaries change periodically in ways that cannot be aligned. In England and Wales in recent years, as well as coding administrative area of residence, the national registration scheme has collected postcodes, which, as discussed in Chapter 10, refer to aggregations of a small number of houses, and hence allow larger areas to be built up in a consistent fashion over time. (They also allow greater flexibility in delineation of study areas and opportunity to analyse risk in areas smaller than administrative units.)

The same issues of need to understand the coding system, consistency of coding, and ability to align different codes, also apply, of course, to age, sex, and cancer site. The first two of these are simple variables which do not generally give rise to problems, and cancer site is usually coded to internationally recognized coding systems—the ICD (WHO 1977) or ICD-O (WHO 1976)—for which bridge coding between revisions is available (e.g. Percy 1987; Percy *et al.* 1990). It is necessary, however, that the investigator be aware of any deviations of the registry from standard ICD/ICD-O coding. For certain common deviations, *Cancer incidence in five continents* gives information on the practice of each registry contributing to the volume (Whelan and Sobin 1987).

In some analyses, further variables may be required. For instance, it is often of interest to know the histology of the tumours or the occupation of individuals.

Interpretation

Several alternative explanations need consideration for geographical patterns found in cancer incidence data. A summary of the possibilities is given here, stressing those aspects that apply particularly to small-area studies. Further detail can be found elsewhere (Swerdlow and dos Santos Silva 1992).

Presentation to medical care, and diagnostic practice

For a cancer to be diagnosed, the patient must present to a doctor or other medical care worker. In areas where individuals tend not to present for medical care, registration rates may be artefactually low, and conversely, in areas where presentation is more complete, rates may appear increased. Thus in parts of developing countries where health care is inaccessible, or in areas where many inhabitants cannot afford medical care, apparent rates of cancer incidence may be low. In places where public awareness campaigns have been organized, rates may be raised (particularly for certain tumours where the campaign may lead to many extra borderline malignant lesions coming to biopsy). Screening programmes, too, may lead to an apparently high risk in an area, by leading to biopsy of borderline and/or asymptomatic lesions. In 'developed' countries, presentation to a doctor is virtually inevitable at death, and therefore artefacts of use of medical care tend to apply particularly to cancer sites with relatively good survival. In 'developing' countries many cancer sufferers may not seek conventional medical care, and special methods may be needed to find them. Rose and McGlashan (1975), in studies delineating the geography of oesophageal cancer incidence in the African population of the Transkei, instituted house to house visiting to find cases who did not seek conventional medical assistance. Cases for whom medical confirmation was not available (e.g. those diagnosed by tribal authorities) constituted 36 per cent of the total oesophageal cancers reported.

The diagnostic methods and categories used by doctors to identify cancers may also introduce geographical artefacts. For instance, differences in the criteria used by pathologists in different areas to define the borderline between malignant and non-malignant lesions, or to define the borderline between two different malignant histologies, may influence apparent risks substantially, as may the preference of an individual doctor for a particular diagnostic terminology.

Completeness and accuracy of data collection

Cancer registration on a national or regional scale will inevitably omit some cases, but good registries can attain completeness of 95 per cent or greater. Of particular concern for small-area studies is that incompleteness might be substantial in a particular small area, for instance the catchment population of a particular clinician or hospital, without this being apparent from data on overall registry completeness. The local knowledge of registry staff is therefore important in assessing apparent small-area variations in risk.

Direct assessment of completeness and accuracy of cancer registration data is not often available. Several indirect measures have been used to try to assess these, for instance mortality to registration ratios as an indicator of completeness (Muir and Waterhouse 1987). These have been used widely and published at registry level, but investigation is needed to determine their value (or whether alternative methods can be used) for smaller-area data.

Occasional errors in data collection or coding may have a disproportionately large effect on small-area analyses based on few cases, and therefore it is desirable to check data on specific cases forming an apparent cluster.

For small-area analyses based on linkage of cancer registration to other data sets, for instance a cohort study of cancer incidence in relation to place of residence at the census, completeness and accuracy of linkage will also be an issue.

Completeness of registration can be affected particularly when patients cross registry boundaries for treatment. This may lead to artefactually reduced registration rates if the registry of residence fails to know of cancer treatment outside its boundaries. Alternatively, it can lead to artefactually raised rates, if both the registry of residence and that of treatment record the cancer, and then in a subsequent amalgamated data set (for instance, a national registry formed from regional registry contributions) both registrations are retained. Similar problems can occur if a patient is treated in two or more hospitals located in different registries' catchment areas, or if a patient is treated in the area of one registry but dies in an area covered by another.

Secular artefacts in small-area data may occur if registry boundaries change, since a change in the registry covering an area may bring changes in completeness of registration, coding systems, policy on inclusion of cases for whom only death certificate data are available, and many other aspects of policy and practice. Similarly, artefacts may occur if comparison is made between cancer risks in small areas covered by different registries.

Duplication of registrations, and multiple cancers

Duplicate registrations are potentially a serious problem for small-area analyses. An apparently significant cluster of a few cases of a rare malignancy at a particular location could be due entirely to inadvertent multiplication of a particular registration (whereas two or three copies of one registration would of itself have negligible effect in regional or national statistics based on far larger numbers). Checking for duplicates is therefore important when assessing apparent local clusters based on few cases. The elimination of duplicates from cancer registration files is complicated, however, by the fact that, unlike mortality data, an individual can correctly be registered twice in cancer incidence files if he/she has had more than one cancer. The distinction between multiple tumours, duplicate registrations, and metastases, is not simple, and for assessment of small-area data it is important to know the cancer registry's policy on discriminating between them. Particularly, this is an issue for multiple tumours occurring in paired organs (for instance breast or testis), multiple tumours of different histologies occurring in one organ, and tumours of mixed histology. As well as understanding the registry's policy on inclusion and exclusion of such cancers from their files, it is necessary also for the study investigator to decide how he/she wishes to regard multiple tumours for the purpose of counting cancers in the analysis.

Coding of place of residence

As noted above, the coding system used by the registry needs to be understood, and the possibility that it has led to small-area artefacts needs to be considered. Incorrect coding of the place of cancer treatment as if it were the place of residence at cancer incidence is one potential source of artefact. (Note that at the time of first diagnosis or first treatment of cancer, patients are unlikely to have moved residence, for instance to a hospice, *because* they are ill with the cancer. This contrasts with the situation for mortality data, where very high rates, which are artefactual from an aetiological viewpoint, can occur in small areas that include a hospice or similar institution; Gardner 1984.) Foreigners who come to a country for treatment may give their hotel address or embassy address as their 'residence', and this, too, can lead to apparent small-area clustering of new cases. Another consideration of greater importance to small- rather than larger-scale geographical studies is the coding system adopted for unknown place of residence. Some registries have coded these to the address of the local post office or to that of the cancer registry (rather than to a 'not known' code). As a result, even though such registrations are few, a small-area analysis might well show very high risk of cancer apparently relating to residence in post offices or in the registry itself!

Late registrations, alterations, and deletions

It can take a considerable period for incident cancers to be registered. Notifications to a registry may be delayed. Case-notes may be unavailable to registry staff in the early period after diagnosis, or definitive decisions on the exact pathological diagnosis may take some time to be made. Similarly, new information regarding an existing registration—for instance, a revision to the diagnosis, or addition of an item of data initially missing—may reach the registry years after the initial registration, leading to alteration, augmentation, or cancellation of the registration. The extent of late registrations and other late changes to the cancer files varies considerably between registries (Swerdlow 1986), and is also likely to do so between small areas. Large variations in apparent risk could therefore arise if data were analysed for too recent data years, still appreciably incomplete.

Accuracy and appropriateness of population denominators

Rates calculated using cancer registration data are dependent on the accuracy of the population denominators as well as of the cancer registration (numerator) data. It is also important for unbiased calculation of rates that the population and cancer data refer to the same population, not just in terms of geographical location, but also with respect to the inclusion and exclusion rules used for individuals temporarily present in, or absent from, an area.

Population data from censuses in Western countries are usually highly reliable for the general population, although they may be less so for certain groups, such as young children and people in poor inner city areas. The errors can become greater for intercensal population estimates, notably for ages born since the last census. Population denominators in developing countries may be far less reliable, or non-existent.

Errors in calculation of rates may occur through differences in definition of place of residence between the cancer registry and the census, for groups such as the armed forces, students, tourists and other visitors, prisoners, others living in institutions, and usual residents of the area who are temporarily away (e.g. are abroad). For data from England and Wales, this has been discussed in greater detail elsewhere (Swerdlow 1986). There is potential for a sizeable artefact in rates in small areas that include an institution such as a university, barracks, or prison, or where there are a large number of visitors, if the census and cancer registry differ in whether to allocate such individuals to the institution/temporary residence or to their more permanent home.

Chance

Random variation is a possible explanation of any geographical pattern of cancer incidence. Assessment of whether chance is a likely explanation of a particular finding is the province of statistical analysis, discussed elsewhere in this volume.

Aetiology

If not due to artefact or chance, patterns of risk by geography may be due to causal factors differing between geographical areas. These may be differences in behaviour or genetic composition between the populations in the locations, or may be differences in the environment in the areas. The further pursuit of these issues is discussed briefly below.

Limitations of small-area cancer analyses using cancer registry data

Cancer registries usually record only one address for the cancer patient, the 'usual' residence at the time of cancer incidence. For health care planning, this is usually the address of interest but for aetiological purposes, it is not, except to the extent that it correlates with the address at an earlier period in life more relevant to aetiology. Therefore, in general, the greater the degree of population mobility and the longer the induction period of the cancer, the less useful will be analyses based on address at incidence.

For analyses relating to an exposure present in an area over a long period, analyses should ideally examine cancer risk in relation to duration of residence in the area, rather than simply to presence or absence in the area at a particular date. Also, the analyses should ideally include past residents of the area, whether or not they still live there at the time of cancer incidence. This can be achieved by conducting a cohort study, taking residential history data as the 'exposure', and relating it to subsequent cancer incidence. It can also be obtained less rigorously by a case-control approach. Thus, Newhouse and Thompson (1965) took residential histories from mesothelioma patients and from control patients with other diseases at a hospital in London. They showed that among subjects with no history of occupational or domestic asbestos exposure, a significant excess of cases had lived within half a mile of an asbestos factory, suggesting that neighbourhood asbestos exposures might be important in aetiology.

When complete residential histories cannot be obtained, it may nevertheless be desirable to obtain information on place of residence at more than one point in time, so that a measure of duration can be imputed from presence or absence on the sequential occasions. For example, we (S. C. Darby, A.J.S, and collaborators) are currently conducting a cohort study of cancer risk in relation to residential radon exposure: we have data on radon levels in specific houses, and by ascertaining the presence or absence of cohort members in these houses at several sequential dates, we can define a subgroup of individuals who are likely to have had long exposure to the radon levels in the houses.

Sometimes, geographical analyses relate to an exposure that occurred over a brief period. In this case the relevant location for small-area analysis will be that at the time of exposure. Thus, the cohort studies of cancer risk in survivors of the Nagasaki and Hiroshima atomic bombs have used information about each individual's exact location at the moment the bomb exploded, to give the best basis available from which to estimate personal radiation doses (Beebe 1979).

As well as limitations relating to residential history, analyses of small-area rates from cancer registry data have other limitations when trying to relate cancer incidence to the distribution of potentially aetiological factors. First, there are the difficulties usual to correlation studies at a population level—that they may not reflect correlations at the individual level (see Chapter 1). Small-area correlation analyses will also be limited by the extent to which the level of the exposure varies between the areal units used for the analysis—if, for instance, variation of exposure is mostly within rather than between such units, real associations might be missed in analyses at unit level.

Lack of information on confounding variables is frequently a major limitation. For instance, in studying the distribution of lung or laryngeal cancers in relation to the geographical distribution of environmental agents, smoking (for lung cancer) or smoking and drinking (for laryngeal cancer) are likely to be major confounding variables, since they are responsible (in the sense of attributable risk) for 80 per cent of these cancers in men in many Western populations (Tomatis *et al.* 1990). If, as is often the case, small-area data on smoking and drinking are not available, the conclusions to be drawn from such small-area analyses must be highly tentative and, particularly if the risks found are small, there may be no aetiological conclusion that can be drawn.

Since most geographical variations in cancer incidence in Western countries so far explained have been due to behaviours or occupation, a likely next step after finding a high incidence in a small area will be to try to obtain data about these. Thus Macbeth's classic observation of high incidence of nasal sinus adenocarcinoma in High Wycombe, England was taken further by Hadfield who noted that work in the furniture industry was a common factor between many of the cases observed (Macbeth 1965; Doll 1975). Similarly, the finding in Oxford cancer registry data of a high risk of nasal cancer in Northamptonshire, was amplified by taking occupational histories to show that risk was raised in boot and shoe operatives (Acheson *et al.* 1970). Some cancer registries have collected variables that can be useful in investigating the reasons for raised risk in small areas—for instance, most registries in England and Wales collect data on occupation. Information on behaviours such as smoking, diet, and drinking, however, are usually beyond the scope of registry data collection (although a rough proxy for them may be obtained from socio-economic variables), and will therefore need special studies. Hence an *ad hoc* study of possible aetiological factors, collecting data on individuals (e.g. a case-control study), is likely to be the next step to pursue a finding of raised risk of cancer in a small-area analysis, if artefact and chance have been deemed unlikely explanations for the finding, and the risk is judged worthy of further investigation.

References

Acheson, E. D., Cowdell, R. H., and Jolles, B. (1970). Nasal cancer in the Northamptonshire boot and shoe industry. *British Medical Journal*, **i**, 385–93.

Beebe, G. W. (1979). Reflections on the work of the Atomic Bomb Casualty Commission in Japan. *Epidemiologic Reviews*, **1**, 184–210.

Burkitt, D. (1962). A 'tumour safari' in East and Central Africa. *British Journal of Cancer*, **16**, 379–86.

Cook, P. J. and Burkitt, D. P. (1971). Cancer in Africa. *British Medical Bulletin*, **27**, 14–20.

Doll, R. (1975). Pott and the prospects for prevention (The 7th Walter Hubert Lecture). *British Journal of Cancer*, **32**, 263–72.

Gardner, M. (1984). Some studies based on the maps in the 'Atlas of Cancer Mortality for England and Wales, 1968–78'. In *Maps and cancer*, MRC Environmental Epidemiology Unit Scientific Report No. 3, pp. 28–32. MRC Environmental Epidemiology Unit, Southampton.

Jensen, O. M., Carstensen, B., Glattre, E., Malker, B., Pukkala, E., and Tulinius, H. (1988). *Atlas of cancer incidence in the Nordic countries*. Puna Musta, Helsinki.

Kemp, I., Boyle, P., Smans, M., and Muir, C. (ed.) (1985). *Atlas of cancer incidence in Scotland 1975–1980. Incidence and epidemiological perspective*, IARC Scientific Publication No. 72. IARC, Lyon.

Knox, G. (1964). Epidemiology of childhood leukaemia in Northumberland and Durham. *British Journal of Preventive and Social Medicine*, **18**, 17–24.

Macbeth, R. (1965). Malignant disease of the paranasal sinuses. *Journal of Laryngology and Otology*, **79**, 592–612.

MacLennan, R., Muir, C., Steinitz, R., and Winkler, A. (1978). *Cancer registration and its techniques*, IARC Scientific Publication No. 21. IARC, Lyon.

Muir, C. and Waterhouse, J. (1987). Comparability and quality of data: reliability of registration. In *Cancer incidence in five continents*, Vol. V, (ed. C. Muir, J. Waterhouse, T. Mack, J. Powell, and S. Whelan), IARC Scientific Publication No. 88, pp. 45–169. IARC, Lyon.

Muir, C., Waterhouse, J., Mack, T., Powell, J., and Whelan, S. (ed.) (1987). *Cancer incidence in five continents*, Vol. V, IARC Scientific Publication No. 88. IARC, Lyon.

Newhouse, M. L. and Thompson, H. (1965). Mesothelioma of pleura and peritoneum following exposure to asbestos in the London area. *British Journal of Industrial Medicine*, **22**, 261–9.

Parkin, D. M. (ed.) (1986). *Cancer occurrence in developing countries*, IARC Scientific Publication No. 75. IARC, Lyon.

Percy, C. (1987). Comparison of the 8th and 9th revisions of the International Classification of Diseases. In *Cancer incidence in five continents*, Vol. V, (ed. C. Muir, J. Waterhouse, T. Mack, J. Powell, and S. Whelan), IARC Scientific Publication No. 88, pp. 33–41. IARC, Lyon.

Percy, C., van Holten, V., and Muir, C. (ed.) (1990). *ICD-O. International classification of diseases for oncology*, (2nd edn). WHO, Geneva.

Rose, E. F. and McGlashan, N. D. (1975). The spatial distribution of oesophageal carcinoma in the Transkei, South Africa. *British Journal of Cancer*, **31**, 197–206.

Stocks, P. (1936, 1937, 1939). *Distribution in England and Wales of cancer of various organs*. 13th, 14th, and 16th Annual Reports of the British Empire Cancer Campaign.

Stocks, P. (1947). *Regional and local differences in cancer death rates*, SMPS No. 1. HMSO, London.

Swerdlow, A. J. (1986). Cancer registration in England and Wales: some aspects relevant to interpretation of the data. *Journal of the Royal Statistical Society, Series A*, **149**, 146–60.

Swerdlow, A. J. and dos Santos Silva, I. M. (1992) *Cancer Research Campaign atlas of cancer incidence in England and Wales, 1968–85*. Oxford University Press, in press.

Teppo, L., Pukkala, E., Hakama, M., Hakulinen, T., Herva, A., and Saxén, E. (1980). Way of life and cancer incidence in Finland. A municipality-based ecological analysis. *Scandinavian Journal of Social Medicine, Supplement*, **19**, 1–84.

Tomatis, L., *et al.* (ed.) (1990). *Cancer: causes, occurrence and control*, IARC Scientific Publication No. 100. IARC, Lyon.

Whelan, S. and Sobin, L. (1987). Coding practices. In *Cancer incidence in five continents*, Vol. V, (ed. C. Muir, J. Waterhouse, T. Mack, J. Powell, and S. Whelan), IARC Scientific Publication No. 88, pp. 26–32. IARC, Lyon.

World Health Organization (1976). *ICD-O. International classification of diseases for oncology*, (1st edn). WHO, Geneva.

World Health Organization (1977). *Manual of the international statistical classification of diseases, injuries, and causes of death*. WHO, Geneva.

6. Cancer incidence data for children

G. J. Draper and D. M. Parkin

In this chapter we consider the special problems and advantages in carrying out small-area studies of the incidence of childhood cancer. We adopt the usual convention in this context that 'childhood' covers the first 15 years of life.

There has been particular interest in, and public concern about, the possible existence of clusters of childhood cancers, usually leukaemias, and these have been extensively studied both in relation to possible environmental causes, especially nuclear installations, and in relation to the possible role of infections (Black 1984; Linet 1985; Caldwell 1990; Kinlen *et al.* 1990) (see also Chapter 25).

Sources of data

Data on childhood cancer incidence are collected routinely by cancer registries throughout the world, since these registries cover all age-groups. These data are published regularly by regional or national registries, and more detailed information will often be available from the original records held by such registries. Many of the registries have contributed to the successive volumes of *Cancer incidence in five continents*, the most recent of which was published in 1987 (Muir *et al.* 1987). Registry data are usually published using the current version of the site-based International Classification of Diseases (ICD) although virtually all registries record both site of tumour and histological type, using the International Classification of Diseases for Oncology (ICD-O) (World Health Organization 1976) or some similar classification system.

In addition, there are a number of specialized children's tumour registries, normally covering the age-range 0–14 years. Since childhood cancer is a rare disease, accounting in Western populations for only about 0.5 per cent of all cancers, these specialized registries can reasonably attempt to achieve a greater degree of completeness in ascertaining cases and more accurate diagnoses than the adult registries. In addition, it will be easier to achieve complete registration of childhood cancers because the majority of cases can be ascertained through paediatric services. It seems probable that, in general, the proportion of cases histologically verified will be greater for children than it is for adults from the same region. For instance, in the US Surveillance, Epidemiology, and End Results (SEER) programme 92.2 per cent of all cases registered in 1973–77 were histologically verified whereas 97.0 per cent of childhood cases (1973–82 registrations) were verified (Parkin *et al*. 1988); similarly in the North West Region of England, 64 per cent of all cases registered in 1979–82 were verified (Muir *et al*. 1987) whereas in the Manchester Children's Tumour registry, covering the same region, 96.1 per cent of cases (1971–83 registrations) were verified (Parkin *et al*. 1988).

It is essential in classifying childhood tumours to use information on tumour morphology in addition to site. Most of the specialized childhood tumour registries publish their data using such a system. Much of the available data from these registries has also been published in the volume *International incidence of childhood cancer* (Parkin *et al*. 1988) which contains data relating to childhood cancer not only from these specialized registries but also from a wide range of national and regional cancer registries, their original data on children having been made available in the form of individual, though anonymized, case records and, where necessary, re-coded to take account of tumour histology.

Diagnostic classification scheme

The data from each registry in the above volume are presented using a standard histology-based classification scheme (see also Birch and Marsden 1987). This scheme, which is based on the ICD-O, is recommended as the standard method for use in publishing data on childhood cancer. It will be revised for future use to take account of the revised coding scheme of the second edition of ICD-O (Percy *et al*. 1990) which will come into general use in 1993, and will also take account of modifications suggested by users (for example, McWhirter and Petroeschevsky 1991).

The 12 major categories in the scheme are as follows:

   I leukaemias;
  II lymphomas and other reticuloendothelial neoplasms;
 III central nervous system (CNS) and miscellaneous intracranial and intraspinal neoplasms;
 IV sympathetic nervous system tumours;
  V retinoblastoma;
 VI renal tumours;
 VII hepatic tumours;
VIII malignant bone tumours;
 IX soft-tissue sarcomas;
  X germ-cell, trophoblastic, and other gonadal neoplasms;
 XI carcinoma and other malignant epithelial neoplasms;
 XII other and unspecified malignant neoplasms.

The definition of these categories in terms of ICD-O topography and morphology codes, and also the subcategories into which they are divided, are given on pp. 13–16 of the volume on childhood cancer edited by Parkin *et al.* (1988). We recommend that epidemiological studies, including small-area studies, should use this classification. Even within the subcategories there will, of course, be diagnostic and, presumably, aetiological heterogeneity: for instance, one subcategory is acute lymphocytic leukaemia, but within this group there are different immunological subtypes that may well have different causes. This further subclassification, however, may not be available even when data from specialized children's tumour registries are used.

Special aspects of the analysis of childhood cancer data for small-area studies

Distinctive features of childhood cancers

Childhood cancers are rare and of different types from those commonly occurring in adults. The incidence of childhood cancer in Western populations is rather more than 1 in 10 000 per year (ranging from about 100 to about 140 per million per year among the population aged 0–14 years); on average, in these populations about 1 in 600 children develop cancer by age 15. About one-third of these cancers are leukaemia, rather more than a quarter are brain tumours, and many of the remainder are distinctive types of 'embryonal' tumours not occurring in adults. The common types of adult cancer, for example carcinomas of lung, breast, colon, rectum, and stomach, are virtually never found in children. The rarity of childhood cancer, the distinctive types which occur, and the public concern about these diseases probably lead to an increased likelihood that apparent clusters will be noted and reported in the media.

Aetiology

Little is known about the causes of childhood cancers. However, what little is known, together with the age distributions—which show a peak incidence early in life for several childhood cancers—and the cell types of some tumours, all suggest that factors operating early in life, including prenatally and even pre-conception, are likely to be important. A large number of possible aetiological factors have been reported but the only external causes identified with any certainty are radiation, including particularly antenatal radiation, and certain forms of chemotherapy used mainly in treating an earlier cancer. Genetic factors are also important: about 40 per cent of cases of retinoblastoma are heritable, and there are a number of associations between childhood cancer and various genetic diseases and congenital abnormalities, that between Down's syndrome and leukaemia being the best known.

Since the time interval between the induction of childhood cancer and diagnosis is necessarily short, it seems reasonable to suppose that the search for aetiological factors should be correspondingly simplified. To date there has been little success in identifying such factors, although there have been a considerable number of aetiological studies, mainly case-control studies. Various explanations are possible: most of the studies may have had insufficient statistical power to detect such factors; on the other hand, it is possible that genetic factors, perhaps multifactorial, are responsible for most cases, or that childhood cancer can be caused by a wide variety of factors that can affect the normal development of the fetus and neonate. Nevertheless, it is reasonable to argue, particularly for childhood cancers, that the existence of a cluster may provide aetiological clues and that clusters, when confirmed as such, should be studied in detail. For children there is a relatively limited life-span to be studied.

Variations in incidence rates

Compared with adult cancers, little information is available about variations in incidence of childhood cancers, either internationally or nationally. One reason for this is that, until recently, relatively few registries had published data on childhood cancer in a form suitable for comparative studies. In addition, the rarity of these tumours means that incidence rates based on small population numbers or short periods of time are subject to relatively large random fluctuations which are difficult to distinguish from true differences in incidence.

International variations in incidence rates

The volume edited by Parkin *et al.* (1988) contains data on childhood cancers from both population-based and hospital-based registries throughout the world, classified according to the system set out on p. 64, and shows that there are substantial variations in incidence for the individual diagnostic groups, although these are considerably smaller than the variations found for adult tumours. Some of the differences in incidence are, no doubt, due to random fluctuations and to varying degrees of completeness of ascertainment, but the magnitude of some of the differences and the consistency within and between different types of population strongly suggest that there are real differences in incidence, although, for instance, the rates for white populations in Europe, North America, and Australia are similar.

Transnational studies

'Transnational' studies are a particular subset of international comparisons, where the geographical units of analysis are not individual countries, but are defined in relation to possible aetiological factors. A current example is the

European Childhood Leukaemia/Lymphoma Incidence Study, with collaborators in 17 European countries (Parkin 1990). The objective of this study is to follow trends in the incidence of childhood leukaemia since 1980, with analysis by geographical subunits defined in terms of the estimated first-year dose of radiation resulting from the accident at Chernobyl in 1986, using estimates of dose given in the UNSCEAR Report (1988). These are relatively large areas, unrelated to national frontiers, so that data collection by small areas, which can be re-aggregated, is required.

Variations in incidence within countries

Little information is available on variations in incidence for small geographical areas. In order to study such variations it is necessary to have some method of allocating the cases on the registry files to the defined set of small areas. Where case addresses are already recorded this may involve some automatic method of allocating each of these addresses to the small area within which it is contained, possibly by first determining a grid-reference. Perhaps the most comprehensive attempt to attach geographical information to disease records is that in Great Britain, where postcodes are being added to the national files of mortality and cancer registration data. It is then possible, as described in Chapter 10, to attach an approximate grid-reference, census enumeration district, and census tract to each address.

For such areas population data are available for both the 1971 and 1981 censuses, and estimates can be made by interpolation for intercensal years; such estimates will be unreliable, but for many purposes it will be necessary to carry out analyses based on aggregations of census tracts, and the errors for such aggregations will be less important provided that the method of interpolation does not introduce any systematic bias. (A census tract has an average child population of around 200.) This system has been used for a series of analyses of the geographical distribution of childhood leukaemia and lymphoma based on data for an 18-year period in Great Britain (Draper 1991). These analyses show some evidence of variations in incidence between different regions which may be, at least in part, attributable to differences in socioeconomic status between the regions.

Some other childhood tumour registries have information on addresses, though this is not usually coded in such detail as for Great Britain. McWhirter and Bacon (1980) calculated rates for childhood acute lymphoblastic leukaemia in the city of Brisbane and the surrounding area, and found higher rates within the city, the difference being statistically significant in the 5–9 year age-group. Craft *et al.* (1985) analysed variations in incidence in electoral wards (having an average child population of around 1000) in the Northern Region of England. Haaf *et al.* (1990) examined regional variations within the Federal Republic of Germany and noted no significant regional variation in leukaemia incidence (based on 4022 cases in 1980–88); the variations noted in CNS tumours (1788 cases)—significantly low in the north and parts of Bavaria—are ascribed to relative under-ascertainment.

Viel and Richardson (1990) analysed childhood leukaemia mortality around the La Hague nuclear waste reprocessing plant in France, grouping electoral wards into those that had half or more of their area within less than 10 km, 10–20 km, or 20–30 km of the plant. They found no evidence of an increased risk in the areas closest to the plant. The authors of this paper commented on the need for cancer registry data. Hatch and Susser (1990) analysed childhood cancer incidence rates in relation to background γ-radiation for 'study tracts', built up from census blocks, in the vicinity of the Three Mile Island nuclear plant in the United States. An association was found between background γ-radiation and total childhood cancer incidence.

Clusters and clustering

A substantial proportion of reported disease clusters are clusters of leukaemia (Caldwell 1990) and there are many reports of childhood leukaemia clusters; some of these have been rigorously investigated. Several theories have been put forward to explain these clusters, some involving a possible viral aetiology (for example, Kinlen et al. 1990). Undoubtedly, the most striking finding to emerge from studies of these clusters is the association reported by Gardner et al. (1990) (discussed in Chapter 25) between childhood leukaemia and paternal pre-conception exposure to radiation, the fathers concerned having worked at Sellafield, the site of a major nuclear fuel reprocessing plant, and the association being sufficient to explain the geographical excess reported in the vicinity of the plant. A study of the Dounreay installation, the only other reprocessing plant in Britain, where a cluster had also been reported, did not find a similar association, but the exposure history of the workforce at this plant was different, and so this study neither supports nor refutes Gardner's finding (Urquhart et al. 1991).

Reports of an increased incidence of childhood leukaemia around a third nuclear site in Britain, the atomic weapons establishments at Aldermaston and Burghfield in Berkshire, have also been examined in detail by the Committee on Medical Aspects of Radiation in the Environment (COMARE) (1989). The committee concluded that there was indeed evidence for a small increase in the incidence of childhood leukaemia in the vicinity of these plants and also (using unpublished data from the Childhood Cancer Research Group) a small increase in the incidence of other childhood cancers. However, neither the exposure of the workers at these plants nor the discharges to the environment seems likely to explain the increased incidence. A case-control study is in progress that should help to resolve the issue of whether there is, in fact, a causal relationship.

Although the three reports referred to here are linked by their association with nuclear installations, the installations themselves are very different, and it may well be that there is, in fact, no connection between the findings reported from the three sites.

These and other reports have raised the question of whether clustering is a general feature of the geographical distribution of childhood leukaemia, and methods have been developed to study this issue. Some of these are discussed and applied to British data in the volume of studies referred to above (Draper 1991); the conclusion of these analyses was that there is some evidence of clustering in acute lymphocytic leukaemia (the most common form of leukaemia in childhood) at least in the age-range 0–4 years (where the peak incidence occurs).

Clustering in relation to place of birth

Most studies of clusters use, inevitably, addresses at diagnosis, since cases come to attention when they are diagnosed. However, for childhood cancer for reasons given in the section on aetiology, it may be more relevant to study incidence by place of birth. One approach would be to look at the places of birth for groups of cancer cases which have been reported to cluster by place of diagnosis; if their home addresses at birth were also close to one other we should be more inclined to believe in the reality of the cluster. This approach is conservative, in that only a proportion of clusters by place of birth would be identified in this way. A different approach is to find the place of birth for every registered case born in a particular group of years. This needs to be done nationally, or at least for a region from which there is little migration, since otherwise cases born in the region but diagnosed elsewhere will not be included. If this can be done it is possible to examine the data, using methods described elsewhere in this volume, for evidence of clustering by place of birth or, more generally, for evidence of variations in incidence rates.

For such analyses to be possible it is, of course, necessary to have appropriate denominators, that is, numbers of births for the different parts of the region. Such data may well be more readily available than the appropriate denominators at the time of diagnosis, i.e. population counts for different age-groups, since number of births will normally be recorded for each year, whereas population counts are only available at the time of a census, with estimates for inter-censal years. Information on place of birth will not normally be available from cancer registries in the required detail, but it may be possible to obtain this information by linking cancer registrations to birth registrations using national record systems; in some cases it may be necessary to do this by clerical methods, but in others it may be possible using computer record linkage (see Chapter 12). The cancer registrations should be linked to birth records that contain area codes corresponding to those used in tabulating the population births, so that the appropriate denominators for an analysis of incidence by birth area will be readily available.

Acknowledgements

The Childhood Cancer Research Group is supported by the Department of Health and the Scottish Home and Health Department. We are grateful to Sue Medhurst for her help with this chapter.

References

Birch, J. M. and Marsden, H. B. (1987). A classification scheme for childhood cancer. *International Journal of Cancer*, **40**, 620–4.
Black, D. (1984). *Investigation of the possible increased incidence of cancer in West Cumbria*. Report of the Independent Advisory Group. HMSO, London.
Caldwell, G. G. (1990). Twenty-two years of cancer cluster investigations at the Centers for Disease Control. *American Journal of Epidemiology*, **132**, S43–S47.
Committee on Medical Aspects of Radiation in the Environment (COMARE) (1989). *Third report. Report on the incidence of childhood cancer in the West Berkshire and North Hampshire area, in which are situated the Atomic Weapons Research Establishment, Aldermaston and the Royal Ordnance Factory, Burghfield*. HMSO, London.
Craft, A. W., Openshaw, S., and Birch, J. M. (1985). Childhood cancer in the Northern Region, 1968–82: incidence in small geographical areas. *Journal of Epidemiology and Community Health*, **39**, 53–7.
Draper, G. J. (ed.) (1991). *The geographical epidemiology of childhood leukaemia and non-Hodgkin lymphomas in Great Britain, 1966–83*, Studies on Medical and Population Subjects No. 53. HMSO, London.
Gardner, M. J., Snee, M. P., Hall, A. J., Powell, C. A., Downes, S., and Terrell, J. D. (1990). Results of case-control study of leukaemia and lymphoma among young people near Sellafield nuclear plant in West Cumbria. *British Medical Journal*, **300**, 423–34.
Haaf, H. G., Kaatsch, P., and Michaelis, J. (1990). *Jahresbericht 1989 des Kinderkrebsregisters Mainz*. Institut für Medizinische Statistik und Dokumentation. Johannes Gutenberg-Universität, Mainz.
Hatch, M. and Susser, M. (1990). Background gamma radiation and childhood cancers within ten miles of a US nuclear plant. *International Journal of Epidemiology*, **19**, 546–52.
Kinlen, L. J., Clarke, K., and Hudson, C. (1990). Evidence from population mixing in British New Towns 1946–85 of an infective basis for childhood leukaemia. *Lancet*, **336**, 577–82.
Linet, M. S. (1985). *The leukaemias: epidemiologic aspects*. Oxford University Press, New York.
McWhirter, W. R. and Bacon, J. E. (1980). Epidemiology of acute lymphoblastic leukaemia of childhood in Brisbane. *Medical Journal of Australia*, **2**, 154–5.
McWhirter, W. R. and Petroeschevsky, A. L. (1991). Childhood cancer incidence in Queensland, 1979–88. *International Journal of Cancer*, **45**, 1002–5.
Muir, C., Waterhouse, J., Mack, T., Powell, J., and Whelan, S. (ed.) (1987). *Cancer incidence in five continents*. Vol. V, IARC Scientific Publication No. 88. International Agency for Research on Cancer, Lyon.

Parkin, D. M. (on behalf of ECLIS Study Group) (1990). The European childhood leukaemia/lymphoma incidence study. *Radiation Research*, **124**, 370–1.

Parkin, D. M., Stiller, C. A., Draper, G. J., Bieber, C. A., Terracini, B., and Young, J. L. (ed.) (1988). *International incidence of childhood cancer*, IARC Scientific Publications No. 87. International Agency for Research on Cancer, Lyon.

Percy, C., van Holten, V., and Muir, C. (1990). *International Classification of Diseases for Oncology (ICD-O)*, (2nd edn). World Health Organisation, Geneva.

UNSCEAR (United Nations Scientific Committee on the Effects of Atomic Radiation) (1988). *Sources, effects and risks of ionizing radiation*, 1988 Report. UN, New York.

Urquhart, J. D., *et al.* (1991). Case-control study of leukaemia and non-Hodgkin's lymphoma in children in Caithness near the Dounreay nuclear installation. *British Medical Journal*, **302**, 687–92.

Viel, J. F. and Richardson, S. T. (1990). Childhood leukaemia around the La Hague nuclear waste reprocessing plant. *British Medical Journal*, **300**, 580–1.

World Health Organization (1976). *International classification of diseases for oncology (ICD-O)*. WHO, Geneva.

7. Congenital anomalies

H. Dolk and P. De Wals

Congenital anomalies include structural defects, chromosomal and monogenic syndromes, and inborn errors of metabolism. Structural defects may be divided into 'major' and 'minor' anomalies, the latter having in themselves little or no medical or cosmetic consequence for the child and being relatively frequent. The dividing line between major and minor anomalies is rather arbitrary, and it is partly for this reason that estimates of the proportion of births affected by major congenital anomalies vary widely from study to study.

For any study of environmental effects on congenital anomaly frequency, two broad categories of causal agents must be defined; the first, mutagenic with pre-conceptional action producing heritable effects, and the second teratogenic with post-conceptional action producing non-heritable effects. A study of Down's syndrome and other chromosomal and monogenic syndromes would require a search for mutagenic agents. For most other anomalies, including central nervous system anomalies, cardiac anomalies, limb anomalies, and facial clefts, attention would also concentrate on environmental factors that act during the 'sensitive period' in the development of the organ concerned (Warkany 1971; Wilson 1977). This usually falls in the first trimester, although the development of the brain continues throughout pregnancy and remains subject to adverse influences (Evrard et al. 1989).

A distinction should be made between the environment of the mother (or external environment) and the environment of the fetus (which includes the mother). The effects of external factors on the fetus are mediated by the mother, and it is possible that exposure of the mother even during her early life to external factors will result in a post-conceptional teratogenic effect (Anderson et al. 1958; Sever and Emanuel 1981), perhaps through a long-term effect on metabolic, hormonal, or nutritional factors.

The effect of any given teratogen will not only depend on the dose and timing, but also on the genetic susceptibility to that teratogen (Wilson 1977). Congenital anomalies with an 'environmental' aetiology are those where the genetic susceptibility varies little, or not at all, in the population. More commonly, the aetiology may be multifactorial (Fraser 1976), where both genetic and environmental aetiological factors vary in the population. The interaction of different environmental factors may also be important. Teratogenic agents which seem to act mainly to potentiate the effects of other environmental exposures have been called 'co-teratogens' (Persaud 1985).

Epidemiological studies of congenital anomalies suffer from a major drawback in that cases are ascertained only after a large proportion of incident cases have been selectively eliminated as early spontaneous abortions (Creasy and Alberman 1976; Kline *et al.* 1990). It is common practice to use the term 'prevalence rate' to refer to the proportion of affected fetuses among all fetuses reaching late pregnancy. The possibility of differential *in utero* survival of cases with different exposure or demographic characteristics should always be considered when making 'causal' inferences (Khoury *et al.* 1989; Kline *et al.* 1990; Hook and Regal 1991).

Cases of congenital anomaly can be identified through *ad hoc* surveys or through routine registration. Routine registration may take the form of a national system of specific notification of congenital anomalies (England and Wales, Finland, Sweden, and Hungary), an information system based on centralized birth notifications (Norway, Belgium, and also Sweden), neonatal discharge records (Scotland and BDMP USA), or specialized (often regional) registries using multiple sources of information (Cole 1983; Weatherall *et al.* 1984). EUROCAT is a network of specialized regional registries in Europe with central co-ordination (Lechat *et al.* 1985; Dolk *et al.* 1991*a*). The International Clearinghouse for Birth Defect Monitoring Systems includes as its members national, multi-hospital, and regional registries (Flynt and Hay 1979; Castillo *et al.* 1986) with different bases for case-ascertainment.

The methodological problems in case ascertainment and accuracy of information belong to three categories:

(1) those pertaining to the nature of congenital anomalies (e.g. late detection, prenatal diagnosis and termination of pregnancy, early fetal deaths);

(2) those pertaining to the use of 'historic' medical records in the absence of standard examination protocols (e.g. variation in diagnostic criteria and in the use of autopsy, karyotype investigation, and ultrasound); and

(3) those pertaining to routine health information systems (e.g. variation in reporting and coding).

Case ascertainment

The sources of information that may be used for case-finding depend on the type of congenital anomaly, and how and when it is generally diagnosed. Possible sources include birth notifications (if mention is made of congenital anomalies), death certificates, maternity records, neonatal and other hospital discharge records, cytology records, pathology records, and records of specialized departments such as paediatric surgery, paediatric cardiology, ophthalmology, and genetic counselling (Dolk *et al.* 1991*a*). Multiple sources of information will generally be necessary to ascertain the full range of con-genital anomalies, and to overcome inevitable gaps in notification or records.

Reliance on special notification from clinicians or other health professionals is more suited to short, intensive *ad hoc* studies, or to the registration of a limited list of very rare conditions, such as is at present carried out by the British Paediatric Surveillance Unit (Hall and Glickman 1988). Routine registration of the full range of congenital anomalies requires the active consultation of medical records, as well as setting up close contacts with clinicians. In a long-term registration system, one of the major problems is to maintain a good level of motivation for case-finding. Various forms of feedback may increase motivation, including sending letters with information on available services to the treating clinicians, organizing seminars, distrib-uting newsletters and reports with results from the registry, running a teratogen or genetic information service in parallel to registration activities, and even supplying items of mutual benefit such as books, journals, computers, or cameras. It is important that the data collected are seen to be of immediate use and of local relevance. This involves regional rather than national registries, and the employment of personnel who can use and evaluate the data as they are being collected.

Although congenital anomalies are, by definition, present at birth, many are not detected until after the neonatal period, notably internal anomalies such as cardiac and urinary tract anomalies. It is essential for the ascertainment of these cases to use sources of information covering the post-neonatal period. The use of post-neonatal sources of information not only ensures a higher overall case ascertainment, but also protects against variations in recorded prevalence caused by a shift in the age at diagnosis. Prenatal and neonatal screening by ultrasound, for example, is leading to the earlier detection of many anomalies which were formally detected only later in life, a phenomenon which was particularly marked in the 1980s for urinary tract anomalies and led to an increase in their reported prevalence in many areas (EUROCAT Working Group 1991a; Lys and Mols 1991).

Prenatal diagnosis and termination of pregnancy is leading to a considerable reduction in the prevalence of conditions such as Down's syndrome, neural tube defects, renal agenesis, and omphalocele (Table 7.1). Since the frequency of prenatal diagnosis varies between regions and over time, it is essential that terminations should be included in the data set, and that some minimal in-formation such as gestational age should be collected for these cases to enable them to be placed in the correct exposure cohorts based on time of conception (EUROCAT Working Group 1988). 'Total' or 'adjusted' prevalence rates can be calculated which include terminations of pregnancy following prenatal diagnosis, on the basis that most of these cases would have reached late pregnancy had there not been prenatal diagnosis.

For many of the more severe anomalies, a large proportion of cases can be expected to be fetal deaths (see Table 7.2). The diagnosis of anomalies in fetal

Table 7.1 Percentage of cases recorded as induced abortions following prenatal diagnosis, 1986–88, eight European regions (based on EUROCAT Working Group 1991*a*)

Registry	Anencephaly	Spina bifida	Renal agenesis	Omphalocele	Down's syndrome
Hainaut, Belgium	94.1	0.0	66.7	50.0	13.8
Paris, France	80.0	56.8	52.4	43.2	33.9
Strasbourg, France	76.9	44.4	40.0	46.2	26.7
Marseille, France	81.8	52.4	58.3	41.7	20.0
Florence, Italy	91.7	70.0	16.7	0.0	20.0
Glasgow, UK	88.4	52.9	31.2	45.8	19.6
Liverpool, UK	86.4	54.5	11.1	40.0	0.0
Belfast, UK	51.5	5.2	7.1	16.7	4.9

deaths, especially those that are internal, requires autopsy examination by a specialized fetal pathologist, and the potential for completeness of coverage of these cases will therefore depend on the extent of autopsy coverage. As the lower limit of fetal viability shifts towards earlier gestational ages, it is necessary to extend data collection to earlier fetal deaths, whether or not they are included in the official birth notifications (as still births). The inclusion of live births but exclusion of fetal deaths at low gestational ages is to be avoided, since it is possible for this distinction to be quite arbitrary (and therefore open to variability) for conditions that severely reduce viability, such as anencephaly. Gestational age, despite the difficulties in its estimation, is a better criterion for inclusion than birthweight, since affected fetuses are often of much lower birthweight than normal fetuses of the same gestational age.

Accuracy of information

The level of accuracy of the data needed for any one study will clearly be a function of the aim and design of the study. However, as a general principle, accurate or good quality data for environmental studies should allow the distinction of aetiological and pathogenetic types, use standard terminology and definitions, use a coding system of high specificity, include an indication of the severity of the condition if this is variable, and exclude false positive diagnoses.

Many of the same factors increasing completeness of ascertainment will also increase the accuracy of the information collected, including the use of multiple sources of information, post-neonatal sources of information, a high coverage by a specialized autopsy service, and maintenance of dialogue with health professionals.

Since the study of pre-conceptional mutagenic effects and post-conceptional teratogenic effects requires different study design and interpretation, it is important to be able to distinguish genetic conditions for separate analysis, as far as this is possible. Identification of genetic conditions relies largely on chromosomal analysis and other techniques for identifying specific genomic mutations, family history analysis, and recognition of well-established syndromes by medical geneticists. It is the *de novo* mutations that are of interest to environmental studies, rather than familial cases of a syndrome. At present, studies of mutagenic effects can most effectively restrict their attention to 'sentinel phenotypes' (Castillo *et al.* 1986; Czeizel and Kis-Varga 1987), i.e. genetic syndromes easily recognizable at birth with dominant inheritance, high penetrance, and a high ratio of sporadic to familial cases. There is currently little literature available evaluating the use of sentinel phenotypes in relation to the accuracy of registration data, although this has been a subject of particular concern to the Hungarian Congenital Anomaly Surveillance System (Czeizel and Kis-Varga 1987). Down's syndrome is commonly analysed as a 'sentinel' for chromosomal anomalies.

Conditions of known environmental aetiology, such as maternal infections or maternal alcoholism, should be distinguishable in the data, all the more so since these conditions show a high variability in time and space.

Careful clinical and pathological examination is needed to distinguish between pathogenetic types. For example, malformations which are sequelae of early amnion rupture are of different aetiological significance to those same malformations without signs of early amnion rupture (Jones 1988). It should at least be possible to separate multiply malformed cases from those with an isolated malformation or sequence (a combination of anomalies originating from the same prior defect; Spranger *et al.* 1982). Multiply malformed cases have a special significance in congenital anomaly studies (Kallen and Winberg 1968; Khoury *et al.* 1987). An isolated anomaly may have a different patho-genesis/aetiology from the same anomaly when associated with other anomalies. Current research aims to investigate to what extent this is true of specific anomalies (Khoury *et al.* 1982; Dolk *et al.* 1991*b*). Experience has also shown that most known teratogens cause multiple anomalies rather than isolated defects, a reflection of the fact that it is easier to detect the relationship between a rare specific pattern of defects and a teratogen than between a more common aetiologically heterogeneous defect and a teratogen, and of the fact that the strongest teratogens may well cause a number of problems at once.

The advantages of gathering diagnostic detail may well be lost in the absence of standard terminology and definitions. It should be recognized that, in this respect, the needs of clinical practice and epidemiology may differ, and a dialogue must be maintained with clinicians.

Coding should also attempt to conserve diagnostic detail. The ICD9 code (WHO 1977) does not include sufficient specificity, and the British Paediatric Association (1979) extension to the ICD code is in common use today. Some specialized registries have developed further extensions to this code, particularly for the coding of syndromes (Weatherall *et al.* 1992). Centralized coding improves the comparability of data, but may be further removed from the original sources of information and reduce its accuracy.

Since the less severe conditions are more likely to escape detection or registration, comparisons of prevalence rates should ideally cover cases of equal severity. This particularly affects conditions that range from major to minor forms, such as microcephaly, hypospadias, and syndactyly, and conditions that involve a sequence of abnormal morphogenetic events with variable expression, such as holoprosencephaly.

False positive diagnoses may be excluded in various ways. Live-borns need to be followed up until the diagnosis is confirmed, changed, or elaborated. Autopsy confirmation of diagnoses in still births should be sought (a particular problem in studies of hydrocephaly; Laurence *et al.* 1967). Diagnoses in induced abortions (following prenatal diagnosis of structural malformation) should also be confirmed by autopsy. A recent study examining the products of induced abortion after prenatal diagnosis by ultrasound found that more than one-third of the original pre-termination diagnoses changed sufficiently to affect genetic counselling (Clayton-Smith *et al.* 1990). Nevertheless, examination of induced abortions is not routine practice in many areas.

Since the methods of investigation may vary according to the type of birth (live birth, still birth, or induced abortion), it may be difficult to achieve complete comparability. For example, it is the practice in some areas (particularly in France) to perform an amniocentesis after prenatal ultrasound detection of structural anomalies in order to exclude the presence of a chromosomal syndrome. Variation in the rate of prenatal diagnosis and termination combined with variation in the rate of amniocentesis after ultrasound will inevitably lead to variation in the reported rate of chromosomal anomalies.

Data 'accuracy' is not an absolute, and depends as much on the state of medical expertise and the resources put into investigation as on the methods of data collection. It can be useful to record information that will allow some standardization to take place. For example, the full description of component anomalies in syndromes can be encouraged in order to estimate the likely extent of underdiagnosis of syndromes on the rates of certain combinations of anomalies. Basic information on whether a karyotype investigation or an autopsy had been performed may allow estimation of the relative accuracy of the case descriptions between different population groups. It may also be useful to collect drawings, photographs, or X-ray pictures and assess these centrally. Information on cases should also be supplemented by a good overview of changes in clinical practice, by recording screening methods and uptake in the population, and by maintaining good communication with clinicians in the collection and interpretation of data.

Prevalence

Prevalence figures for congenital anomalies are, of course, affected by the factors discussed above, which determine the completeness of ascertainment and accuracy. In addition, they may be affected by selection bias, especially in single- or multi-hospital studies which selectively include (or exclude) high-risk pregnancies.

The relative frequency of different anomaly groups, as well as the relative frequency of fetal deaths and induced abortions following prenatal diagnosis, are shown for selected congenital anomalies in Table 7.2. Figures are based on EUROCAT data for 18 European registries for the period 1980–88 (EUROCAT Working Group 1991*a*). Among the 18 registries there is variation in ascertainment, as well as apparently true variation in risk and variation in prevalence linked to demographic factors. Table 7.2 therefore serves as a comparative

Table 7.2 Average total prevalence rates per 10 000 births of selected anomalies in Europe, and distribution by type of birth (based on EUROCAT Working Group 1991*a*)

Anomaly	Rate	%LB	%FD	%IA
Nervous system[1]	29.8	62	18	20
Neural tube defects[1]	17.7	49	21	30
Anencephaly[1]	7.0	19	35	46
Spina bifida[1]	8.8	72	11	17
Encephalocele[1]	1.6	54	17	29
Hydrocephaly[1]	4.9	64	21	15
Microcephaly[1]	3.3	91	6	3
Arrhinencephaly/holoprosencephaly[1]	0.7	–	–	–
Eye[1]	6.0	94	4	2
Anophthalmos[1]	0.3	74	–	–
Microphthalmos[1]	1.4	92	–	–
Cataract[1]	1.2	98	1	1
Ear[1]	6.8	87	5	8
Anotia/microtia[1]	0.8	81	17	2
Congenital heart disease[1]	47.7	93	4	3
Hypoplasia left heart[1]	2.0	90	3	7
Common truncus[1]	0.9	84	9	7
Transposition great vessels non-corrected[1]	3.2	95	4	1

Table 7.2   (*cont.*)

Anomaly	Rate	%LB	%FD	%IA
Facial clefts[1]	15.1	90	6	4
Cleft lip with or without palate[1]	8.8	89	7	4
Cleft palate[1]	6.3	92	6	2
Digestive system[1]	13.9	88	7	5
Pyloric stenosis[1]	7.5	100	0	0
Tracheo-oesophageal fistula, oesophageal atresia, and stenosis[1]	2.9	92	6	2
Ano-rectal atresia and stenosis[1]	3.5	86	8	6
Atresia and stenosis of small intestine[1]	2.3	93	4	3
Internal urogenital[1]	17.7	80	9	11
Renal agenesis[1]	3.9	66	16	18
Cystic kidney disease[1]	3.1	78	7	15
External genital[1]	15.3	95	3	2
Hypospadias[1]	11.6	98	1	1
Indeterminate sex[1]	0.9	67	16	17
Limb[1]	60.8	94	4	2
Limb reduction[1]	6.1	84	10	6
Polydactyly[1]	8.4	93	4	3
Syndactyly[1]	6.4	92	4	4
Musculoskeletal and connective tissue[1]	29.0	81	9	10
Omphalocele[1]	2.7	57	21	22
Gastroschisis[1]	0.9	62	16	22
Anomalies of diaphragm[1]	3.0	85	9	6
Chromosomal syndromes[1]	20.0	79	5	16
Down[1]	13.8	86	3	11
Other[1]	2.8	65	14	21
Other syndromes[2]	12.8	88	7	5
Multiple anomalies (2 or more)[2]	17.1	82	11	7
Multiple anomalies (3 or more)[2]	6.2	77	15	8

LB, Live births; FD, fetal deaths from 20 weeks' gestation; IA, induced abortions following prenatal diagnosis.
[1] 18 EUROCAT registries, 1980–88.
[2] 15 EUROCAT registries, 1986–88.

guide to the frequency of different anomalies rather than as a statement of the expected rate of any one anomaly type.

Neural tube defects are probably the best known example of a geographically varying congenital anomaly, where the variation may be due to environmental

H. Dolk and P. De Wals

factors, possibly combined with differences in genetic predisposition (Elwood and Elwood 1980). Within Europe alone, prevalence rates were 2–3 times higher in the United Kingdom and Ireland than in Continental Europe in the 1980s and rates varied also within the British Isles (EUROCAT Working Group 1991*b*). Various environmental factors, such as water quality and nutritional factors, have been studied in relation to neural tube defect risk as well as proxies for environmental factors, such as socio-economic characteristics and seasonal variation in prevalence (Elwood and Elwood 1980).

The prevalence of cleft lip also varies geographically, but this is thought to be more closely linked to genetic factors than is the variability in neural tube defect prevalence (Leck 1984).

Demographic factors explain the geographical variation of some anomalies, notably Down's syndrome for which the major known risk factor is maternal age. Table 7.3 shows for 18 European populations the proportion of births to women of 35 or over, the proportion of affected fetuses/babies to mothers in this maternal age-group, and the prevalence of Down's syndrome. Twofold

Table 7.3 Relation of maternal age structure of the population to the prevalence of Down's syndrome in 18 European populations, 1980–88 (based on EUROCAT Working Group 1991*a*)

Registry	Number of cases (LB + FD + IA)	Prevalence rate per 10 000	Percentage of mothers 35 years and over		
			Cases (LB + FD + IA)	Cases (LB)	All births
West Flanders, Bel.	68	10.0	NA	21.9	4.8
Hainaut, Bel.	70	9.4	21.4	19.0	4.6
Odense, Denmark	48	11.3	29.2	17.9	6.3
Paris, France	459	16.0	49.5	23.9	14.7
Strasbourg, France	121	13.2	39.7	26.6	8.0
Marseille, France	114	16.2	49.1	40.7	10.6
Florence, Italy	120	14.9	51.7	43.0	10.7
Umbria, Italy	69	11.7	NA	30.9	7.6
Em. Romagna, Italy	243	13.3	NA	37.3	11.8
Dublin, Ireland	352	17.2	52.8	53.4	14.0
Luxembourg, GDL	28	12.7	NA	27.6	7.1
Groningen, NL	103	13.9	33	23.0	7.0
Glasgow, UK	132	11.3	31.1	22.2	6.4
Liverpool, UK	180	11.0	31.1	25.5	6.9
Belfast, UK	329	14.8	45.3	42.7	11.6
Zagreb, Yugoslavia	52	16.5	NA	13.5	4.8
Malta	29	18.0	44.8	44.8	13.9
Switzerland	18	7.4	NA	21.4	10.8

LB, Live births; FD, fetal deaths from 20 weeks' gestation; IA, induced abortions following prenatal diagnosis; NA, not applicable (induced abortions following prenatal diagnosis not registered).

differences in prevalence are found within Europe due to differences in maternal age distribution alone. Other relationships have been suggested between fertility patterns and the prevalence of congenital anomalies. For example, a reduction in average family size may have the effect of increasing the proportion of total births to relatively infertile women, who may be at higher risk of certain congenital anomalies. This has been suggested as an explanation for the variation in rates of hypospadias across the world (Kallen *et al.* 1986). Increased spacing between children may also affect the risk of congenital anomaly, but in general these types of demographic factors have been insufficiently studied. Changes in fertility patterns by socio-economic group have been suggested as playing a role in the decline of neural tube defect rates in the British Isles (Jongbloet 1981).

The trend in prenatal diagnosis is towards more extensive coverage and earlier testing during pregnancy. This will in itself lead to apparent geographical and temporal variation in the prevalence of anomalies which have high early spontaneous abortion rates, such as Down's syndrome (Kline *et al.* 1990). Prenatally diagnosed cases will include a large number of cases which would normally have been eliminated as early and often undiagnosed spontaneous abortions. Prevalence rates which include a high proportion of early induced abortions will therefore be overestimated in comparison with those in populations where most diagnosed cases are live births and still births.

It has been suggested that differences between the *in utero* survival of affected fetuses in different populations contribute to differences in prevalence at birth. This has been investigated for neural tube defects, but there is, as yet, no strong evidence to support the hypothesis (Elwood and Elwood 1980; Byrne and Warburton 1986). For Down's syndrome, a discussed (and disputed) suggestion is that maternal smoking increases the likelihood of spontaneous abortion of an affected fetus (Hook and Cross 1988; Cuckle *et al.* 1990; Hook and Regal 1991) which would, hypothetically, lead to a higher prevalence in populations with low maternal smoking rates.

Geographical resolution

The most commonly recorded geographical information is residence of the mother at birth of the affected child, and this is also the most readily usable information since it can be related to birth statistics, normally also available by residence of the mother. The adequacy of this information depends on the time of the relevant exposure, and the level of maternal migration between the time of exposure and the time of delivery. The single most useful geographical variable (but one not currently available in denominator statistics) may be residence at conception, since periconceptional and first trimester exposures are particularly important. Few estimates have been made of maternal migration between conception and delivery.

The limit of geographical resolution will tend to be the limit of resolution of denominator statistics. In England and Wales, births are recorded with post-codes (*c.* 14 households). In Belgium, the 118 000 annual births are recorded by commune on vital statistics (589 communes, or an average of 200 births per commune) but on medical records, the place of residence is usually recorded with the postal code (1161 codes, or an average 100 births per code). The boundaries of postal codes and communes do not always coincide.

A further constraint on resolution will be the availability of information on exposure or confounding variables at a small-area level for births. Although the birth notification may be a potentially valuable source of information without the problems of extrapolation between censuses, it is more limited than census information. Certain variables may need to be derived from census information, with the lowest limit of geographical resolution then being the census unit. If census information is to be used, further study will be required to examine the correlations between the characteristics of total populations and the characteristics of pregnant women, taking into account also the fact that important characteristics, such as employment outside the home, smoking, or nutrition, may change during pregnancy.

Role of special surveys and *ad hoc* studies

There is a conflicting requirement in making data available for small-area studies between the need to limit the size of the registry in order to collect complete and accurate data, and the need to obtain coverage across extensive geographical areas in order to allow geographical comparisons, and ensure that all localized risks will have available local health outcome information. Where a national birth defect monitoring system is in place, small specialized registries may be useful in addition to assess, on detection of a cluster, the possible role of incomplete ascertainment, or to provide background epidemiological data needed to interpret the cluster and suggest hypotheses for investigation. Some specialized regional registries can serve to 'calibrate' the national system (Knox *et al.* 1984; De Wals *et al.* 1988; Dutton *et al.* 1991) but this is not an easy objective to achieve, since reporting to the national system and to the specialized registry will not usually be independent.

At present, large geographical areas in Europe have no information system covering congenital anomalies, and it is not clear that putting resources into more complete geographical coverage, rather than increasing data quality in 'representative' regions, would be advisable, keeping in mind also that environmental studies are only one of the uses of a congenital anomaly in-formation system. Inevitably, therefore, many small-area studies will have to be conducted on an *ad hoc* basis, while requiring extensive background epidemiological information from both specialized registries and special additional surveys. Special additional surveys could include the systematic karyotyping of a cohort of fetuses/babies, the systematic pathological examination of a cohort of fetal and neonatal deaths according to a standard protocol, or the screening of neonates for selected non-life-threatening conditions.

Special surveys or *ad hoc* studies will also be needed for congenital anomalies in early fetal deaths and for minor anomalies, for which no permanent information systems of any scale currently exist, and for which medical records are not an adequate source of information.

Studies of early spontaneous abortions are needed to estimate the type and degree of bias that may be expected in studies of births (Khoury *et al.* 1989; Hook and Regal 1991). Also, in investigations of specific environmental exposures, the sensitivity of the study may be increased by including spontaneous abortions (Kline *et al.* 1977). These studies will be complex and costly, since not all spontaneous abortions are covered by hospitals, nor are they routinely investigated for congenital anomalies except for research.

Minor anomalies are characterized by great diagnostic variability and an understandable variability in detection and reporting, since they are, in themselves, of limited significance. Nevertheless, minor anomalies are important in the recognition of genetic syndromes (e.g. Down's syndrome) and environmental embryopathies (e.g. fetal alcohol syndrome) and have a certain predictive value for underlying major pathologies of various types (Pinsky 1985; Holmes *et al.* 1987; Leppig *et al.* 1987). They may well be more sensitive indicators of environmental insults than major anomalies. Since minor anomalies are more frequent, exhaustive population coverage may be replaced by sampling, which suggests the opportunity to restrict coverage to a limited number of centres with personnel trained in standardized examination and description. As yet, research into minor anomalies is at an early stage. Counting the total number of babies with minor anomalies is unlikely to be effective, and efforts are being made to determine which minor anomalies, or combinations of minor anomalies, are most predictive of environmental insults during pregnancy, or whether 'scoring' systems can be developed.

Small-area studies and congenital anomalies

Congenital anomaly surveillance was given its main impetus by the thalidomide tragedy in the early 1960s. Monitoring systems were set up for the early detection of increases in congenital anomaly frequency. It has been recognized that there are fundamental problems in reliance on routine monitoring (Khoury and Holtzman 1987; Kallen 1989) since 'epidemics' may be restricted to small, exposed subgroups of the population, or to very specific defects or defect patterns. Statistical monitoring of many population groups for many different defects results inevitably in the detection of a large number of random clusters in time, from which it is difficult to distinguish 'true' clusters which may be caused by environmental changes.

Added to this statistical problem is the problem of variation in case ascertainment and case definition. Even with the most thorough case-finding methods, such variation may be expected due to changes in medical practice (e.g. introduction or expansion of screening, increased differentiation of pathogenetic entities or recognition of syndromes, changes in cytogenetic and autopsy services). When operational problems in case-finding are added, it can be seen that the ascertainment factor alone can explain many variations over time in the frequency of specific defects, and this is, indeed, the experience of most congenital anomaly surveillance systems.

The same problems in the detection and interpretation of clusters or patterns of variation in time may be expected when analysis is made in the spatial dimension, and in each case it is necessary to consider the strength and specificity of the prior hypothesis when interpreting the results.

It may be theoretically justifiable in the first stage of small-area studies to sacrifice to some extent completeness and accuracy of data to comparability between small areas. In practice, it is likely to be difficult to ensure comparability of incomplete and inaccurate data, and the safest method to increase comparability is to attain high completeness and high accuracy.

It is often believed that congenital anomalies are an easier area of study than cancer because of the shorter delay between exposure and outcome. Although this is to some extent true, the complexities of exposure assessment and the importance of the time dimension should not be ignored.

First, exposure to an external environmental factor may have occurred well before the study pregnancy; for example, for mutagenic effects, or for the teratogenic effects of exposure to a substance with a long half-life in the body, or an exposure that entails long-term changes in the maternal environment.

Secondly, whereas a dose–response effect in cancer studies can be constructed from assessment of cumulative exposure of the individual, in the case of congenital anomalies it is the timing of exposure that is crucial. Each developmental event occurs in only hours or days, and for toxins with a short half-life in the body the dose-rate during these few days will be the relevant consideration.

Thirdly, whereas the assumption that cancer is a stochastic effect with a linear dose–response curve over a wide dose range may be a reasonable simplification, and allows the effective use of average exposure levels, it is not nearly so clear that this would be a reasonable assumption for teratogenic effects. There has been some debate over whether a 'threshold dose' for teratogenic agents should always be assumed (Brent 1986; Gaylor et al. 1988). In most cases the genetic and environmental variability in the population may be so great that the presence of threshold doses for individuals cannot be discerned in a population study. However, it is important to keep in mind for teratogenic effects that the dose-response curve may be far from linear, and that analyses of observed or expected effects in relation to the average dose may give very different results from analyses that take into account the variation in dose.

Taking a hypothetical example of geographical studies of pesticide exposures and assuming a short half-life of pesticides in the maternal body, a powerful study will be able to define the cohorts in time which have been exposed during the sensitive period of development to aerial spraying (which may occur during only one week of the year). Relative levels of exposure should then be determined not only from the average annual amount of pesticide used in each area, but from the degree of concentration of pesticide use at certain times of the year. Some attention may be required in future to the provision of suitable exposure information for congenital anomaly studies (Dolk *et al.* 1989).

Finally, where there is a short delay between exposure and outcome, this increases the likelihood of short and well-defined epidemics in response to environmental factors, and therefore necessitates a simultaneous analysis of the space and time dimensions.

Small-area studies are not new to congenital anomaly epidemiology, including the detection and investigation of individual clusters (Edmonds *et al.* 1975; Dorsch *et al.* 1984, Wrensch *et al.* 1990), analyses of epidemicity or generalized clustering (Knox 1963; Leck 1966; Roberts *et al.* 1975), and the investigation of possible effects of localized environmental contaminants (Mastrioacovo *et al.* 1988). However, this field remains underdeveloped at present, partly because of the daunting difficulties in achieving sufficient diagnostic and methodological standardization to allow valid comparison. Few environmental factors with strong localized geographical components (such as pesticide use, or air or water quality) have been subjected to intensive study. As is the case with monitoring in time, the routine detection of patterns or clusters in space will, at present, only be able to check for the presence of very large localized increases in risk, of an order that might normally be picked up by the local community or 'alert clinician'. The success of small-area studies will come from the formulation and testing of specific hypotheses, and the integration of small-area studies with other approaches to the study of environmental risk factors and the study of the aetiology of congenital anomalies.

References

Anderson, W. J. R., Baird, D., and Thomson, A. M. (1986). Epidemiology of stillbirths and infant deaths due to congenital malformation. *Lancet*, **1**, 1304–6.

Brent, R. L. (1986). Editorial comment: Definition of a teratogen and relationship of teratogenicity to carcinogenicity. *Teratology*, **34**, 359–60.

British Paediatric Association (1979). *British paediatric classification of diseases*. British Paediatric Association, London.

Byrne, J. and Warburton, D. (1986). NTD in spontaneous abortions. *American Journal of Medical Genetics*, **25**, 327–33.

Castillo, E., *et al.* (1986). Methodology for birth defects monitoring. *Birth Defects: Original Article Series*, **22**, (5), 1–43.

Clayton-Smith, J., Farndon, P. A., McKeown, C., and Donnai, D. (1990). Examination of fetuses after induced abortion for fetal abnormalities. *British Medical Journal*, **300**, 295–7.

Cole, S. K. (1983). Evaluation of a neonatal discharge record as a monitor of congenital malformations. *Community Medicine*, **5**, 21–30.

Creasy, M. R. and Alberman, E. D. (1976). Congenital malformations of the central nervous system in spontaneous abortions. *Journal of Medical Genetics*, **13**, 9–16.

Cuckle, H. S., Alberman, E., Wald, N. J., Royston, P., and Knight, G. (1990). Maternal smoking habits and Down's Syndrome. *Prenatal Diagnosis*, **10**, 561–7.

Czeizel, A. and Kis-Varga, A. (1987). Mutation surveillance of sentinel anomalies in Hungary, 1980–1984. *Mutation Research*, **186**, 73–9.

De Wals, P., Vincotte-Mols, M., Lys, F., Borlee, I., and Lechat, M. F. (1988). Evaluation de l'enregistrement des anomalies congenitales dans les statistiques belges d'Etat Civil. *Archives Belges Médecine Sociale*, **45**, 441–5.

Dolk, H., De Wals, P., and Lechat, M. F. (1989). Dose information needed to assess the effect of exposure to radiation *in utero*. *British Medical Journal*, **298**, 1710.

Dolk, H., Goyens, S., and Lechat, M. F. (1991*a*). *EUROCAT registry descriptions 1979–90*. Report EUR 13615, Luxembourg.

Dolk, H., *et al.* (1991*b*). Heterogeneity of NTD in Europe: the significance of site and presence of other major anomalies in relation to geographic differences in prevalence. *Teratology*, **44**, 547–59.

Dorsch, M. M., *et al.* (1984). Congenital malformations and maternal drinking water supply in rural South Australia: a case-control study. *American Journal of Epidemiology*, **119**, 473–86.

Dutton, S. J., Owens, J. R., and Harris, F. (1991). Ascertainment of congenital malformations: a comparison of two systems. *Journal of Epidemiology and Community Health*, **45**, 294–8.

Edmonds, L. D., Falk, H., and Nissim, J. E. (1975). Congenital malformations and vinyl chloride. *Lancet*, **2**, 1098.

Elwood, J. M. and Elwood, J. H. (1980). *Epidemiology of anencephalus and spina bifida*. Oxford University Press, Oxford.

EUROCAT Working Group (1988). Preliminary evaluation of the impact of the Chernobyl radiological contamination on the frequency of central nervous system malformations in 18 regions of Europe. *Paediatric and Perinatal Epidemiology*, **2**, 253–63.

EUROCAT Working Group (1991*a*). *EUROCAT Report 4. Surveillance of congenital anomalies 1980–88*. Department of Epidemiology, Catholic University of Louvain, Brussels.

EUROCAT Working Group (1991*b*). The prevalence of neural tube defects in 20 regions of Europe and the impact of prenatal diagnosis, 1980–86. *Journal of Epidemiology and Community Health*, in press.

Evrard, P., Saint-Georges, P., Kadhim, H. J., and Gadisseux, J.-F. (1989). Pathology of prenatal encephalopathies. In *Child neurology and developmental disability* (ed. P. H. Brookes).

Flynt, J. W. and Hay, S. (1979). International Clearinghouse for Birth Defect Monitoring Systems. In *Contributions to epidemiology and biostatistics*, (ed. M. A. Klingberg and J. A. C. Weatherall), vol. 1, pp. 44–52. Karger, Basel.

Fraser, F. C. (1976). The multifactorial/threshold concept – uses and misuses. *Teratology*, **14**, 267–80.

Gaylor, D. W., Sheenan, D. M., Young, J. F., and Mattison, D. R. (1988). The threshold dose question in teratogenesis. *Teratology*, **38**, 389–91.

Hall, S. M. and Glickman, M. (1988). The British Paediatric Surveillance Unit. *Archives of Disease in Childhood*, **63**, 344–6.

Holmes, L. B., *et al.* (1987). Predictive value of minor anomalies: II Use in cohort studies to identify teratogens. *Teratology*, **36**, 291–7.

Hook, E. B. and Cross, P. K. (1988). Maternal cigarette smoking, Down Syndrome in live births, and infant race. *American Journal of Human Genetics*, **42**, 482–9.

Hook, E. B. and Regal, R. R. (1991). Conceptus viability, malformation, and suspect mutagens or teratogens in humans. The Yule–Simpson Paradox and implications for inferences of causality in studies of mutagenicity or teratogenicity limited to live-births. *Teratology*, **43**, 53–9.

Jones, K. L. (1988). *Smith's recognizable patterns of human malformation*, (4th edn). W. B. Saunders, Philadelphia.

Jongbloet, P. H. (1981). NTD. *Lancet*, **2**, 1291.

Kallen, B. (1989). Population surveillance of congenital malformations. Possibilities and limitations. *Acta Paediatrica Scandinavica*, **78**, 657–63.

Kallen, B. and Winberg, J. (1968). A Swedish register of congenital malformations: Experience with continuous registration during 2 years with special reference to multiple malformations. *Pediatrics*, **41**, 765–76.

Kallen, B., *et al.* (1986). A joint international study on the epidemiology of hypo-spadias. *Acta Paediatrica Scandinavica*, **324**, (Suppl.), 1–52.

Khoury, M. J. and Holtzman, N. A. (1987). On the ability of birth defects monitoring to detect new teratogens. *American Journal of Epidemiology*, **126**, 136–43.

Khoury, M. J., Erickson, J. D., and James, L. M. (1982). Etiologic heterogeneity of NTD: clues from epidemiology. *American Journal of Epidemiology*, **34**, 980–7.

Khoury, M. J., Adams, M. M., Rhodes, P., and Erickson, J. D. (1987). Monitoring for multiple malformations in the detection of epidemics of birth defects. *Teratology*, **36**, 345–53.

Khoury, M. J., Flanders, W. D., James, L. M., and Erickson, J. D. (1989). Human teratogens, prenatal mortality, and selection bias. *American Journal of Epidemiology*, **130**, 361–70.

Kline, J., Stein, Z., Strobino, B., Susser, M., and Warburton, D. (1977). Surveillance of spontaneous abortions: Power in environmental monitoring. *American Journal of Epidemiology*, **106**, 345–50.

Kline, J., Stein, Z., and Susser, M. (1990). *From conception to birth*. Oxford University Press, Oxford.

Knox, E. G. (1963). Detection of low intensity epidemicity. Application to cleft lip and palate. *British Journal of Preventive and Social Medicine*, **17**, 121–7.

Knox, E. G., Armstrong, E. H., and Lancashire, R. (1984). The quality of notification of congenital malformations. *Journal of Epidemiology and Community Health*, **38**, 296–305.

Laurence, K. M., Carter, C. O., and David, P. H. (1967). Major central nervous system malformations in South Wales. I Incidence, local variations and geographical factors. *British Journal of Preventive and Social Medicine*, **21**, 146–60.

Lechat, M. F., de Wals, P., and Weatherall, J. A. C. (1985). European Economic Communities concerted action on congenital anomalies: The EUROCAT project. In *Prevention of physical and mental congenital defects. Part B: Epidemiology, early detection and therapy, and environmental factors* (ed. M. Marois), pp. 11–15. Alan R. Liss, New York.

Leck, I. (1966). Incidence and epidemicity of Down's Syndrome. *Lancet*, **2**, 457–60.

Leck, I. (1984). The geographical distribution of NTD and oral clefts. *British Medical Bulletin*, **40**, 390–5.

Leppig, K. A., Werler, M. M., Cann, C. I., Cook, C. A., and Holmes, L. B. (1987). Predictive value of minor abnormalities. I Association with major malformations. *Journal of Pediatrics*, **110**, 531–7.

Lys, F. and Mols, M. (1991). Increase in urinary tract abnormalities in South Hainaut, Belgium, and use of ultrasound scanning. *European Journal of Epidemiology*, abstract, in press.

Mastrioacovo, P., Spagnolo, A., Marni, E., Meazza, L., Bertollini, R., and Segni, G. (1988). Birth defects in the Seveso area after TCDD contamination. *Journal of the American Medical Association*, **259**, 1668–72.

Persaud, T. V. N., Chudley, A. E., and Skalko, R. G. (1985). *Basic concepts in teratology*. Alan R. Liss, New York.

Pinsky, L. (1985). Informative morphogenetic variants: Minor congenital anomalies revisited. In *Issues and reviews in teratology*, (ed. H. Kalter), vol. 3, pp. 135–70. Plenum Press, New York.

Roberts, C. J., Laurence, K. M., and Lloyd, S. (1975). An investigation of space and space-time clustering in a large sample of infants with neural tube defects born in Cardiff. *British Journal of Preventive and Social Medicine*, **29**, 202–4.

Sever, L. E. and Emanuel, I. (1981). Intergenerational factors in the etiology of anencephalus and spina bifida. *Developmental Medicine and Child Neurology*, **23**, 151–4.

Spranger, J., *et al.* (1979). Errors of morphogenesis: Concepts and terms. Recommendations of an international working group. *Journal of Pediatrics*, **100**, 160–5.

Warkany, J. (1971). *Congenital malformations*. Year Book Medical Publishers.

Weatherall, J. A. C., de Wals, P., and Lechat, M. F. (1984). Evaluation of information systems for surveillance of congenital malformations. *International Journal of Epidemiology*, **13**, 193–6.

Weatherall, J. A. C., Lys, F., and Gillerot, Y. (ed.) (1992). *EUROCAT Guide 5. Classification and coding of congenital anomalies*, in press.

WHO (1977). *International Classification of Diseases*, (9th edn). World Health Organization, Geneva.

Wilson, J. G. (1977). Current status of teratology. In *Handbook of teratology I. General principles and etiology*, (ed. J. G. Wilson and F. C. Fraser), pp. 47–74. Plenum Press, New York.

Wrensch, M., *et al.* (1990). Pregnancy outcome in women potentially exposed to solvent-contaminated water in San Jose, California. *American Journal of Epidemiology*, **131**, 283–300.

8. Specialized registers

A. Ahlbom and N. Hammar

All epidemiological investigations, regardless of their specific objectives, require information on the number of cases of the health event under study and on the population and time period that have generated the cases. In many countries information on the size of the population by age and sex and by geographical region is available, or can be estimated. Information on the number of incident disease cases, however, is only readily available for a limited number of diseases in any country. Typically, cancer and some infectious diseases are registered, and in some countries birth defects. For most diseases, incidence has to be studied by means of proxy variables or by information collected in *ad hoc* fashion. Thus, there is a need for methods by which diseases not covered routinely can be investigated. The objective of this chapter is to present and evaluate some of the available options. Clearly, these options vary depending on the disease, the country, and the aim of the specific investigation in which the disease information is to be used. As an example, we present a method for setting up a disease register for epidemiologic investigations of myocardial infarction, based on our experience in Sweden.

General considerations

Case ascertainment and study base

Epidemiological investigations usually compare disease rates across populations defined by demographic, sociological, temporal, or exposure related variables. For this exercise to be valid, there needs to be correspondence between the number of cases and the population and time period that have generated the cases. Miettinen (1985) has coined the term *study base* for this population and time experience. Since the information about the cases and the population often originates from different sources, the correspondence between cases and study base is far from guaranteed.

Consider an attempt to evaluate an alleged disease cluster in a defined geographical area, located, say, around a waste site. If the geographical area is defined using standard administrative boundaries, it is possible in many countries to estimate the size of the population and (possibly in cruder fashion) the number of person-years lived in the area during an observation period. Of the possible cases, only those originating at a time when the person contributes to the number of person-years should be eligible, and it requires fairly detailed information about all these possible cases to determine accurately which are to be included and which are not. Extra information may be available about some of these cases but may have to be disregarded. For example, people might actually not have spent time in the area even though they have been registered there; or, alternatively, cases known to have spent a considerable time in the area may not be included since they did not contribute to the number of person-years over the period of study.

An even more difficult situation arises when the area is not defined by administrative boundaries, but, for example, by levels of some exposure. Such a situation usually calls for an *ad hoc* study with information specifically collected for the purpose of the study.

Incidence and prevalence

The underlying objective of the comparisons of disease rates across populations variously exposed to some environmental pollutant is to evaluate whether the risks of disease differ. In many cases the natural study design would be a cross-sectional study using an interview or questionnaire, possibly followed by a clinical examination of everyone in the study or an appropriate subsample. For the objectives under consideration in this book, however, incidence rather than prevalence is the relevant measure of disease occurrence, even though it may not be feasible to carry out a study in which it can be observed.

Thus the relative risk, defined as the ratio of the incidence rate in one population to the incidence rate in another is usually the measure of choice by which morbidity is compared across populations. In some instances, it might be acceptable to measure the prevalences in the two populations, since the prevalence odds ratio is an estimate of the relative risk under fairly general conditions (Rothman 1986). However, this method of estimation does not take into account the possibility that diseased people, i.e. the prevalent cases, elect to move out in order to avoid further exposure, e.g. as might happen in the case of asthma and air pollution. Under these circumstances, cross-sectional studies are prone to underestimate relative risks.

Case ascertainment and proxy methods

In any country, information about the incidence of most diseases is difficult to come by. There is no standard, straightforward method available; indeed, whatever approach is being used requires careful evaluation.

Proxy methods of case ascertainment include indicators of treatment, consequences of the disease, and economic compensation. Some of the sources of information that have been used are as follows:

(1) Treatment:
   (a) inpatient, outpatient or emergency care, and general practice consultations;
   (b) drug prescription or drug sale;
   (c) surgical procedures.
(2) Consequences:
   (a) mortality;
   (b) disability.
(3) Economic compensation:
   (a) sick leave compensation;
   (b) pension.

In attempting to use one or several of these sources of information it should be appreciated that they are intended for purposes other than epidemiological investigations and usually merely for administrative purposes. For any disease, each of these information sources would cause some difficulties and in some cases these could be devastating. For example, no one would consider using in-patient hospital care information for investigation of the occurrence of back disorder. On the other hand, these sources might work satisfactorily for other diseases, e.g. the occurrence of lung cancer is well described by lung cancer mortality.

The problems are of a number of different kinds. Some of them pertain to the quality of the information. Some registries may have a high coverage rate, such as the mortality registry in many countries, while this is not necessarily true for others, such as out-patient care registries. The diagnostic information may be of varying quality; this problem is, of course, amplified by the lack of universally accepted diagnostic criteria for most diseases.

Other problems relate to the fact that the information recorded in these registries is usually not cases of disease but something that is more or less closely related to disease. Not everyone with a certain disease is admitted to hospital and this proportion depends on the disease, the hospital, and social, geographical, and other circumstances. Highly relevant information, such as disease onset, may well be lacking in a registry that is kept in order to provide economic support to the patients.

Myocardial infarction in Stockholm: an example

Method

In Sweden almost all hospital care is provided by the county councils, and most of these have computerized information systems in which data on hospital discharges are stored. For each discharge record, the unique personal identification number of the patient is stored, as well as the diagnoses, the hospital department, and the dates of the hospital stay. However, the hospital discharges can not be used directly, not even as proxies, for the identification of events of myocardial infarction, since one event may give rise to a varying number of hospital stays, depending on treatment policy and the organization of the hospital departments, as well as on the condition of the patient, the development of the disease, and the possible presence of other disorders.

To overcome this problem a special algorithm has been developed which translates hospital stays into events of myocardial infarction. The algorithm takes advantage of the unique personal identification number that is used in Sweden, and creates individually based records, with all hospital stays for each individual in one record. The length between one admission and the next is the basis for the algorithm—it usually requires a distance of 4 weeks from one admission to the next for a new event of myocardial infarction to be considered. The algorithm uses information on type of hospital department and a few other factors, which sometimes make exception to this 4-week rule. The personal identification number also makes it possible to perform record linkage to the cause of death registry. Thus, the hospital discharges can be combined with mortality information to enable the inclusion of non-hospitalized fatal cases: the algorithm treats deaths in similar fashion to hospital stays.

The validity of this method of creating a myocardial infarction registry depends on a large number of factors, including the coverage of the discharge registrations and the accuracy of the diagnoses accompanying the hospital stays and the deaths. We have addressed several of the potential sources of error in various ways. Thus, we have used samples of medical records with the objective of estimating the proportion of false positive diagnoses, and more such studies are under way (Ahlbom 1978). Furthermore, we have made a comparison with some WHO-coordinated myocardial infarction registries in Sweden in order to assess the agreement between the two methods (Ahlbom and Nordlander 1979). Although these efforts to validate our system have indeed indicated several difficulties with the method, overall it should be sufficiently accurate for a number of purposes.

Thus, for Stockholm county, and some other counties in Sweden, it has been possible to create a comprehensive, population-based myocardial infarction registry from routine information that is collected for other reasons. For certain purposes this registry can be used to address the same type of issues as the widely available cancer registries. That is, the myocardial infarction registry might be used as a source of end-point information in cohort studies and as a source of cases in case-control studies; it is currently being used for both these purposes in studies in Stockholm. The registry may also be used as the source of cases in several kinds of descriptive epidemiological studies to investigate time trends, geographical differences, etc.

Some applications

A, perhaps trivial, test of the usefulness of the myocardial infarction registry is the assessment of age- and sex-specific incidence rates, as in Ahlbom (1978).

These incidence rates show a good agreement with the corresponding rates from a WHO myocardial infarction registry in Gothenburg, Sweden.

Changes in myocardial infarction incidence rates have attracted great interest. In many Western countries, such as the USA, the incidence has declined over several decades. In Stockholm, however, a significant increase was noticed during the 1970s, which then turned into a similarly significant decrease (Alfredsson and Ahlbom 1983; Hammar and Ahlbom 1987; Hammar and Gillström 1990; Hammar *et al.* 1991). These changes are shown in Fig. 8.1 for 30–89-year-old men and women.

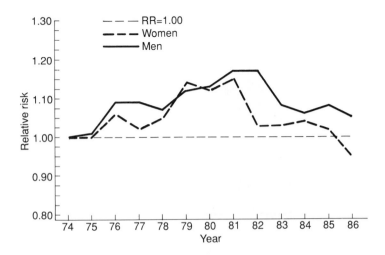

Fig. 8.1 Yearly age-adjusted relative risk of myocardial infarction in Stockholm county, 1974–86. 1974 is used as the reference year. Men and women aged 30–89.

For the purpose of this book, geographical variations are of special interest. The population registries in Sweden provide sufficient information to divide cases as well as populations into parishes which contain between 5000 and 40 000 inhabitants. The parish-specific information may then be aggregated into groups of parishes by use of extra information, such as socio-economic data. Such work is in progress in Stockholm. Analyses of communities in Stockholm county revealed large differences in the incidence of myocardial infarction for middle-aged men in 1979–86. In Fig. 8.2, the communities have been grouped with respect to the risk of myocardial infarction relative to Stockholm city, by far the largest community in the county. In the community with the highest incidence a middle-aged man had, on average, a 75 per cent greater risk of the disease than a man of the same age in the community with the lowest incidence. These differences were clearly related to a number of socio-economic conditions in the community, including median income, percentage of manual workers, and percentage of persons on social welfare.

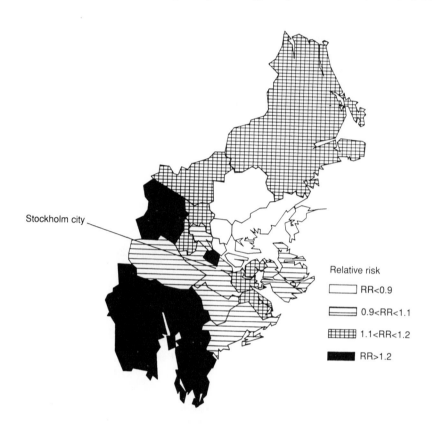

Fig. 8.2 Age-adjusted relative risk of myocardial infarction in 1979–86 in different municipalities of Stockholm county relative to Stockholm city. Men aged 30–64.

Some remarks

Although the method that has been presented here may seem rather straight-forward, a considerable amount of work was required to develop and evaluate it. We believe it to be a very useful resource with great potential for epidemio-logical research. Nevertheless, we warn against application of the method in other settings without careful evaluation of the primary data. Similarly, we warn against application to other diagnoses without even more careful evaluation. One reason why the method seems to work well with myocardial infarction is that almost all non-fatal cases, save the silent ones, are treated by in-patient care and that, after all, the diagnostic criteria are reasonably standardized for this disease. For most diseases these conditions are not normally met.

References

Ahlbom, A. (1978). Acute myocardial infarction in Stockholm – a medical information system as an epidemiological tool. *International Journal of Epidemiology*, 7, 271.

Ahlbom, A. and Nordlander, R. (1979). Application of diagnostic criterial in the diagnosis of myocardial infarction. *Scandinavian Journal of Social Medicine*, 7, 67–72.

Alfredsson, L. and Ahlbom, A. (1983). Increasing incidence and mortality from myocardial infarction in Stockholm county. *British Medical Journal*, 266, 1931–3.

Hammar, N. and Ahlbom, A. (1987). Recent trends in mortality and incidence of myocardial infarction in Stockholm, Sweden. *British Medical Journal*, 294, 609–10.

Hammar, N. and Gillström, P. (1990). Trends and regional differences in mortality from and incidence of myocardial infarction in Stockholm county 1974–86. *Paper presented at the Healthy Cities Symposium, Stockholm, Sweden 24 September.*

Hammar, N., *et al.* (1991). Identification of cases of myocardial infarction: hospital discharge data and mortality data compared to myocardial infarction community registers. *International Journal of Epidemiology*, 20, 114–20.

Miettinen, O. S. (1985). *Theoretical epidemiology. Principles of occurrence research in medicine*. John Wiley and Sons, New York.

Rothman, K. J. (1986). *Modern epidemiology*. Little, Brown and Co., Boston.

9. Population counts in small areas

I. Diamond

Calculation of disease rates in small areas requires an accurate estimation of the population exposed to risk. As the area of interest becomes smaller the problem becomes more acute and small changes in the population can have large effects on the resulting rates. These errors can be magnified many times if the small-area rates are then generalized to larger areas or populations. Unfortunately, the relative accuracy of a small-area population estimate is inversely proportional to the square root of the population size. This problem is similar to those faced in survey sampling (for a review see Kish 1965).

For census years, reasonably accurate population counts are available, but outside of these years it is necessary to make some kind of estimate or forecast —the term 'population estimate' is used for intercensal years (in this chapter we use 'estimate' to refer to a population estimate) and 'population forecast' (or projection) for years since the last census or into the future. These estimates are typically based either on statistical models or on a component approach—a method that accounts in turn for each of the components of population change; mortality, fertility, and migration. In the short term the former approach may be satisfactory, but in the longer run it is usually more accurate to base the estimate on the component approach.

This chapter reviews the data available for estimating the populations of small areas and then considers a number of common methods of estimation.

Data

Ideally, small-area estimates should be based on continuously updated counts of the population, such as those found in population registers. However, as such registers are relatively rare, many small-area estimates rely on two main sources: censuses and vital registration. In addition, estimates may be improved by ancillary information from large surveys, although it is rare for surveys to be large enough to permit the accurate adjustment of estimates of population counts at a very low level of aggregation.

Population registers

Population registers are continuously updated records of the population of some area. They usually contain basic demographic information, such as age, sex, place of birth, and marital status. Sometimes they include occupation and, for those still in education, current educational status. These registers are updated by data from vital registration and by notifications of change of address which residents are obliged to report to the registration authorities. These registers are primarily compiled for administrative purposes such as taxation, health and social services, or electoral registration but, where available, they have great potential for epidemiologists. A good overview can be found in Redfern (1989).

Table 9.1 summarizes the availability of population registers in much of Western Europe. The local registers have a long history in many countries—dating back to the seventeenth century in Finland and Sweden—but the development of national registers that link the data from local sources is largely confined to the past 40 years.

Table 9.1 Availability of population registers in Western Europe (adapted from Redfern 1989)

	Local population registers	Central population register
Belgium	X	X
Denmark	X	X
Finland	X	X
Luxembourg	X	X
Norway	X	X
Sweden	X	X
France	–	X
Netherlands	X	–
Portugal	–	X
Spain	X	X
Federal Republic of Germany	X	X
Greece	X	X
Italy	X	X
Ireland	–	–
UK	–	–

A notable exception in Table 9.1 is the UK. Although permanent registers have been proposed a number of times (e.g. Mallett 1929), they have never found favour outside of the periods of the First and Second World Wars. The last National Register in the UK was abandoned in 1952, as Redfern (1989) describes: 'in a post war spirit of "set the people free"'.

It has been suggested that the National Health Service Central Register (NHSCR) serves as a register. This includes all residents of the UK except a very small percentage who were born abroad and have never registered with a doctor in the UK. However, it serves only the National Health Service and cannot be exploited by other agencies. In addition, it suffers from three major drawbacks which limit its potential use for epidemiologists:

(1) many data do not include an individual's identity number and so cannot be linked into the NHSCR. This is particularly true of death registrations.
(2) Addresses are only changed when an individual moves to a new doctor, which will typically preclude moves over a short distance. Furthermore, moves to a new doctor often take a long time to reach the register.
(3) Information on a woman's change of name on marriage (or divorce) only reaches the NHSCR by chance, for example when she registers her new name with a different doctor.

One further source worthy of mention, although as yet little used for geographical epidemiology, is the Office of Population Censuses and Surveys (OPCS) Longitudinal Study (LS). This is a 1 per cent sample of the population which was started with the 1971 census and has been updated using the 1981 census data, death records, births to female members of the sample, subsequent infant mortality, and cancer registrations. This data set is similar to the French Panel Démographique and has been used widely to study topics such as occupational differentials in mortality (see, for example, Fox and Goldblatt 1982). For epidemiologists interested in estimating the size of small socio-economic groups this is an increasingly useful source. However, for reasons of preserving anonymity it is not possible to use the LS to estimate the populations of geographically small areas.

In summary, registers are potentially the most valuable source of small-area population data, and where they exist their use is strongly recommended. However, in countries such as the UK and the USA alternative sources are required.

Census data

Any population estimate requires a base population as a starting point. In many countries the most reliable base population comes from the decennial census. Censuses have been held throughout Western Europe and North America since the late eighteenth/early nineteenth century and consist of a count of the population on a particular day. Increasingly, census data are becoming available throughout the rest of the world and form the base for most, if not all, population projections and estimates.

Census data are necessarily restricted to demographic characteristics and basic socio-economic information. This is due both to financial restrictions and to the need to ask questions which are relevant to the majority of the population and which will be answered accurately. In the UK, cost considerations have led to a large reduction in the size of the census questionnaire in both 1981 and 1991 relative to those of 1961 and 1971. In addition, the large mid-censal population survey introduced in 1966, which gave important information on internal migration, seems likely never to be repeated.

The major advantage of census data is that population counts are available at very low levels of aggregation. In the UK the basic enumeration district consists, on average, of around 170 households. These can then be progressively aggregated to larger geographical areas. Data are published in the UK down to electoral ward level (around 5 000 persons) and below that census data are available through computers using a specially prepared package—SASPAC (1981).

The information that one could typically expect from a census include age, sex, marital status, household size, type of housing, dependants, occupation, education, ethnicity, and, in most countries except the UK, income. The census is also tremendously important as a source of data on migration. These are obtained by asking individuals about their usual address some time before the census. In the UK there used to be two questions—on residence 1 year and 5 years before the census, respectively. Unfortunately, the question on residence 5 years before the census has been left out of the 1981 and 1991 censuses.

It should be pointed out that in The Netherlands the 1981 census was cancelled due to poor response in 1971 and a poor field test. The then Federal Republic of Germany also experienced serious problems in 1981 due to boycott movements and that census finally took place in 1987. However, in general, census data have not experienced too many problems and are, without doubt, the most reliable national source of small-area population data. This is not to say that censuses are completely accurate. All censuses will undercount the population to some extent. Post-enumeration surveys are held to assess the extent of the undercount. These can be used to adjust the census data, and the methods by which this is done will be reviewed later in this chapter. The message of these analyses is that reasonable estimates of undercounts can be made where the local areas are 'average' areas but that, as with any regression-like technique, there are greater problems when the local areas are towards the extremes of the distribution or have particular socio-economic characteristics.

Census data are also subject to inaccuracy in areas where there are special populations; in particular, students, the armed forces, or other mobile groups present problems. For example, there has been much discussion over the determination of usual place of residence for students. In the UK the census has dealt with this by choosing a date in the student vacation.

For epidemiologists the presence of a large institution in some relatively small area may inflate rates of both morbidity and mortality. In the UK the borough of Castle Morpeth in the North-east has a standardized mortality ratio (SMR) for women which is very much higher than that anywhere else in the UK. Castle Morpeth is not a repository for strange and severe diseases, merely it is a relatively small area with a large regional geriatric speciality.

Vital registration data

Outside the census years it is necessary to estimate the populations of small areas. To do this it is usual to use vital registration data—registrations of births, marriages, and deaths. These data are published at small-area level in most countries, although they do not contain many socio-economic data and so are mainly used simply to adjust census counts.

Special surveys

Small-area population counts may be inferred from data available from large-scale sample surveys which are routinely undertaken for other purposes. For example, in all European Community (and many other) countries Labour Force Surveys are taken regularly. These surveys do not normally provide population estimates below regional level but they can be used to give an idea of trends in population size. Ratio methods (discussed in the next section) can then be used to adjust census distributions in order to estimate population size.

However, there are many situations when important data are simply not available from standard sources. For example, in noise pollution studies the population exposed to particular levels of noise may not be known and special acoustical surveys will be required. Again, when estimating the number of households exposed to some risk factor, specially commissioned social surveys may be the only sensible strategy. However, the cost of such surveys means that they should only be used when all other possibilities have been exhausted. For an example of a study linking social and acoustical surveys, see Diamond et al. (1989).

Small-area population estimates and projections

There are two basic strategies for computing population size in small areas: regression models and component projections. Both usually start with census data and then adjust the base census population using data from another source. They are outlined briefly below.

Regression estimates

Regression models have, for many years, been widely used for making small-area estimates (see, for example, Morrison and Relles 1976). A good review is provided by Purcell and Kish (1979) and the comprehensive set of papers by Platek et al. (1987). The basic framework is that

$$\widehat{\mathbf{P}}_2 = f(\mathbf{X}_1, \mathbf{X}_2, \widehat{\mathbf{P}}_1) \tag{1}$$

where $\widehat{\mathbf{P}}_1 = (\widehat{P}_{11}, \ldots, \widehat{P}_{1k})'$ is population at time t_1, in k small areas;

$\hat{\mathbf{P}}_2 = (\hat{P}_{21}, \ldots, \hat{P}_{2k})'$ is the estimated population at time t_2; and $\mathbf{X}_1, \mathbf{X}_2$ are vectors of characteristics of the k small areas at times t_1 and t_2, respectively. One may also have a separate $f(.)$ for each subgroup.

Regression models can take on varying degrees of complexity, but they have to conform to a number of conditions, the most fundamental of which is that

$$\sum_{i=1}^{k} \hat{P}_{2i} = \sum_{i=1}^{k} P_{2i},$$

i.e. that the estimated populations of the small areas should add to the overall population size—which can often be estimated very accurately. A good review of these conditions is provided by McCullagh and Zidek (1987). The simplest form of regression model is to estimate a rate of growth for each small area based on the characteristics that can be observed. This can be done using the formula

$$r_i = \log \left[\frac{x_{2i}}{x_{1i}} \right] \frac{1}{t_2 - t_1}.$$

Then the population at the time t_2 in small area i can be estimated as

$$P_{2i} = P_{1i} r_i^{\beta} \tag{2}$$

where β is the regression coefficient which must be estimated.

In general, there will be $K(>1)$ characteristics in the regression equation and Equation (2) will become

$$P_{2i} = P_{1i} \sum_{j=1}^{K} r_{ij}^{\beta_j} \tag{3}$$

This is the basic form of the model proposed by Morrison and Relles (1976) and is described by Swanson and Tedrow (1984). Good practical examples of these models are provided by Ericksen and Kadane (1987) and Lundström (1987).

One final approach should be mentioned. This is a synthetic method which assumes that small areas have the same characteristics as given larger areas that contain them. Purcell (1979) proposed a sophisticated synthetic method, using a categorical data approach known as Structure Preserving Estimates (SPREE). Here one has data, say from a census, that can be categorized into a multiway contingency table. A subsequent survey, say a Labour Force Survey, gives marginal totals at a higher level of aggregation, such as region. Purcell (1979) assumes a superpopulation model for the relationship between the distribution of the number of individuals in each small area over time; SPREE estimates are then calculated by adjusting the data from t_1 to t_2 subject to the new marginals and maintaining the structure in the multiway table at t_1. The estimation is made using iterative proportional fitting. This approach, although not used widely, has been shown to work well by Feeney (1987), Lundström (1987), and Pujadas (1983).

Component projections

Component projections are essentially accounting techniques based on the standard population balancing equation:

$$P_2 = P_1 + B - D + I - E$$

where P_1 = population at time t_1;
  P_2 = population at time t_2;
  B = births between t_1 and t_2;
  D = deaths between t_1 and t_2;
  I = immigrants between t_1 and t_2;
  E = emigrants between t_1 and t_2.

Many of these techniques were developed before 1950, but the increasing need for small-area projections in local and central government has led to a huge increase in their use, with a commensurate increase in the variety of methods used to calculate them. Full reviews of projection strategies are found in Joshi and Diamond (1990) and Diamond et al. (1990). These reviews describe many approaches but the vast majority use some variation on the cohort survival model. This has four steps:

(1) identify the base population at t_1 categorized by, say, age and sex;
(2) calculate the number of survivors of this population at time t_2 using mortality rates or vital registration;
(3) calculate the survivors of the births between t_1 and t_2;
(4) adjust for migration.

There has been a lot of work on the accuracy of component projections at a national level (e.g. Long 1990) but less for small areas. Simpson (1989), who studied projecting educational rolls, suggests that for short time horizons the accuracy may be fairly good. Epidemiologists will typically be interested in relatively short time horizons and so reasonable accuracy should be possible. For short time horizons the major problem is estimating migration. Fertility is more of a problem in long-term projections, while mortality has been thought not to be a major problem, although recently Murphy (1990) has argued that major changes in expectation of life may require a rethink on this issue. For a review of current trends in each of these areas see Lutz (1990).

For fairly large areas migration flows can be estimated reasonably accurately, but as the areas become smaller so the need for local knowledge becomes essential. Table 9.2 provides a review of the appropriate methods for areas of different sizes. Woodhead and Dugmore (1990) divide these approaches into three groups:

1. *Demographic trend models* (single-area or multi-area cohort models). This approach is the one described above. In the single-area model, migration is extrapolated from recent trends.

2. *Causal hypothesis models.* These models first adjust the base population for mortality and fertility, then local information on housing developments or employment opportunities is used to estimate the total population. Net migration is then the difference between the two. Note that if all that is required is a population count then these models could be used without a base population categorized by age and sex. A count from the census year could be adjusted using changes in the housing or employment stock to give a subsequent count.

3. *Ratio models.* These are used for very small areas and are calculated by first estimating population change for a large area and then assigning this change to smaller levels according to some criteria such as the ratio of population levels at the census. This approach is similar to the synthetic ratio estimation proposed by NCHS (1968) and described by Purcell and Kish (1979).

Table 9.2 Appropriate projection strategies for areas of different population sizes (adapted from Woodhead and Dugmore 1990)

Area	Strategy				
	Single-area cohort	Multi-area cohort	Employment	Housing capacity	Ratio
Nation	X	X			
Region	X	X	X		
County	X	X	X	X	
City-region	X	X	X	X	
Local authority district	X	X		X	
Service catchment[1]		X		X	X
Neighbourhood				X	X

[1] Service catchment refers to the catchment population for some public service, such as health or education.

It should also be noted that governments typically provide some subnational projections. For example, the Australian Bureau of Statistics provides state-level projections, and in the UK projections are made for local authority areas and national health service districts. If such nationally produced data are available for the epidemiologist's required area then it is recommended that they are used. For smaller areas the experience of Joshi and Diamond (1990) and Diamond *et al.* (1990) suggests that local authority projections and those made by university research groups tend to cover most areas and are reliable. In summary, only make your own projection if you really need to!

Summary

This chapter has reviewed data sources for small-area population counts and methods for estimation in years when counts are not available. In countries where local population registers are available then these provide the best source and it is recommended that they should be used, particularly when a central register makes different levels of aggregation easy to assess.

When population registers are not available, census data provide the best and most reliable source. However, census data are subject to undercounts and it is recommended that adjustments should be made before use. When an area has a large mobile or institutional population, the use of census and vital registration data may lead to inaccuracies. There is no formal method of adjusting for these, other than the accounting methods adopted by census authorities. Epidemiologists should simply be aware of the nuances of the area they are studying and take appropriate care.

In years when there is no census then the standard approaches are regression models and component projections. Component projections are probably the most widely used and, for short- and medium-range projections, their accuracy is good. It should be noted that each of these methods is dependent on accurate ancillary data for their success. If such data do not exist, then the epidemiologist will have to struggle to obtain reliable estimates.

Finally, in the UK and several other countries, there are now good population estimates available for small areas which have been produced by local and central government, as well as by a myriad of research organizations. The epidemiologist should make his/her own estimates only if it is absolutely clear that no counts exist for the particular area or subgroup of interest.

References

Diamond, I. D., Ollerhead, J. B., Bradshaw, S. A., Walker, J. G., and Critchley, J. B. (1989). *A study of disturbance due to general and business aviation.* Department of Transport, London.

Diamond, I. D., Tesfaghiorghis, H., and Joshi, H. (1990). The uses and users of population projection in Australia. *Journal of the Australian Population Association,* **7**, 151–70.

Eriksen, E. P. and Kadane, J. B. (1987). Sensitivity analysis of local estimates of undercount in the 1980. US Census. In *Small area statistics*, (ed. Platek *et al.*), pp. 23–45. Wiley, New York.

Feeney, G. A. (1987). The estimation of the number of unemployed at the small area level. In *Small area statistics*, (ed. Platek *et al.*), pp. 198–218. Wiley, New York.

Fox, A. J. and Goldblatt, P. O. (1982). *Socio-demographic differentials in mortality 1971–75*, OPCS Series LS, No. 1. HMSO, London.

Joshi, H. and Diamond, I. (1990). Demographic projections: who needs to know: In *Population projections: trends, methods and uses*, OPCS occasional paper, No. 38, pp. 1–22. HMSO, London.

Kish, L. (1965). *Survey sampling*, pp. 50–1. Wiley, New York.

Long, J. (1990). Relative effects of fertility, mortality and immigration on projected age structure. In *Future demographic trends in Europe and North America*, (ed. W. Lutz), pp. 503–22. Academic Press, London.

Lundström, S. (1987). An evaluation of small area estimation methods: the case of estimating the number of nonmarried cohabiting persons in Swedish municipalities. In *Small area statistics*, (ed. R. Platek *et al.*), pp. 239–56. Wiley, New York.

Lutz, W. (1990). *Future demographic trends in Europe and North America*. Academic Press, London.

McCullagh, P. and Zidek, J. V. (1987). Regression methods and performance criteria for small area population estimation. In *Small area statistics*, (ed. R. Platek *et al.*), pp. 62–76. Wiley, New York.

Mallett, Sir Bernard (1929). Reform of vital statistics: outline of a system of national registration. *Eugenics Review*, **21**, 87–94.

Morrison, P. A. and Relles, D. A. (1976). A method of monitoring small area population change in cities. *Public Data Use*, **3**, 10–15.

Murphy, M. (1990). Methods of forecasting mortality for population projections. In *Population projections: trends, methods and uses*, OPCS occasional paper, No. 38, pp. 87–102. HMSO, London.

NCHS (1968). *Synthetic estimates of disability*, PHS publication 11759. US Government Printing Office, Washington DC.

Platek, R., Rao, J. N. K., Sarndal, C. E., and Singh, M. P. (ed.) (1987). *Small area statistics: an international symposium*. Wiley, New York.

Pujadas, L. (1983). Small area estimation. Unpublished M.Sc. thesis. University of Southampton.

Purcell, N. J. and Kish, K. (1979). Estimation for small domains. *Biometrics*, **35**, 365–84.

Purcell, N. J. (1979). Efficient domain estimation: a categorical data approach. Unpublished Ph.D. thesis. University of Michigan, Ann Arbor.

Redfern, P. (1989). Population registers: some administrative and statistical pros and cons. *Journal of the Royal Statistical Society, Series A*, **152**, 1–41.

SASPAC (1981). *Small area statistics package manual*. Office of Population, Censuses and Surveys, London.

Simpson, S. (1989). School roll forecasts: their uses, their accuracy and educational reform. *Journal of the Royal Statistical Society, Series A*, **152**, 287–304.

Swanson, D. A. and Tedrow, L. M. (1984). Improving the measurement of temporal change in regression models for county population estimates. *Demography*, **21**, 273–89.

Woodhead, K. and Dugmore, K. (1990). Local and small area projections. In *Population projections: trends, methods and uses*, OPCS occasional paper, No. 38, pp. 65–76, HMSO, London.

10. Use of routine data in studies of point sources of environmental pollution

P. Elliott, I. Kleinschmidt, and A. J. Westlake

As was discussed briefly in Chapter 2, an important application of small-area methods is in the investigation of possible health effects around point sources of environmental pollution. Traditionally, these studies were costly and time-consuming since health data relevant to a particular location had to be assembled and analysed *ad hoc*. We discuss here how the rapid initial investigation of health around sources of industrial pollution can now largely be automated using routine data, and describe our experience in setting up such a system in the UK.

Although routine statistics have often been used to display and analyse geographical variations in disease (e.g. Teppo *et al.*, 1980; Gardner *et al.* 1983), their use in small-area analyses has been limited. For example, health data are usually aggregated for reporting purposes to administrative areas which are often inappropriate for detailed statistical analyses related to a point source. Not only can the area of concern cross administrative boundaries, but the size of the administrative units is likely to swamp truly local effects. Ideally, a system is required that can store and handle disaggregated data and then rapidly retrieve, assemble, and analyse the data relevant to a particular area. Essential components of such a system are as follows:

1. There should be accurate data on health events, which must include mortality and preferably some morbidity data (for example, from a national cancer registry). The whole data set must be of high quality with high levels of ascertainment if errors in the estimation of local rates of disease are to be minimized.

2. Each event needs to be located geographically by place of residence (and/or place of birth) using either the individual's address or, for reasons of confidentiality and ease of computation, an address code identifying a small geographical area or a limited set of addresses.

3. Population data are required (e.g. from national census) to provide denominators for the calculation of disease rates. The data should be as disaggregated as possible while preserving the rights and confidentiality of individuals. If possible, intercensal small-area population estimates should also be available.

4. Geographical links are needed to match the address codes on the events (numerators) with the population data (denominators).

5. Appropriate computer and information technology is required to allow rapid access to the relevant event and population data, and to carry out the statistical analyses.

We are fortunate in the UK that all the above conditions are met. We outline below the application of a routine data system for the UK which has been implemented in the Small Area Health Statistics Unit (SAHSU) at the London School of Hygiene and Tropical Medicine, and (for England and Wales) in the Environmental Monitoring Project at the Office of Population Censuses and Surveys (OPCS). The system automatically assembles and displays data around any point, compares the observed number of cases with those expected from national or regional rates, and takes account of the socio-economic distribution of areas around the point of interest.

The Small Area Health Statistics Unit

Following the report of an increased incidence in childhood leukaemia around the nuclear reprocessing plant at Sellafield (described in detail in Chapter 25), the Government set up an independent enquiry under the chairmanship of Sir Douglas Black (Black 1984). Recommendation 5 of the report called for an organization: 'to coordinate centrally the monitoring of small area statistics around major installations producing discharges that might present a carcinogenic or mutagenic hazard to the public. In this way, early warning of any untoward health effect could be obtained.'

Subsequently, SAHSU was established and funded by Government departments of health and environment, and the Health and Safety Executive. SAHSU works closely with the Environmental Monitoring Project at OPCS. The two groups have set up a parallel system involving joint staff appointments and the exchange of data, programs, and computer expertise. There are also close working relationships with the Information and Statistics Division of the Scottish Health Service, the Welsh Office, Northern Ireland, and the various cancer registries which provide cancer incidence data.

Requests for investigation by SAHSU from Government or other sources are directed to a steering committee, representing the funding departments and their independent scientific advisers. While funded by the Government, SAHSU works independently and is free to publish its findings. Its terms of reference are as follows:

1. To examine quickly reports of unusual clusters of disease, particularly in the neighbourhood of industrial installations, and to advise authoritatively as soon as possible.
2. In collaboration with other scientific groups, to build up reliable background information on the distribution of disease amongst small areas so that specific clusters can be placed in proper context.
3. To study the available statistics in order to detect any unusual incidence of disease as early as possible and, where appropriate, to investigate.

4. To develop the methodology for analysing and interpreting statistics relating to small areas.

Most of our attention has focused on methods for the study of point sources. We have been particularly concerned with the study of disease around multiple sites, either to replicate an enquiry conducted *post hoc* around one site (by studying other sites in Britain producing similar discharges; see Chapter 29) or to test hypotheses related to emissions from particular industrial processes. The various components of the SAHSU system are described below.

Geography

In the 1970s the Post Office introduced a comprehensive system of postcodes, covering the whole of the UK, to improve the efficiency of delivering mail. Postcodes are allocated through a hierarchy. In the UK there are 120 postal areas, and approximately 2700 districts, 9000 sectors, and 1.6 million unit postcodes, representing 22 million postal addresses. Unit postcodes uniquely define areas containing on average only 14 households each. The geographical extent of the postcode depends on whether the location is urban or rural, whether the buildings are commercial or residential, and whether there are private houses or multi-tenanted apartment blocks.

Many health events in the UK are now routinely postcoded (e.g. deaths, cancer registrations, congenital malformations). Although the postcode relates to too small an area for analyses in its own right, it serves as the key to the entire system: it can be used to locate events either in standard geographical areas, such as local government districts, or in arbitrarily constructed areas, such as a circle around a point source of pollution. Standard directories give a map grid reference (accurate to 100 m) for each postcode and approximate geographical links to census enumeration districts (EDs) and hence to the relevant population data. (EDs are the smallest area for which population data are available. In Scotland, there are direct links between postcodes and EDs; in England and Wales following the 1991 census, the census office will be able to assign postcodes directly to EDs, although some postcodes will span more than one ED).

Health events

Postcoded data sets held by SAHSU and OPCS include:

1. Deaths, live births, and still births for England and Wales from 1981; SAHSU also has mortality data for Scotland from 1974 and for Northern Ireland from 1986. The information on births provides accurate year-by-year denominator data for perinatal

and childhood events. OPCS (but not SAHSU) has link files that enable information on infant mortality to be collated for particular individuals.

2. Cancer registrations for England and Wales from 1974. These were originally collected by the 12 regional cancer registries, and enhanced by a large retrospective postcoding exercise undertaken by the Environmental Monitoring Project at OPCS. SAHSU also holds Scottish cancer data from 1975, and data on childhood leukaemia and non-Hodgkin's lymphomas in Great Britain from 1966, supplied by the Childhood Cancer Research Group in Oxford.

3. Congenital malformations from 1983.

4. Abortions from 1984 (cases where there was a substantial risk that the baby would be born handicapped) held only by OPCS.

In addition, the Environmental Monitoring Project at OPCS holds some data items which for legal and confidentiality reasons cannot be passed to SAHSU, including names and dates of birth; SAHSU holds age in years and months, and an identifier allowing OPCS to link to individual records. A similar system is in place for Scottish data.

Populations

The population data come mainly from the decennial census. Population statistics were published for wards in 1971 and at the level of ED in 1981. There are approximately 10 000 wards and 130 000 EDs in Britain, each ED containing on average about 170 households and 400 individuals. A system of 'census tracts' based on 1981 geography links areas between the two censuses. Similar data from the 1991 census will be published for EDs together with some small-area aggregated postcode data. Standard directories are available to relate EDs to wards and higher-level administrative units, such as local government districts and parliamentary constituencies.

Denominators for calculating diseases rates are obtained from the census small-area statistics. Currently, SAHSU holds tables that contain sex and age counts (in five-year groups) for 1981 EDs and 1971/81 census tracts; data for 1991 EDs will be added when they become available. Year-by-year population estimates for local authority districts have also been acquired (from OPCS) as well as estimates of population for 1986 at ED level, obtained from CACI Ltd (89 Kingsway, London WC2B 6RH).

Tables giving socio-economic information for EDs have been abstracted from the small-area statistics as described in Chapter 11 (e.g. car ownership, proportion unemployed) and a neighbourhood classification based on census characteristics is available for EDs (ACORN; from CACI Ltd). These data allow some control for social and demographic confounding variables in the statistical analyses. In addition, two years' data from the General Household Survey are available giving, for example, data at the level of ED on smoking prevalence and alcohol consumption by ACORN type.

Computer hardware and software, and data storage

The SAHSU system runs under Unix on a RISC (Reduced Instruction Set Computer) Digital (DEC) 5500 super-microcomputer, with about 24 mips of processing power and installed data storage of about 10 500 Mbytes. We use the Oracle relational data-base management system and implement algorithms in 'C' with 'embedded' SQL for access to the data-base. Further analysis is done in the statistical packages Gauss, 'S', and SAS.

Table 10.1 shows the data storage requirements. The event data are added to each year and make the largest contribution (particularly deaths) whereas the postcode table and (except following a census year) the population census data are stable requirements. Births require similar amounts of data storage as the death file. Note that indexing constitutes a large overhead in storage.

Table 10.1 Computer storage requirements for the Small Area Health Statistics Unit

		Data	Indexes		Total
Table	Rows	Mb	Number	Mb	Mb
Events					
Cancer	2 584 000	200	2	150	350
(1974–84)					
Deaths	6 011 483	370	2	320	690
(1981–89)					
Population (EDs)					
Counts	130 000	6	4	16	22
Socio-economic	130 000	35	1	16	51
Postcode	1 600 000	102	4	172	274
Other		5	7	5	10
Totals		718		679	1397

Mb, Megabytes.

Figure 10.1 shows the structure of the SAHSU data-base. Links between two sets of data (referred to as tables) are established through common attributes ('foreign keys') as indicated by the lines joining the tables. Geography is determined by the map coordinates of the postcode (represented as a point location) and by the hierarchy of membership of administrative units, which (as indicated in the figure) is made up mainly of one-to-many relationships.

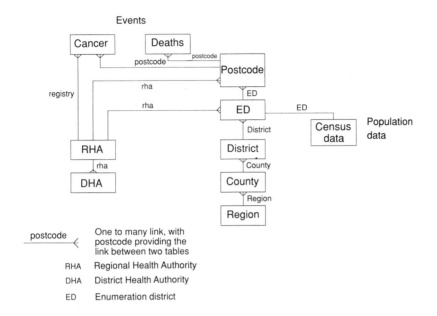

Fig. 10.1   Outline of the Small Area Health Statistics Unit data-base showing links between events and population data, and the administrative geography.

Since administrative areas and postcodes change with time, the data-base needs to hold updates of postcode changes, and multiple versions of tables defining the membership of areas.

Data access and retrieval

Data retrieval for an arbitrary geographical area is discussed for the simplest case, namely a circle with an arbitrary centre and radius (although extension to other mathematically defined areas is possible). The centre of the circle may be given as a grid reference or as a full postcode. Response times are generally acceptable and depend on the number of cases and on the population captured in the specified area (i.e. about 5 minutes per 100 000 population for rare diseases).

Calculation of numerators

The system is required to retrieve all cases defined by ICD code (WHO 1977) occurring in a specified time period whose postcodes of residence have their 'centroids' within a specified circle. To achieve rapid response times, we first divided Britain into a set of 1 km grid squares, and having indexed each post-code on its corresponding 1 km square, the following steps (illustrated in Fig. 10.2) are carried out:

1. Determine the coordinates of the (smallest) covering square that completely contains the circle and coincides with the boundaries of the 1 km grid squares (square A, Fig. 10.2).
2. Compute the set of 1 km squares that are contained within this square (table *sqs*, see below).
3. Run through the list of squares, reject those that lie entirely outside the circle (B, Fig. 10.2) and mark those that are wholly within the circle (C, Fig. 10.2).
4. Do a distance calculation on each postcode in the set of unmarked squares, i.e. those that straddle the circumference of the circle (D, Fig. 10.2), and select the postcodes that lie within the circle. Add this list to all postcodes that are already marked as being within the circle (step 3, above) to get the target list of postcodes (table *pcs__temp*, see below).

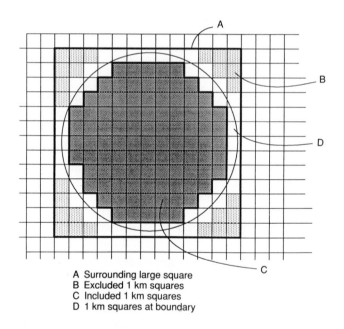

A Surrounding large square
B Excluded 1 km squares
C Included 1 km squares
D 1 km squares at boundary

Fig. 10.2 Diagrammatic illustration of the algorithm to locate postcodes within a circle.

Steps 1 to 3 above can be performed entirely by computation (without scanning the data-base) and hence are rapid operations, carried out in 'C'. Calculation of distances between individual postcodes and the circle centre (step 4) is done in SQL and involves access to the data-base (i.e. the Central Postcode

Directory); this is manageable since the temporary table *sqs* is small. A join operation between *pcs_temp* and the indexed event table (deaths, cancers) produces the numerator set for the specified circle, which can then be aggregated for cross-tabulation purposes, e.g. by five-year age-group and by sex.

Calculation of denominators

As discussed, the ED (containing on average about 14 postcodes) is the lowest level at which the denominator data are available, whereas the event data (and the circle algorithm) are based on postcodes; we therefore need to allocate ED populations to postcodes for those EDs that straddle the boundary of the circle. At present, this is done according to the proportion of constituent postcodes that lie within the circle, but later we may be able to refine this method (for example, when data on the number of households per postcode are available from the 1991 census).

Calculation of national and regional rates and standardized ratios

The expected number of cases is obtained by applying regional or national age- and sex-specific rates (calculated from within the data-base) to the population data for the circle (i.e. indirect standardization). This standardization procedure has been extended to include stratification by socio-economic variables at the level of EDs. Typically, calculating standard rates is expensive in computer time (2–3 hours per run) but the values obtained can be stored for future use.

Further developments

We are currently restricted to spatial queries related to circles or administrative units, although the algorithm is sufficiently general to apply (with modification) to any mathematically defined area. The flexibility of the system will be further enhanced by the addition of a Geographic Information System (GIS), which will extend the range of spatial enquiries (for example, to correspond with pollutant dispersion patterns) and provide a mapping facility both as a means of defining search areas and for presentation purposes. The GIS will need to link in with the relational data-base around which the present system has been developed.

Conclusions

Advances in computer technology and the availability of high-quality national data sets with high resolution information, have enabled the initial screening and analysis of health data around point sources of industrial pollution to be largely automated. If cause for concern around a particular site is confirmed, the data will need to be checked and validated (for completeness, diagnostic accuracy, etc.). Replication around sites with similar discharges (if such can be found) can be carried out from within the data-base, or alternatively, disease around multiple sites can be studied (and if necessary replicated around other sites) to investigate the risks associated with a particular industrial process. Confirmatory field studies may then be required, to include environmental measurements and assessment of possible confounding factors, such as smoking, alcohol consumption, housing quality, and occupational histories. An example of an enquiry around multiple sites using the SAHSU data-base is given in Chapter 29.

References

Black, D. (chairman) (1984). *Investigation of the possible increased incidence of cancer in West Cumbria*. Report of the Independent Advisory Group. HMSO, London.
Gardner, M. J., Winter, P. D., Taylor, C. P., and Acheson, E. D. (1983). *Atlas of cancer mortality in England and Wales, 1968–1978*. John Wiley and Sons, Chichester.
Teppo, L., Pukkala, E., Hakama, M., Hakulinen, T., Herva, A., and Saxén, E. (1980). Way of life and cancer incidence in Finland. A municipality-based ecological analysis. *Scandinavian Journal of Social Medicine, Supplement*, **19**, 5–84.
World Health Organization (1977). *Manual of the International Statistical Classification of Diseases, Injuries, and Causes of Death*. WHO, Geneva.

11. Socio-economic confounding

D. J. Jolley, B. Jarman, and P. Elliott

Suppose that the incidence of lung cancer is elevated in the population living around an industrial installation suspected of emitting hazardous substances. Can the increase in rates be attributed to the installation? People living near an industrial site do not constitute a random sample of the general population. Rather, they have chosen (or been selected by economic forces, employment, or family circumstance) to live in what is often a disadvantaged area, subject not only to ambient atmospheric or other sources of environmental pollution resulting from local industry, but also to a myriad of social disadvantages related to poor housing, overcrowding, poor economic performance, and the like. How do these factors relate to disease?

Measures of the social class of individuals have long been known to predict disease incidence and mortality (Farr 1875; Vernon 1939; Logan and Brooke 1957), while similar findings for residential areas have been reported using socio-economic data to classify areas by levels of deprivation (Jarman 1983; Townsend *et al* 1988; Carstairs and Morris 1991). For most diseases displaying a social class gradient, the more disadvantaged individuals experience higher risk (Leon 1988). Socio-economic factors are therefore likely to confound (usually in a positive direction) the relationship between disease and proximity to a point source, and if unaccounted for, may seriously bias that relationship. Thus, in the hypothetical example above, an increased incidence of lung cancer could be due entirely to confounding by socio-economic factors, which in themselves might be related to smoking rates.

In this chapter, methods used to quantify ecological differences in the socio-economic status of areas are reviewed with reference to the literature on inequalities in health in Britain and elsewhere. Local variation in socio-economic characteristics is examined near an industrial source and an approach to the adjustment of socio-economic confounding at the small-area level is presented.

Measures of socio-economic differences

The study of socio-economic differentials and health has been carried out since the nineteenth century in Britain (Fox 1989, 1990) and more recently in many other countries (UN/WHO/CICRED 1984). Internationally, there are considerable variations both in the extent to which data are available to measure social stratification, and in the validity of such measures within a particular country, although there are a number of variables which are common to many countries. Because people live in communities which, to a large extent, share the same social milieu, indicators of social difference can be defined and measured at several levels: the individual, the family or household, the neighbourhood, the local community, and even at the regional or national level.

For *individuals*, a number of measures has been used to describe social status, over and above the standard demographic variables (age, sex, ethnic group). Income is an obvious example, and studies in the USA in particular (Goldberger *et al.* 1920; Kitagawa and Hauser 1973) have demonstrated a relationship between income and disease incidence or mortality. Another example, occupation, was first classified during the middle of the nineteenth century by William Farr (1875) in his analysis of all-cause mortality in England and Wales; it remains perhaps the most common measure of socio-economic status internationally, and has been used in many countries, e.g. France, Germany, Australia, and Norway (UN/WHO/CICRED 1984). Level of education has also been used to measure socio-economic status of individuals. Examples include Finland (Valkonen 1982) and France (Desplanques 1984); and employment status, in particular unemployment, has been shown in the national longitudinal studies in both Britain (Leon 1988) and France (Desplanques 1984) to be an important predictor of health outcome.

Household indicators of socio-economic status have a history that can be traced to an analysis of the 1911 census of Britain (Stevenson 1928) and include density of accommodation, housing tenure, basic amenities, and access to a car. Single-parent families and elderly people living alone are also important household characteristics (Moser *et al.* 1988). In the USA (Rosenberg and McMillen 1984), family income is a common measure of household status; mobility and migration are also usually family or household characteristics. It is also common practice for the individual characteristics of the 'head of household', such as occupation, ethnicity, or education, to be used to classify the entire household.

Some socio-economic factors are most naturally measures at the level of *neighbourhoods* or local communities: examples include housing stock, educational opportunities, employment, and access to health care. For example, studies in Finland (Teppo *et al.* 1980) have demonstrated a relationship between cancer incidence and urbanization, population density, and industrialization.

At the *regional* or *national* level, large differences may exist in economic development or gross national product, and in diet, life-style, and any number of social and cultural factors.

Socio-economic differences in Britain: recent developments

Over the past 20 years, a number of indices have been developed to measure socio-economic variation across small geographical areas in Britain. These originated in cluster analyses using 1971 UK census data (Craig and Driver 1972; Webber and Craig 1976) which were made possible by the rapid developments in computing power. This methodology has been applied successfully in the field of commercial marketing, including the targeting of advertising and financial services based on socio-economic profiles, particularly at the postcode level. Similar area classification schemes have been developed for scientific research (mainly into primary health care delivery and social deprivation) using a number of indicators of socio-economic status selected a priori from the small-area census statistics (rather than using the data-driven approach of cluster analysis).

The Underprivileged Area (UPA) score

The Acheson Committee Report (London Health Planning Consortium 1981) into general practitioner (GP) services in the UK called for a method to identify so-called 'underprivileged areas', i.e. where there were high numbers of patients who were thought to increase the workload or pressure on the services of GPs. A questionnaire was sent to a random sample of GPs throughout the UK, which was used to obtain statistical weights for the calculation of a composite index of underprivileged areas, based on GPs' perceptions of workload and patient need (Jarman 1984). Respondents were asked to score a number of possible indicators of the pressure of work, using a scale from 0 (no problem) to 9 (very problematical). The eight census-derived indicators making up the final UPA index are shown in Table 11.1, along with their

Table 11.1 Census-derived variables contributing to the Underprivileged Area (UPA) score, and their relative weights

Indicator	Weight
% elderly living alone	6.62
% children under 5 years old	4.64
% persons in households with an unskilled head	3.74
% unemployed	3.34
% persons in households with single parent	3.01
% persons living in overcrowded households	2.88
% persons who moved house in last year	2.68
% persons in households with ethnic minority head	2.50

relative weights. The index is calculated at census ward level, an area comprising approximately 5000 people.

All indicators are expressed as percentages. The denominator is the total number of residents in private households, except for 'unemployed' (when it is all economically active residents) and 'moved house' (all residents). The eight census variables are then transformed by an angular transformation to make their distribution more symmetrical; standardized (by subtracting the mean and dividing by the standard deviation of the transformed values), weighted (Table 11.1), and summed to give the UPA score of the ward.

Department of the Environment (DoE) index

The DoE's Inner Cities Directorate (1983) published an index of 'Urban Deprivation' designed to assess the relative levels of deprivation in local authorities in England. Based on the 1981 census, the DoE index had three dimensions of deprivation: social, economic, and housing. A seventh un-classified indicator was the percentage of residents whose head of household was born in the New Commonwealth or Pakistan (Table 11.2).

Table 11.2 Dimensions of deprivation and census-derived variables contributing to the Department of the Environment's Urban Deprivation Index

Dimension	Variable
Social	% households with single parents % pensioners living alone
Economic	% persons unemployed % persons unskilled
Housing	% households overcrowded % households without amenities
(Unclassified)	% households whose head was born in New Commonwealth or Pakistan

Percentage of population change (1971–81) and the all-cause standardized mortality ratio (SMR) were also to be included, but were unavailable at the level of census enumeration districts (EDs) at the time of publication of the index. (An ED contains approximately 400 individuals.) The percentage of unskilled workers, measured as the proportion of heads of households falling into social class V (based on the Registrar General's classification of occupations), similarly was unavailable. The DoE basic index comprised a weighted sum of these indices, with all weights set to unity, except '% unemployed', which received a double-weighting to compensate for absence of '% unskilled'.

To accommodate the skewed nature of the distributions for most of these indicators at the small-area level, logarithmic transformations were adopted; the standardized scores (zero mean and unit variance) were then weighted and summed to give a score for the electoral ward or census ED.

Townsend's index

The index proposed by Townsend *et al.* (1988) comprises unemployment, absence of a car, housing tenure, and overcrowding. Again, indicators are expressed as percentages, but the denominator is all private households, except for unemployment for which percentage of economically active persons is used. Townsend's index is thus household- rather than person-based (and might be subject to biases stemming from unequal numbers of persons per household).

Townsend specifically rejected indicators that were thought to reflect the characteristics of the deprived, rather than of deprivation itself; these include the elderly, non-white heads of households, and single parents. Townsend's percentages were normalized and standardized, and unit weights were used to create the combined index, as this was considered the least biased option.

Carstairs' index

Carstairs and Morris (1991) developed an index for Scotland which was similar to Townsend's index of deprivation, but avoided the use of households as denominators. The variables used were: persons in households with more than one person per room; persons in households where the head is economically active and from social class IV or V; economically active males seeking work, and persons in private households without access to a car. The indicators were standardized and equally weighted to sum to the index of deprivation. There was no attempt to correct for skewing of the distributions.

Relative to the Townsend index, apart from the change in focus from the household to the individual, Carstairs' score has replaced a housing tenure indicator with one based on the Register General's classification of social class by occupation.

Relation of socio-economic indices of areas to disease incidence

There have been several studies that have established a link between a number of diseases and the measures of deprivation and GP workload described above (Carstairs and Morris 1989, 1991; Mays and Chinn 1989). For example, Fig. 11.1 shows standardized registration ratios (SRRs) of lung cancer for men and women in Great Britain, 1979–83, by Carstairs' index. The scores were calculated for each of the 130 000 census EDs in Britain, and used to group EDs into 20 equal-sized categories of increasing 'deprivation'. SRRs for each

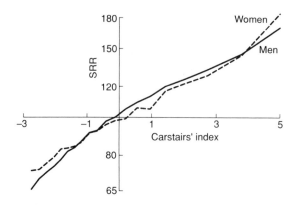

Fig. 11.1 Standardized registration ratios (SRRs) relating lung cancer incidence to Carstairs' score; men and women, Great Britain, 1979–83.

stratum were calculated using rates for Great Britain (1979–83) as standard, and plotted against the median Carstairs' index of the stratum. Each SRR is based on lung cancer registrations of about 4000 men or 1300 women, with a sampling error of less than 5 per cent. As can be seen (Fig. 11.1), the SRR is two- to threefold higher on comparing those living in the most deprived 5 per cent of EDs with those in the most advantaged 5 per cent (as classified by Carstairs' index).

Not all diseases show a steep positive socio-economic gradient with Carstairs' score, as seen with lung cancer. Leukaemia, for example, has a weak inverse relationship (Carstairs and Morris 1990).

Potential for socio-economic confounding

The definition of a confounding variable is that it should be related both to the exposure and to the disease of interest. We have already seen that, at least for some diseases, the socio-economic status of areas is a powerful predictor of disease risk. It remains for us to examine to what extent socio-economic status of areas can vary near an industrial site.

As an example, we consider the docklands area at Barrow-in-Furness in Cumbria, northwest England. Barrow is a small coastal town (population around 50 000 at the 1981 census) in which one industrial site (the docks) supports most of the economy. Carstairs' index was calculated for the 156 census EDs which fall within a 10 km radius of the dockyard. Figure 11.2 shows a scatterplot of these Carstairs' scores plotted against the distance between the dockyard and the centroid of each ED. A smoothed curve (heavy line) shows median Carstairs' index with distance, and the dotted lines delineate the interquartile range.

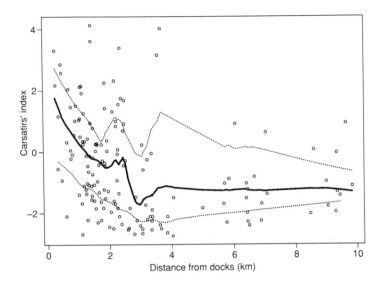

Fig. 11.2 Scatterplot of Carstairs' index with distance from Barrow docks. Each point represents the centroid of an enumeration district (ED). The heavy line represents the smoothed median score with distance, the dotted lines delineate the interquartile range. Carstairs' score could not be obtained for two EDs.

From this figure, it is clear that Carstairs' index varies markedly with distance from the dockyard. Within the first 3 km, there is a transition from relatively deprived EDs (i.e. higher Carstairs' scores on average) close to the source, towards more advantaged areas as one moves away from the docks.

Methods of adjustment

Various methods could be used to adjust for socio-economic confounding. A regression approach, for example, might introduce the deprivation score for each small area as a covariate, so that tests for trend in disease with distance from putative source could be carried out on the residuals, after adjustment for other variables. Another approach is to extend the usual indirect age-standardization method by stratifying on socio-economic status of areas. If appropriate discrete strata based on social differences can be defined, so that age- and sex-specific incidence or mortality rates can be calculated within these strata, then (assuming the age–sex-specific population structure of the area is known) an adjusted SRR, or standardized mortality ratio (SMR) may be calculated.

Continuous measures of small-area socio-economic status (such as UPA, Townsend, or Carstairs') may be used to create strata by defining appropriate cutpoints; these may usefully be, for example, quintiles or even deciles of the national distribution. One difficulty with this approach is the method of stratification. For a continuous measure, the selection of cutpoints is essentially arbitrary; in the case of age, five-year grouping is considered standard, but no such natural scale is available for deprivation scores. It is easy to choose too many strata, particularly for the study of rare diseases, when even the national stratum-specific rates will be based on relatively few cases. In addition, the number of simultaneous confounders that can be controlled for by this method is limited.

The Small Area Health Statistics Unit at the London School of Hygiene and Tropical Medicine is currently using the stratification method outlined above (see Chapter 29). National standard rates are being compiled by cause of death and cancer registration site as enquiries proceed. Strata now used routinely for each analysis are sex (two levels), age (five-year groups, 18 levels), and socioeconomic band (six levels). The latter is currently determined by quintiles of Carstairs' score, at ED level; the sixth band is made up of those EDs that cannot be classified by Carstairs' index, usually because they contain too few 'permanent households' (standard census units), i.e. fewer than five. This sixth band with missing deprivation scores comprises around 5 per cent of all EDs in Great Britain (though 0.7 per cent of the population), and includes hospitals, old peoples' homes, armed forces barracks, etc. On average, it has much higher age-specific disease rates than the most deprived of the classifiable bands.

Summary

Social and socio-economic factors are powerful predictors of disease at both the individual and ecological (small-area) level. Sources of industrial pollution tend to be located in relatively disadvantaged areas, characterized, for example, by poor housing and high unemployment. Local variation in the socio-economic status of areas may be large within distances consistent with hypotheses of environmental risk. Under these circumstances, there is marked potential for confounding in small-area analyses of health data near sources of environmental pollution. An analysis of disease incidence close to a point source that does not take account of this potential confounding could be seriously biased, and result in misleading or false conclusions about the possible effects of pollution on health.

Acknowledgements

DJ is supported by the Victorian Health Promotion Foundation.

References

Carstairs, V. and Morris, R. (1989). Deprivation: explaining differences in mortality between Scotland and England. *British Medical Journal*, **299**, 886–9.

Carstairs, V. and Morris, R. (1990). Deprivation and health in Scotland. *Health Bulletin (Edinburgh)*, **48**, 162–75.

Carstairs, V. and Morris, R. (1991). *Deprivation and health in Scotland*. Aberdeen University Press, Aberdeen.

Craig, J. and Driver, A. (1972). The identification and comparison of small areas of adverse social conditions. *Applied Statistics*, **21**, 25–35.

Desplanques, G. (1984). La mortalité selon le milieu social en France. In *Socioeconomic differential mortality in industrialized societies*, (ed. UN/WHO/CICRED), Vol. 3. CICRED, Paris.

Farr, W. (1875). *Supplement to the thirty-fifth annual report of the Registrar General in England*. HMSO, London.

Fox, A. J. (1989). *Health inequalities in European countries*. Gower, Aldershot.

Fox, A. J. (1990). Socio-economic differences in morbidity and mortality. *Scandinavian Journal of Social Medicine*, **18**, 1–8.

Goldberger, J., Wheeler, G. A., and Sydenstricker, E. (1920). A study of the relation of family income and other economic factors to pellagra incidence in seven cotton-mill villages of South Carolina in 1916. *Public Health Reports*, **35**, 2673–714.

Jarman, B. (1983). Identification of underprivileged areas. *British Medical Journal*, **286**, 1705–9.

Jarman, B. (1984). Underprivileged areas: validation and distribution. *British Medical Journal*, **289**, 1587–92.

Kitagawa, E. M. and Hauser, P. M. (1973). *Differential mortality in the United States: a study in socioeconomic epidemiology*. Harvard University Press, Cambridge, Mass.

Leon, D. (1988). *Longitudinal Study: Social distribution of cancer*, OPCS Series LS, No. 3. HMSO, London.

Logan, W. P. D. and Brooke, E. M. (1957). *The survey of sickness 1943 to 1952*, Studies on medical and population subjects, No. 12. HMSO, London.

London Health Planning Consortium (1981). *Primary health care in Inner London*. Department of Health and Social Security, London.

Mays, N. and Chinn, S. (1989). Relation between all-cause SMR and two indices of deprivation at regional and district level in England. *Journal of Epidemiology and Community Health*, **43**, 191–9.

Moser, K., Pugh, H., and Goldblatt, P. (1988). Inequalities in women's health: looking at mortality differentials using an alternative approach. *British Medical Journal*, **296**, 1221–4.

Rosenberg, H. M. and McMillen, M. M. (1984). New research directions on socio-economic differential mortality in the United States of America. In *Socio-economic differential mortality in industrialized societies*, (ed. UN/WHO/CICRED), Vol. 3. CICRED, Paris.

Stevenson, T. H. C. (1928). The vital statistics of wealth and poverty. *Journal of the Royal Statistical Society*, **91**, 207–30.

Teppo, L., Pukkala, E., Hakama, M., Hakulinen, T., Herva, A., and Saxén, E. (1980). *Way of life and cancer incidence in Finland*. Finnish Cancer Registry, Helsinki.

Townsend, P., Phillimore, P., and Beattie, A. (1988). *Health and deprivation: inequality and the North*. Croom Helm, London.

UN/WHO/CICRED (1984). *Socio-economic differential mortality in industrialized societies*, Vol. 3. CICRED, Paris.

Valkonen, T. (1982). Psychosocial stress and sociodemographic differentials in mortality from ischaemic heart disease in Finland. *Acta Medica Scandinavica, Supplement,* **660**, 152–64.

Vernon, H. M. (1939). *Health in relation to occupation*. Freedom Press, London.

Webber, R. and Craig, J. (1976). Which local authorities are alike? *Population Trends,* **5**, 13–19.

12. Use of record linkage in small-area studies

E. Pukkala

Record linkage is the combination of data items, often from different files, for a certain unit of observation. The data may originally have been collected for some other purpose, without knowledge of the future uses to which the data might be put. In epidemiology, record linkage is usually used to connect data for a particular individual. It is often used for causal research and is applied when the data on causes (treatment, exposure, etc.) are to be related to the effect (survival/risk of the disease).

Although record linkage was only exploited once automatic linking of computerized files became possible, its concept and aims do not require that linkages necessarily be carried out automatically. The issue is largely one of magnitude: computerized record linkage can handle much larger data sets more rapidly and at minimal cost compared with manual linkage, which usually involves visual comparisons of two sets of data.

To carry out record linkage, files to be linked must contain a common key which has a unique value for each observation. The key can either be a single variable or a combination of several variables. For record linkage for individuals, the personal identification number system used, for example, in all the Nordic countries is ideal. If personal numbers cannot be used, the main keys can be time and place of birth, sex, and name. In this case several problems arise: many persons of the same sex are born on any day, even in the same area, and possibly with the same name. This may lead to the records of two different persons being combined. If a person's name is changed during the follow-up period or the spelling of the name varies, records which belong together may not be linked. If the logical relationship between the key variables is complicated, a non-automatic linking procedure may be safer. In practice, especially when the data sets to be linked are large, a computer-assisted record linkage system may, in any case, be the only possible solution.

The routine system of the Finnish Cancer Registry provides a comparison of the accuracy of manual and computerized record linkage. Until 1974, the follow-up for annual death files was performed manually by comparing the alphabetical list of persons who died during the year (about 40 000 names) with an alphabetical list of cancer registry patients not known to have died (80 000 names). The possible previous surnames were taken into account as well. The comparison was made by those secretaries at the Finnish Cancer Registry who

E. Pukkala

were known to be most thorough. From 1975, the linkage has been done automatically, using person-number as a key. A linkage of the whole cancer registry against the population central register provided the means to evaluate the accuracy of the original linkages. Figure 12.1 shows the proportion of deaths missed in the original manual and in the automatic record linkage.

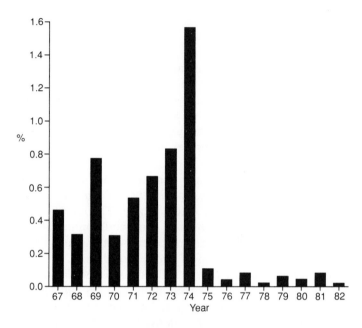

Fig. 12.1 Failures in record linkage between cancer registry data and death certificate data carried out manually using names (1967–74) or automatically using the person-number (1975 onwards).

Manual record linkage did not succeed for about 50–100 cases annually (out of some 10 000) even though Finnish names are ideal for this kind of record linkage—names are always written exactly as they are pronounced, so that no system like the soundex system in the English-speaking world is needed (cf. Baldwin *et al.* 1987). The small proportion of mismatches since 1975 (0.05 per cent) represents typically those with incorrect cancer registration or even cancer notification missing at the time of record linkage.

Epidemiologists in the Nordic countries are fortunate in having access to high-quality health and population data which can be linked by means of a unique personal identifier. Elsewhere, even when high-quality data exist, linkage may be difficult because of the lack of unique identifiers, or impossible because of confidentiality restrictions. Thus, some of the examples discussed below indicate what is possible under ideal conditions.

Record linkage of individual health data

In most countries, there are usually several registers, both manual and computerized, containing individual health data. In fact, the first data on individual health are recorded before birth, i.e. those obtained during pregnancy. Further data on the health of individuals are often recorded at the time of birth, when individuals receive medical treatment in school, when they use the national health system (if one exists), and at time of death. For some diseases there are special registers; in Finland, congenital malformations, cancers, certain heart diseases, tuberculosis, and some other diseases are registered for the whole country. A registration system for causes of death has been in operation for hundreds of years. There are also countrywide records on some intervention procedures, such as mass screening for cancer of the cervix or breast. All hospital discharges, with codes of treatment for individual diseases, are registered centrally.

In addition to countrywide health information systems, there may also be health surveys based on population samples. In record linkage studies, only the linked part of different samples can be used. Therefore, the sampling rules should be the same whenever possible for all studies on the same population. For example, if everybody born on a certain day in any month is to be studied, then it may be best to use the day selected by other research groups.

A system which provided the life-long history of the health of any individual whenever needed for generally accepted and scientifically important studies would be optimal. In practice, this kind of a system, if ever possible, would do better to build on linkable specialized registries rather than use a huge all-in-one data-base. First of all, in a centralized system it might not be possible to have all the expertise needed to maintain data quality, which is usually the case with specialized registers. Secondly, the privacy of the registered individuals is protected better if only the data actually required for each specific study are put together.

Data on exposures

For epidemiological research, health data alone—even if all possible elements of health data could be linked together—are not usually sufficient. Data sets containing information about risk determinants and potential risk factors are required and may also be linkable. In some countries, socio-demographic data for all citizens may be available from population registers, censuses, etc., and it may be possible to extract approximate histories of occupation, for example, from these resources if they have been in operation for a long time. However, the data in general population registers are limited, the classification may be imprecise, and the data may not be continuous over time. In addition, essential data, such as those on diets and smoking, are available only for samples of the population, and researchers may be forced to use averages calculated for subgroups of the population instead of the individual values of the variables. Furthermore, automatic record linkage is not usually possible with files created before, say, the 1960s. For diseases with a long delay between cause and onset, the most relevant risk factor data may only be available from manual files. For detailed risk factor analysis the only acceptable source file is a cohort containing exact information about the risk factors under study, such as occupational histories with exposure data, or results of blood samples taken from a sample of the healthy population a long time ago.

The variables may also be indirectly linked, for example, the population register may include a house code for every person. It may be possible to link this to a register of houses which gives the exact coordinates of each house. These coordinates can be used to determine distance from a point source of exposure, amount of natural radon radiation, strength of electromagnetic fields due to power lines, etc. If such a chain of linkages, connecting the individuals to their exact places of residence and work, is available—perhaps even with data on life-events and work history—this then becomes a powerful tool for studies on the spatial patterns of diseases.

The most typical example of a study based on record linkages is a cohort study on disease risk. In Finland it often starts from a file originally collected for some other purposes (e.g. the pay-roll register of a company, a list of persons exposed to certain chemicals, drugs, radiation, etc.).

Usually, the cohort first has to be linked with the central population register to find out the correct identification data (up-to-date person-number, or information that there is no such person in the population register) and possibly time of death or emigration. If complete person-numbers are available, the linking is easy and accurate. If names and at least one of the data items: date (year) of birth, place of birth, or place of residence can be used, the Population Register Center of Finland is still able to run a computerized record linkage, with the percentage of correct matches varying from 50 to 100 per cent (depending on the amount and accuracy of the key variables). The price of the record linkage without person-number is more than $US1 per case, which is roughly fiftyfold higher than the linkage based on person-numbers. If there is no centralized population registration system, as was the case in Finland before 1967, the only possibility is a manual record linkage with local population registries—in Finland mainly run by the religious congregations—which is slow and expensive.

In this kind of a study the quality of the registers to be linked, especially the accuracy of the key variables, and the carefulness of the linking procedure are critical. Occasionally combining unlinked records is less harmful than not combining records that belong together, since the latter type of error causes a systematic bias in results. If the key variable in any of the linked files is erroneous, no data on death will be found. This increases the number of person-years available, especially in the oldest age-groups. Because the incidence of many diseases increases strongly with age, even a small addition of person-years due to failure in record linkage may cause a relatively large artefactual addition to the expected number of cases.

The second record linkage needed for a cohort study is that between the cohort and a disease registry. For those members of the cohort with invalid key variables, no observed cases will be found. Thus, where there is incomplete record linkage, the risk estimates calculated as ratios of too few numbers of observed cases and too large numbers of expected cases are systematically too low.

Examples

The cohorts analysed by record linkage methods can be large, which makes it possible to study rare diseases. The biggest cohort analysed by the Finnish Cancer Registry is the total population of Finland as defined in the census of

Table 12.1 The observed numbers of cases (Obs) and standardized incidence ratios (SIR) of lung cancer among 25–64-year-old Finnish males in 1971–80. Selected occupations with consistently high or low SIR in two subsequent periods (1971–75 and 1976–80). SIR for economically active population = 1.00

Occupation	Obs	SIR
Cigarette-makers	2	14.25*
Asphalt-roofers	11	3.96***
Insulaters	31	3.83
Miners	58	2.45
Chimney sweeps	15	1.77
Concrete-shutterers	54	1.71***
Plumbers	95	1.71***
Sheet-metal-workers	72	1.70***
Bricklayers	88	1.68***
Forestry workers	331	1.60***
Assistant housebuilding workers	258	1.56***
Medical doctors	4	0.25***
Fire-fighters	2	0.22*
University teachers	2	0.18**
Judges	1	0.17*
Priests	2	0.12***

* $p < 0.05$; ** $p < 0.01$; *** $p < 0.001$.

31 December 1970 (4.8 million persons). The follow-up for death and cancer for the years 1971–85 was done in two subsequent computerized record linkages. Cancer risks were then calculated by social class, education, and occupation (Pukkala *et al.* 1983; Pukkala and Teppo 1986). A typical example of this kind of tabulation—a small piece of an enormous information bank—showing the occupations with highest and lowest lung cancer risks in working ages, is given in Table 12.1. This kind of background information should always be at hand when possible environmental risks are to be evaluated, e.g. what is the appropriate reference risk level?

For those concerned about the privacy of the individuals registered, it is worthwhile remembering that in this type of study, the names or other identification data of the persons in the linked files are never revealed, not even to the researchers performing the study. This is not possible with manual record linkage. Only if an error occurs is it necessary to find out the identity of some of the study subjects, a fact that further underlines the need for high quality data files to be linked.

Air pollution and lung cancer in Helsinki

An example of the use of record linkage to define risks of a disease in small areas is a study of the association between cancer risk and air pollution within the city of Helsinki. This study was done by the health authorities of the City of Helsinki and the Finnish Cancer Registry in the mid-1980s, and repeated in 1990 (Pönkä *et al.* 1992). Using data stored in a local population register, the population of Helsinki (0.5 million) was divided into 33 small areas, each with an average population of 15 000 and area of 5 km^2, for which concentrations of SO_2 and NO_2 in ambient air were estimated. Statistics for various confounding factors, such as socio-economic structure, were available. After record linkage with the Finnish Cancer Registry, the observed numbers of lung cancers for these areas were calculated by sex and age. Expected numbers of lung cancer cases were simply estimated by multiplying the number of person-years by the incidence of lung cancer in the whole city.

The standardized risk ratios among the subareas of Helsinki varied from 0.6 to 1.4 in males and from 0.3 to 3.2 in females. Most of this variation could be accounted for by the average educational level (known to indicate different smoking habits) in each subarea. Only a very slight association between lung cancer and SO_2 concentration could be demonstrated. The major weaknesses of this study were the lack of residential history of each citizen of Helsinki and the lack of confounder data (smoking, occupation, etc.) on an individual basis, although these data (except data on smoking which are not registered in any of the population-based registries in Finland) could, in principle, have been obtained from national registries by means of record linkage if the crude analysis had indicated cause for concern.

High-voltage power lines and cancer

A cohort study on the cancer risk of populations living close to high-voltage (110–400 kV) power lines in Finland is based entirely on record linkages. The risk ratios expected are so low, and cancer types studied so rare that no other methods to detect possible associations are realistic.

The coordinates of the power lines were first defined. Then the areas within the electromagnetic fields of the power lines were defined as a function of distance from, and type of the power line. The houses within this area (a 100–300 m wide 'corridor' along the power line) were searched in a record linkage with the central house register.

In the Finnish population register there are links to all residences since the early 1970s, with dates of moving in and out. Therefore it was possible to identify persons who had been living in houses with increased electromagnetic fields and even to calculate the times of exposure and cumulative doses of radiation for them. At the same time, a reference cohort of persons who had never been living in houses closer than 300 m from the power lines was identified. The follow-up for death and emigration was taken from the population register at the same time.

The final record linkage will be with the Finnish Cancer Registry. The incidence rates of cancers of interest will be calculated according to the duration and level of the electromagnetic radiation. After adjustment for potential confounders (e.g. urban–rural status and socio-economic status) it might be possible to give not only the risk ratio of cancer for those living close to the power lines, but even estimates of the dose–response relationship between electromagnetic radiation and cancer risk. Although the whole study is based on the quickest possible method, i.e. a chain of automatic record linkages, the results are not expected to be ready before the end of 1992.

References

Baldwin, J. A., Acheson, E. D., and Graham, W. J. (ed.) (1987). *Textbook of medical record linkage*, Oxford Medical Publications. Oxford University Press, Oxford.

Pönkä, A., Pukkala, E., and Hakulinen, T. (1992). Lung cancer risk and ambient air pollution in Helsinki, to be published.

Pukkala, E. and Teppo, L. (1986). Socioeconomic status and education as risk determinants of gastrointestinal cancer. *Preventative Medicine*, **15**, 127–38.

Pukkala, E., Teppo, L., Hakulinen, T., and Rimpelä, M. (1983). Occupation and smoking as risk determinants of lung cancer. *International Journal of Epidemiology*, **12**, 290–6.

13. Confidentiality

M. J. Quinn

This chapter covers definitions of confidentiality and security, describes the legal and other safeguards for individuals in the UK, outlines the procedures currently adopted by the Office of Population Censuses and Surveys (OPCS) for some of the wide range of data it holds, summarizes the methods used to ensure confidentiality, and briefly refers to physical and other security measures. Many of the examples relate directly to the problems encountered in examining statistics of disease in small areas.

It is generally accepted that any items of demographic or medical data which would permit the identification of an individual person are *confidential*, i.e. they should be kept secret so that, directly or indirectly, information about an individual is not revealed. Personal identification data include name, full date of birth (and death, if dead), and unique reference numbers of various types, e.g. NHS and National Insurance numbers. However, in certain circumstances, other types of data may enable individuals to be identified, particularly if they have a rare disease and live (or have lived) in a sparsely populated area. Both medical researchers and the staff of national data collection offices, such as OPCS, must be aware of the need to preserve confidentiality in connection with or during the process of collection, transmission, storage, use, and dissemination of data. For medical data, the same standards of confidentiality as customarily apply to the doctor–patient relationship must be maintained, and this obligation does not cease with the death of the person concerned. *Security* denotes measures that may be taken to ensure the preservation of confidentiality. In the computing context, security also covers the integrity and availability of data. It should be noted that a secure system does not guarantee confidentiality, for example there may be misuse of data by authorized users.

Confidentiality is of importance for three main groups of people. For *data subjects*, i.e. individuals on whom information has been collected, the protection of confidentiality is of paramount importance—information must not reach unauthorized third parties (i.e. anyone other than the data subject and the collecting agency). It is essential for *data suppliers*, e.g. clinicians reporting a case of cancer to a registry, to know that arrangements for maintaining the confidentiality of data in the registry are at least as stringent as those maintained by the persons or institutions supplying the data. Clearly, any breaches of confidentiality could adversely affect the willingness of providers of data to continue to do so. The supply of data to *users* should be for specified purposes related to the benefit of those with the particular disease, to the control of disease in the general population, to medical audit, and for other bona fide medical research.

Legal and other guidelines on confidentiality

There are many guidelines, codes of good practice, and other such documents. Some are governmental and some are professional. Some are principally concerned with classified information or physical and/or computing security, but others touch on privacy, confidentiality, or data protection. In the UK, these include: the International Statistical Institute, *Declaration on professional ethics*; the *Government statistical code of practice on the handling of data obtained from statistical inquiries* (Cmnd. 9270); *Responsibility in the use of personal medical information for research, principles and guide to practice*, Statement by the Medical Research Council; Royal College of Physicians of London, *Guidelines on the practice of ethics committees in medical research*; *Security of the census of population* (Cmnd. 5365); *1981 Census of population: confidentiality and computing* (Cmnd. 8201); *Computers and privacy* (Cmnd. 6353); *Computers: safeguards for privacy* (Cmnd. 6354); the Data Protection Act 1984; and the Data Protection Registrar's guideline booklets 1–8: booklet number 4 deals with the eight, statutory, data protection principles.

In addition, supranational bodies such as the European Community (EC) and the Council of Europe have established principles and recommendations about the confidentiality of individual data (see *The confidentiality of medical records—the principles and practice of protection in a research-dependent environment*, report of a working party of the Advisory Panel for Social Medicine and Epidemiology in the EEC, 1983; and Recommendation No. RE(81)1 of the Council of Europe Committee of Ministers of 23 January 1981, on the regulations applicable to automated medical data banks). There are also draft EC measures on data protection [COM(90)314 FINAL-SYN 297–299] that are expected to have implications for the way in which personal data are handled.

A code of confidentiality, such as that produced (in draft) by the International Association of Cancer Registries, cannot, of course, absolutely guarantee that individuals will not inadvertently or otherwise be identified, or ensure that providers of data supply information of high quality, or ensure that the best possible use is made of the data.

Until recently, Section 2 of the Official Secrets Act 1911 made it a criminal offence for a civil servant to disclose any information acquired in the course of his or her duties to any person other than someone to whom he or she was authorized to communicate it. Many government departments, including

OPCS, were able to refer to Section 2 as one of the ways of reassuring the public that the information they had given would be safeguarded and kept in confidence. In recent years, Section 2 was widely considered by the public, politicians, and the press to have fallen into disrepute because of its wide-ranging 'catch all' effect and as a result of several well-publicized prosecutions of serving or former civil servants. Consequently, Section 2 was repealed and replaced by the Official Secrets Act 1989. This does not give official information the blanket protection of Section 2, although some OPCS data is still protected by other legislation such as the 1920 Census Act and the Population (Statistics) Acts. OPCS has, therefore, drawn up a 'code of practice' on confidentiality of personal information. The signing of this code by existing and future staff (whether legally binding or merely declaratory) would make clear OPCS policy on confidentiality, should have a deterrent effect, and would be evidence in disciplinary proceedings. Each division of OPCS also has a divisional code that provides specific guidance on the data handled by the division. All items of data are assigned to a 'data custodian' who is responsible for their confidentiality.

In addition, the revision of the civil service code of conduct is at an early stage. It is likely that in place of Section 2 it will place a general duty of confidentiality on all past or present civil servants with regard to official information not covered by the 1989 Act but which must be protected. Information on individuals which has been received in confidence would be one such category.

Consideration has also been given to the creation of a new statutory test of breach of confidence for certain categories of information, including personal information, to replace the existing civil actions in the courts (*Law Commission Report on Breach of Confidence*, Law Com. No. 110, Cmnd. 8388), but no action has been taken since the report was published in 1981.

Penalties for unauthorized disclosure of information by civil servants fall into three main categories: criminal, civil service disciplinary, and civil. As noted above, repeal of Section 2 has removed some of the criminal remedies. The new civil service code may be relevant in some cases, and in others civil law may apply—but for some cases no redress may be available.

Medical researchers who receive information but are not civil servants are asked by OPCS to sign an undertaking not to make unauthorized disclosures. For example, the Medical Statistics Division has a set of eight such declarations, relating to different data sets including deaths, cancer registrations, and still births. These contain different combinations of conditions depending on the information to be released, the medium (paper or magnetic), the recipient, and the purpose. The conditions generally include that: the information would be used only for the purposes of the approved research; the data would be stored with proper safeguards; no contact would be made with any individuals (unless specifically agreed in the protocol, and then usually only with the general practitioner's agreement); the information would not be released to anyone else (except, of course, in the form of statistical tables or conclusions);

any reports or papers published would not identify individuals, or enable individuals to be identified; all records would be destroyed on completion of the project; and anyone replacing the researcher would complete the same declaration.

Researchers who apply for use of the National Health Service Central Register (NHSCR) are sent a copy of an explanatory booklet on such use, and have to complete a lengthy, standard protocol. The NHSCR's *Code of guidance* describes four strictly limited exceptions to the general principle that identifiable personal information should never be disclosed to third parties without the patient's consent. These are: where the law requires a disclosure to be made (e.g. under the Public Health Acts or under subpoena); for the prevention or detection of serious crime and the apprehension or prosecution of serious offenders; where disclosure is clearly to the advantage of the patient concerned; and for medical research and follow-up purposes. The NHSCR recognizes that medical research may be of direct benefit to existing or future patients or lead to an improvement in the health of the community, and thus that access by bona fide researchers should not be hampered unnecessarily. But there must be appropriate safeguards, and normally data would be made anonymous, or the patient's informed consent to release must be obtained; otherwise a detailed case must be made for approval by an appropriate ethical body. Applicants for details of cancer registrations must supply a detailed protocol for submission via OPCS to the British Medical Association Central Ethical Committee.

It is not clear whether any breaking of the conditions of such declarations would enable a successful civil action, for breach of contract or breach of confidence, to be mounted. For researchers, loss of reputation represents an adequate deterrent and penalty.

Confidentiality of census, demographic, and medical data

Census information proper is protected by the census legislation, and the Census Confidentiality Act 1990 extended protection to data from test censuses and post-enumeration checks. Under the provisions of the Public Records Acts the censuses are subject to a 100 years' closure rule (Lord Chancellor's Instrument No. 12, 1966). In addition, OPCS has given written assurances on the census forms, leaflets, and other publicity material, that information supplied will be kept strictly in confidence. No names or addresses are fed into the computer. Oral assurances are also given during parliamentary debates (and recorded in *Hansard*). It is the practice to commission independent reviews of security arrangements for the census, and results have been published (White Papers Cmnd. 5365 and Cmnd. 8201).

The OPCS statement on policy and practice with regard to protecting the confidentiality of census data covers the collection, analysis, and storage of data; legal safeguards and measures and instructions to staff on protection of information; and safeguarding confidentiality in census tables. On the last of these, the precautions do not guarantee that inferences about individuals cannot be made, but (taking into account the work that would be involved in attempting to make such inferences) make the possibility extremely unlikely. In statistics produced for areas smaller than local authority districts (of which there are over 300 in England and Wales, with average population about 150 000) three special measures are applied:

(1) the non-zero cells of standard tables produced from 100 per cent of the data are modified by $+1$, 0 or -1;

(2) tables derived either from 100 per cent or from a sample of the data will not be released if the number of households or persons in the area are below certain thresholds; and

(3) statistics produced according to customer specifications will be subject to rounding to the nearest multiple of 5 where the procedure at (1) is inappropriate.

OPCS receives and processes a large amount of information on births, still births, deaths, marriages, divorces, and adoptions. In addition, the Longitudinal Study (LS) has linked 1 per cent of records from the 1971 census with those for 1981, together with health and other 'event' data between the two censuses, and there are plans to link these with the 1991 census. Most of the information is protected by legislation; written undertakings have been given to Ministers of State that LS records will not leave OPCS, and two reports have been published on LS confidentiality (Studies on Medical and Population Subjects No. 25; and *Setting up and operation of the LS for England and Wales*). There is a comprehensive standards manual covering the release of individual and summary data, and access to and release of computer files. For birth, still birth, and death draft entry forms there are three levels of release. Level 1 covers that information which is in the public domain. Level 3 relates to data covered by the Population Statistics Act and hence may not be released. Level 2 covers data not in levels 1 or 3, and is subdivided according to the sensitivity of the data. Summary data may be published by OPCS or produced in response to an *ad hoc* request. Sensitive summary data, such as deaths from AIDS at ward level, are never released. Summary data are considered to be potentially sensitive if they relate to certain data items (e.g. illegitimacy, AIDS, suicide); and have a count of 1 or 2; and relate to an area below that of District Health Authority (DHA, of which there are nearly 200 in England and Wales) or with a population of less than 60 000. Where sensitivity is a problem, groupings or variables are collapsed until aggregated cells total 3 or more.

The chief concern with hospital episode statistics (HES) is to protect sensitive patient information. No names, addresses, or other direct identifiers of patients are held. Nevertheless, the combination of unusual variables could lead to the identification of an individual patient, which could cause embarrassment or distress. From the files, it is also possible to derive information about the workload of individual doctors, and the medical profession would regard the leakage of such information as a serious breach of confidentiality. HES data items are divided into three categories according to the confidentiality and sensitivity of the data. Category 1 items are not sensitive and may be released to DHAs for patients treated or resident in their area, and to others connected with the health service. Data in category 2 are considered to be sensitive and may only be released to the Regional Health Authority (RHA) at the 100 per cent level. All other requests for category 2 data need written authority from the Deputy Chief Medical Statistician. Category 3 data can not generally be released without special permission. Data with 'expanded area codes' (based on postcode of home address) are in a special class: area codes down to RHA are treated as category 1, down to DHA as category 2, and at ward level as category 3. All researchers must sign a confidentiality declaration before HES data are released to them.

Some of the data on medical statistics topics, such as abortions, cancer registrations, congenital malformations, thyrotoxicosis, morbidity statistics from general practice (MSGP), and infant and perinatal mortality, are very sensitive. Disclosure of much of the information is covered by abortion, births and deaths registration, population statistics, and National Health Service legislation. In addition, there are a number of written agreements, e.g. with the Royal College of General Practitioners on MSGP and on the release and/or protection of sensitive information on mortality (such as duration of illness, cause of death) and congenital malformations. Release of original death certificates (310s) and congenital malformation forms (SD56s) is permitted to genuine researchers. Abortion notification forms are definitely not available to any researcher. Mortality data which are not released include primary records with registration details, ward, postcode (with the exception of data passed to the Small Area Health Statistics Unit—see Chapter 10), occupational status, or original cause; cause data for areas smaller than county district or London borough; data by social class other than published figures; and mortality at postcode level. Abortions summary data are not released if any cells of tables have small counts, for DHA of determination, for areas smaller than DHAs containing fewer than 80 000 people, and for individual hospitals. The Chief Medical Officer at the Department of Health personally authorizes named individuals in OPCS who alone may have access to personally identifiable abortion data. Requests for other data, e.g. notifications of infectious diseases, cancer registrations, MSGP, are not met if cross-tabulations, particularly of small-area data, would lead to small counts in the cells of the table.

Cancer registration

With the expansion of cancer registration in many countries around the world (see Chapters 5 and 6), the increasing use of cancer registries for a variety of clinical and aetiological research—sometimes involving linkage with records collected for other purposes—and in view of public concern over individual privacy, many cancer registries have formally elaborated rules on confidentiality.

Effective cancer registration requires the collection of data about individuals with cancer, often from several different sources over a number of years. It is essential that personal identifying information be collected to eliminate multiple counting of a single tumour; to ensure that data are accurate, can be readily checked and, if necessary, corrected; to enable the production of survival statistics; and to enable epidemiological studies of cancer to be carried out.

By matching the notifications sent to a cancer registry with death certificates it is possible to assess the survival of *all* people with cancer in a defined population. Survival for the population as a whole is frequently quite different from that for selected series of patients. Case-control and cohort studies can assist in identifying possible causes of cancer. Cancers occurring in members of a cohort can be detected by matching files of the cohort with cancer registry files and/or death certificates—this is an extremely efficient, economical, and confidential method of uncovering risk (see Chapter 12). Although such linkage requires individual identity to be known, any published reports must present only anonymous aggregated data.

The International Association of Cancer Registries considers that restrictions —such as a requirement that patients give written or oral consent for data about their cancer to be entered into a registry—produce uncontrollable selection and unacceptable losses in, and distortion of, cancer incidence data. Adequate safeguards of the individual's right to privacy can be obtained by adherence to an appropriate code of conduct in the operation of the registry and hospital records systems. The maintenance of confidentiality by a registry is not restricted to information on cancer patients. Other data in which individuals may be identifiable include lists of members of industrial or other cohorts, death certificates, medical records, and interview records stored in, or provided to, the registry.

Cancer registries do not generally inform individuals whether or not there are data about them in the registry, unless required by law. Requests made for purposes such as pension schemes, sickness reimbursement, life insurance, etc., are usually passed to the data source concerned (the patient, the doctor, or the relevant health service).

The Medical Director of the registry (or equivalent) is responsible for the authorization of the disclosure of confidential information. All the regional cancer registries in England and that in Wales, and in Scotland the Information and Statistics Division of the Scottish Health Service, have a formal process to deal with such requests. This includes declarations of confidentiality, similar to those used by OPCS. In addition, for international studies, most registries do not forward data to other countries in a form that would permit any individuals to be identified. For verification purposes, each study subject is usually allocated an identifying number which allows tracing in the cancer registry of origin. Any data transferred between countries should be subject to the rules of confidentiality in both—and therefore, in effect, conform to the stricter of the requirements.

Security

In addition to the almost universally adopted procedures whereby passwords are required for access to data files held on mainframe computers, a wide range of measures can be taken to preserve confidentiality in the storage and transmission of data.

On *storage*, all magnetic media (including back-up tapes or cartridges produced at the end of each working day) should be kept in a secure and properly managed file library and, where appropriate, in a locked fire-proof safe. Similar procedures should apply for remote storage and for floppy disks containing personal data. Although much of the data stored on computers is not readily accessible to the uninitiated, many organizations also hold a considerable amount of data on paper, which is easily read, and so this information should be kept as secure as possible. Measures that can be taken include defining who has access to the premises and the issue of security passes; defining which particular personnel have access to some rooms where especially sensitive data may be held; putting material into locked cabinets at the end of each day; and ensuring that unauthorized staff (e.g. cleaners) are not able to examine records (including carbon copies or waste paper). Where files are kept for a fixed period, e.g. for 2 years after a cancer patient has died, their destruction (after possible microfilming) should normally involve shredding.

For the *transmission* of data by mail, protective measures include the use of registered post, sending lists of names (and other identifying information) separately from the other medical data, use of plain envelopes or double envelopes with the exterior having only a general address and the interior marked 'to be opened by X only'. If a commercial courier service is used, a written guarantee on confidentiality should be obtained. When information is sent on magnetic media (tape, cassette, or floppy disk), measures should be taken to ensure that they do not leave the premises of the organization without authority, that they do not go astray, and that they cannot easily be read by third parties. Precautions may include the encrypting of names and other sensitive data, and (as with paper records) the preparation of separate tapes for the identifying and other information. The telephone is frequently used, for example by cancer registries to seek additional information on a registered case. Although convenient, breaches of confidentiality could easily arise. No confidential information should be given over the telephone unless the caller is an authorized recipient and has given proof of identity (a common procedure involves calling the enquirer back, after verification). Increasing amounts of data are being transmitted over public or dedicated telephone lines. Security precautions can include the use of user numbers and passwords (which should not appear on screens), tokens and biometrical verification, the recording of the times of use of those authorized to have access, the frequent checking of audit trails produced by the system, the changing of passwords at frequent intervals, and encryption of the data.

Acknowledgements

I am grateful to my colleagues at OPCS, particularly Mr R. McLeod and his staff who carried out the review of confidentiality policies and procedures on which much of this chapter is based; and Mr. B. Meakings for valuable comments on the draft; also Dr M. Cotter, Mrs S. M. Gravestock, Dr D. Pheby, and Ms J. Warner who jointly responded with OPCS on behalf of the cancer registries in England, Wales, and Scotland to the draft guidelines on confidentiality produced by the International Association of Cancer Registries.

14. Practical approaches to disease mapping

M. Smans and J. Estève

Disease mapping has a long history (Howe 1989), and it is not surprising that this method of descriptive analysis was first used for communicable diseases in an attempt to identify the sources of infection, and to describe the rate of spread. Mapping of chronic diseases probably started with the recognition that environmental factors play an essential role in their aetiology. One of the first cancer maps can be found in a Swiss atlas (Bureau Fédéral de l'Intérieur 1914), which describes the crude rate of cancer mortality by district for the years 1901–10. Stock (1928) produced a map showing cancer prevalence by counties in England and Wales for 1919–23. He was probably the first to use mapping as a way of demonstrating the geographical variation of cancer risk as opposed to quantifying the cancer burden. It was, however, later (Howe 1963) that the real extent of methodological difficulties associated with cancer mapping was recognized. As well as the variation of age distribution in the various regions, which has to be taken into account, the geographical variation in population density is responsible for additional difficulties; it leads to undue attention being drawn to sparsely populated areas while dense populations will have little influence on the map; moreover, the less precise estimates often associated with sparsely populated areas have a tendency to produce the more extreme estimates of risk. The resolution of these problems is made difficult by the conflict between the desire to provide unbiased information and that of describing the geographical pattern of disease in such a way that its main characteristics are immediately perceived (for example, see lung cancer map in Howe 1989).

This chapter presents some of the ideas that have been developed at the International Agency for Research on Cancer (IARC) while preparing or participating in the production of several cancer atlases (Becker *et al.* 1984; IARC 1985; Rezvani *et al.* 1985; Carstensen and Møller Jensen 1986; Cislaghi *et al.* 1986a; OFS 1987; Møller Jensen *et al.* 1988; Zatonski and Becker 1988; Ménégoz *et al.* 1989; RTV 1991). Our personal preference is to describe the risk of cancer using a geographically based map, and our discussion will be limited to this approach. This personal preference may be justified on the basis of better communicability as outlined above; it is also our belief that recent advances in smoothing methodology, added to increased availability of information on small areas, can overcome to a large extent the danger of providing biased information. In order to reach this ideal goal, a number of decisions must be made before undertaking the production of a map. Although they are interrelated, we shall nevertheless discuss them separately for the sake of clarity.

Risk estimation

The main purpose of cancer mapping is to describe the geographical variation of cancer risk in an attempt to obtain new hypotheses on its aetiology or, more simply, to demonstrate that a particular cancer is caused by risk factors that have a spatial structure. It is therefore of prime importance to have, for each region, an unbiased and precise estimate of risk.

Because cancer risk is strongly dependent on age, standardization is necessary. It must be borne in mind in this context that, for a disease with marked time trend, the cross-sectional age curve may be a poor representation of the age-specific risk in the various regions. If the prevalence of risk factors responsible for the trend have begun to change at different periods in each region, standardization may average out the most interesting features. However, when the cross-sectional age curves in each unit of the map are proportional, all standardization methods will give similar and realistic pictures of risk variation. When the standard set of age-specific rates is appropriate, the indirect method of standardization has the advantage of providing the maximum likelihood estimate (MLE) of the risk ratio. This latter property, however, only leads to optimal estimates when the risk in only one region is being estimated. When, as is the case in mapping, several risks have to be estimated together, the MLE is generally not the 'best' estimate. The 'best' estimate of a set of risk parameters is not the same as the 'best' estimate of each parameter taken alone (James and Stein 1961). This somewhat counter-intuitive statement may be understood if we realize that the observed dispersion of the risk estimates gives us some information on risk variability in the country, and this information can be used to eliminate some of the random variation present in the MLE estimate. This is especially relevant when the areas of the map have grossly different population sizes, leading to estimates of very different precision from region to region. Thus an extreme estimate of low precision should be made less extreme to be consistent with the estimate of the risk variability obtained from the more precise estimates. The appropriate method for correcting the MLE is described in Chapter 18. We shall only note here that the final estimate of the risk in the region is a compromise between the 'univariate' estimate (e.g. MLE) and the average risk. It can be thought of as a mean of these two statistics weighted by their precision. This method may be refined if it is known a priori that the risks are spatially autocorrelated. It is then useful to take into account the mean risk in the neighbouring areas to further correct the estimate. These principles of estimation have been used successfully by various authors (Tsutakawa *et al.* 1985; Clayton and Kaldor 1987; Manton *et al.* 1987; Mollié and Richardson 1991), and an example showing the resulting improvement of the risk description for cancer of the gallbladder in France is shown in Plates 1(a) and 1(b). The example was first described by Mollié (1990).

Categorization of risk estimates

When the risks in the various areas of the map have been properly estimated, it is necessary to define a finite number of risk categories which will be used for describing graphically the risk variation: it seems that all attempts to link a continuous variable to a continuous system of representation have failed so far (see below). It is therefore necessary to decide on the number of categories, the choice of cut points (including the choice of an arithmetic or logarithmic scale) and, in the case of a set of several maps, on whether or not these choices will differ from map to map.

The number of classes is chosen to preserve as much information as possible, and the choice will depend on whether or not the scale is 'data-dependent'. When the standardized mortality ratio (SMR) has to be categorized, the scale may be the same for all maps (i.e. independent of the risk distribution), but the number of categories has to be sufficiently large in order to allow an informative description (e.g. nine classes of length 0.20, from 0.30 to 1.70+, as in the French mortality atlas, Rezvani *et al.* 1985). When no obvious scale is evident, the alternative is to describe the variability present in the data, and to choose to have the same number of categories whatever the range of risk may be (e.g. five categories presenting the quintile of the distribution), or, in an even more data-dependent way, one may prefer to choose the cut points according to the shape of the risk distribution (e.g. Scottish cancer atlas, IARC 1985).

It is clear that the latter approaches emphasize the need to give the reader the maximum available information, whereas the former emphasizes the need for comparability. Our belief is that both approaches are useful and may be used. In some atlases the number of categories has been increased to show separately elevated risks which are significantly different from the average, and elevated risks which are not, in an attempt to combine level of risk and statistical significance. This approach is unsatisfactory from several points of view. In particular, it imposes a linear order on quantities that are not comparable, and creates a confusion between identification of high (low) risk regions and risk estimations. It is evident that only risk estimation requires supporting map information. It is now accepted among statisticians that the way around this problem is, as discussed above, to produce a smoothed and down-weighted estimate of the risk in each area of the map which takes into account the risk estimates in other areas.

Colour design

The choice of map colour or hatching patterns requires careful consideration, in order to be sure that the numerical information produced in the previous steps is transformed into an informative picture. The use of a 'wrong' set of colours can easily convey a very different impression from that which should emerge from the data after allowing for our mechanisms of visual perception.

The final goal is to give the reader the idea of the progression of risk with the change of colour or hatching pattern. To this end, one may be tempted to produce a continuous set of patterns (e.g. hatches with spacing inversely proportional to the risk). This, however, does not produce satisfactory results because the eye tends to perceive the differences before the similarities. Thus, two adjacent areas of similar risk will be seen to be more different than they actually are, because the eye will exaggerate the slight difference in hatching pattern. As mentioned before, this emphasizes the need to categorize the data, and consequently to establish a finite set of patterns or colours for coding risk categories.

Perception of colours can be expressed simply in three dimensions, consisting of hue, lightness, and saturation (Munsell 1941; Rogers 1985). Two of these parameters, hue and saturation, can be represented on a disc using concentric circles to describe hue variation, and radii to show the degree of saturation from pale to intense (Plate 2). The presentation of the third dimension could be performed by showing several discs of different lightness. Only hue and saturation are important for our argument.

A colour scale is represented on the disc by a number of points along a path drawn on the disc. Once two colours corresponding to the end points of the scale are chosen, the representation of the categories will be obtained from the points on the disc which correspond to a regular subdivision of the chosen path. This will ensure minimal visual effort to skip from one colour to the next. The choice of a colour scale is then equivalent to the choice of a path between two end points. Going from the centre to the periphery will suggest change from low value to high value. Following a circle will depict contrast between the central value and the end points, and will give an adequate representation of low- and high-risk relative to the average situation. Combination of both gives us adequate flexibility for a good representation.

Scales C and D (shown in Plate 2) are well adapted to stress departure from an average situation. The path chosen in B is too long and makes it difficult to perceive the progression of risk. We suggest that only two of the primary colours (red, green, blue) are used. The hue variation being circular, the use of all three will fail to give a sense of the direction of gradation. The path chosen in A is too steep on the saturation scale, resulting in white as the average, an unfortunate choice (Plate 2).

Colour is necessary if we want to contrast high/low-risk areas with the average. Black-and-white may be sufficient if we only need to describe progression of risk from low to high values. In the past, the use of systems of hatching introduced various unfortunate side-effects which hampered the legibility of the map (hatching at different angles, single hatching, cross-hatching, etc.) and distracted the reader's attention away from the important information. Recently, the availability of good-quality printers has made possible the use of dot patterns of various densities to convey very effectively the grey scale well suited to this type of map.

Interpretation of the geographical pattern

As noted earlier, the aim of cancer mapping is to help in answering whether the risk of a particular cancer has spatially defined determinants; it is obviously of no use if the risk of cancer is homogeneous over the set of regions under study. The classical homogeneity tests are, however, irrelevant in this context since they do not take into account the information on contiguity or even proximity of the regions. However, in most cases this question is of academic interest, since the variation observed in the point estimates provides adequate information about the geographical variability. For some rare cancers, however, it is useful to have some method available to decide whether or not the small variation observed is statistically significant, in order to help assess the need for further research in the suspected high-risk areas. In addition, it may be that after elimination of a gradient at a larger scale, some further research is needed to see if any geographical variation exists at a finer scale (Cislaghi *et al.* 1986*b*).

The full Bayesian treatment of the data described in Chapter 18 has the ability to deal with most of these questions. We shall describe here simpler methods which may help to assess the heterogeneity of the risks and their spatial autocorrelation. Table 14.1 gives the test statistics which may be used in this context with their mean and variance under the hypothesis of the absence of spatial autocorrelation. Unfortunately, these parameters cannot be used if risks are estimated by age-standardized statistics for populations of various sizes (Besag 1989; Smans 1989); since it is very likely that population sizes are spatially, positively autocorrelated, the precision of the estimates will have the same property. Therefore, any indices from Table 14.1 calculated on these estimates will show a positive autocorrelation even if the underlying risks are the same for all regions. The more precise estimates will be closer to this common risk because of the very fact of their greater precision, and they will be closer to each other because of the spatial autocorrelation of the precision. The true distribution of the statistics may be obtained by simulation. An example is shown in Table 14.2, where a test of the homogeneity of testis

Table 14.1 Test statistics for spatial autocorrelation

Statistic[1] D	Mean[1] $E(D)$	Second moment[2] $E(D^2)$	References
$\dfrac{n \sum\limits_{i\neq j} W_{ij}(R_i - \bar{R})(R_j - \bar{R})}{S_o \, \Sigma (R_i - \bar{R})^2}$	$-\dfrac{1}{n-1}$	$\dfrac{n^2 S_1 - n S_2 + 3 S_o^2}{(n-1)(n+1) S_o^2}$	Moran (1950) Cliff and Ord (1981)
$\sum\limits_{i\neq j} W_{ij} C_{ij}$; $C_{ij} = 1$ if same colour $= 0$ if otherwise[3]	$\dfrac{S_o C_o}{n(n-1)}$	$\dfrac{S_1 C_1}{2 n^{(2)}} + \dfrac{(S_2 - 2S_1)(C_2 - 2C_1)}{4 n^{(3)}}$ $+ \dfrac{(S_o^2 + S_1 - S_2)(C_o^2 + C_1 - C_2)}{n^{(4)}}$	Ohno and Aoki (1981) Mantel (1967) Walter (1974)
$\sum\limits_{i\neq j} W_{ij} T_{ij}$ $T_{ij} = \text{Rank}(R_i) - \text{Rank}(R_j)$	$\dfrac{S_o T_o}{n(n-1)}$	same as above with C replaced by T	Smans (1989) Mantel (1967)
$\dfrac{(n-1) \sum\limits_{i\neq j} W_{ij}(R_i - R_j)^2}{\Sigma (R_i - \bar{R})^2}$	1	$1 + \dfrac{(2S_1 + S_2)(n-1) - 4 S_o^2}{2(n+1) S_o^2}$	Geary (1954)

[1] R_i is the risk in region i; n, number of regions; W_{ij} measures the proximity of regions i and j; $S_o = \sum\limits_{i\neq j} W_{ij}$, identical definition for C_o, T_o.

[2] $S_1 = \frac{1}{2} \sum\limits_{i\neq j} (W_{ij} + W_{ji})^2$; $S_2 = \Sigma (W_{i.} + W_{.i})^2$, identical definition for C_i and T_i; $n^{(i)} = n(n-1) \cdots (n-i+1)$

[3] Twice the number of pairs close in space and of the same colour.

Table 14.2   Incidence of testicular cancer in the French Département of Isère

Method	SMR estimates		Test	*p*-value[1]
	Min.	Max.		
MLE	0	629	Homogeneity[2]	0.295
Empirical Bayes[3] (a priori: gamma)	96.9	101.3		
Spatial autocorrelation			Smans	0.02 (0.001)
			Moran (SMR rank)	0.006 (0.002)
			Moran (log SMR)	0.01 (0.001)
Empirical Bayes[3] (a priori: CAR)	95.4	162.0		

[1] The *p*-values are obtained by simulations ($N=10^4$) based on the multinomial distribution. The incorrect probability obtained from a normal approximation using the moments of Table 14.1 are shown in parentheses.

[2] Likelihood ratio test.

[3] Method of Clayton and Kaldor (1987) using an a priori distribution of risk which is either the gamma distribution or the conditional normal autoregressive process (CAR). The SMR estimates given are the a posteriori means.

cancer incidence in the French Département of Isère is reported. This southeastern Département of France is covered by a cancer registry which recorded 88 cases of testicular cancer distributed in 45 'cantons' during the period 1979–84. The test of homogeneity, which was performed by Colonna (1991), was obviously non-significant; in addition, none of the SMRs (MLE) were significantly different from 100. Despite that, the strong spatial autocorrelation present in the data makes it possible to demonstrate the heterogeneity and to identify the high-risk area (Fig. 14.1). As a rule, the direct use of Moran statistics with the rank of the SMR seems to be more robust against autocorrelated population sizes but less powerful than D (Colonna *et al.* 1991).

The detection of spatial autocorrelation implies heterogeneity and is a powerful test against the null hypothesis of the absence of geographical variation. In that case, it is also easy in practice to identify the high/low-risk area. However, when no spatial structure exists, the problem of identifying high/low-risk regions is made difficult by the low power of the heterogeneity test and the multiple decision problem associated with the testing of each SMR against one. Use of the credible interval which comes from a full Bayesian treatment may provide a solution which will become acceptable when efficient computer programs for implementation of this methodology are available, provided the idea is viewed favourably among professional epidemiologists.

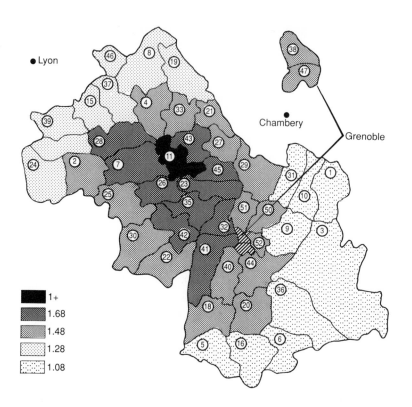

Fig. 14.1 Cancer of the testis in the French Département of Isère, male, 1979–84. Empirical Bayes estimate with a priori correlated risks (from Colonna 1991).

Conclusion

Maps convey instant visual information on the geographical distribution of diseases, and are becoming an indispensable tool for the epidemiologist. The ideal data to use as input for this kind of descriptive epidemiological procedure would be incidence data obtained at a small-area level. These data are rarely available, and we often have to use mortality data from medium-sized areas. The information provided by the map will never be better than the data available to produce it.

For mapping rare cancers, it is important that risks are standardized and smoothed in an appropriate manner in order to avoid conveying false information. Without such a methodology, spuriously elevated risks will be produced, resulting in unjustified concern in the corresponding population.

To carry out smoothing of risks, our preference is for statistically driven methods. Besides leading to better risk estimates, smoothing also provides some information on their precision and retains the possibility of carrying out statistical modelling and inference. The most modern computer technology is necessary to meet all the requirements of this methodology.

References

Becker, N., Frentzel-Beyme, R., and Wagner, G. (1984). *Atlas of cancer mortality in the Federal Republic of Germany.* Springer Verlag, Berlin.
Besag, J. E. (1989). Discussion of a paper by J. Cuzick and R. Edwards: Spatial clustering for inhomogeneous populations. *Journal of the Royal Statistical Society, Series B*, **52**, 100.
Bureau Fédéral de l'Intérieur (1914). *Statistiques de la Suisse, 191ème livraison.* Bureau de Statistique du Bureau Fédéral de l'Intérieur, Bern, Switzerland.
Carstensen, B. and Møller Jensen, O. (1986). *Atlas over Kroeftforekomst i Denmark 1970–79.* Danish Cancer Registry, Danish Cancer Society, Environmental Protection Agency.
Cislaghi, C., Decarli, A., La Vecchia, C., Laverda, N., Mezzanotte, G., and Smans, M. (1986a). *Data, statistics and maps on cancer mortality, Italia, 1975/1977.* Pitagora Editrice, Bologna.
Cislaghi, C., Mezzanotte, G., La Vecchia, C., Decarli, A., and Vigotti, M. A. (1986b). Geografia del cancro: Analisi dei trend territoriali e individuazione delle zone anomale. *Epidemiologia e Preventione*, **29**, 15–49.
Clayton, D. and Kaldor, J. (1987). Empirical Bayes estimates of age-standardized relative risks for use in disease mapping. *Biometrics*, **43**, 671–81.
Cliff, A. D. and Ord, J. K. (1981). *Spatial processes models and applications.* Pion, London.
Colonna, M. (1991). Analyse de la Distribution Spatiale du Cancer:Problèmes posés par l'Etude de Faibles Incidences. Thèse, Grenoble.
Colonna, M., Smans, M., and Estève, J. (1991). Comparison of the efficiency of several indices of autocorrelation used in cancer mapping, in preparation.
Geary, R. C. (1954). The contiguity ratio and statistical mapping. *The Incorporated Statistician*, **5**, 115–45.
Howe, G. M. (1963). *National atlas of disease mortality in the United Kingdom.* Nelson, London.
Howe, G. M. (1989). Historical evolution of disease mapping in general and specifically of cancer mapping. In *Recent results in cancer research – cancer mapping*, (ed. P. Boyle, C. S. Muir, and E. Grundmann). Springer Verlag, Berlin.
IARC (1985). *Atlas of cancer in Scotland, 1975–1980. Incidence and epidemiological perspective*, IARC Scientific Publications, No. 72. International Agency for Research on Cancer, Lyon.
James, W. and Stein, C. (1961). Estimation with quadratic loss. In *Proceeding of the Fourth Berkeley Symposium*, Vol. 1, pp. 361–79. University of California, Berkeley.
Mantel, N. (1967). The detection of disease clustering and a generalized regression approach. *Cancer Research*, **27**, 209–20.
Manton, K. G., Stallard, E., Woodbury, M. A., Riggan, W. B., Creason, J. P., and Mason, T. J. (1987). Statistically adjusted estimates of geographic mortality profiles. *Journal of the National Cancer Institute*, **78**, 805–15.

Ménégoz, F., Colonna, M., Lutz, J. M., and Schaerer, R. (1989). *Atlas du Cancer dans le Département de l'Isère*. Registre du Cancer de l'Isère, Grenoble.

Møller Jensen, O., Carstensen, B., Glattre, E., Malker, B., Pukkala, E., and Tulinius, H. (1988). *Atlas of cancer incidence in the Nordic countries*. Nordic Cancer Union, Helsinki.

Mollié, A. (1990). Représentation géographique de faux de mortalité: modélisation spatiale et méthodes bayésiennes. Thèse de doctorat de Université Paris VI.

Mollié, A. and Richardson, S. (1991). Empirical Bayes estimates of cancer mortality rates using spatial models. *Statistics in Medicine*, **10**, 95–112.

Moran, P. A. P. (1950). Notes on continuous stochastic phenomena. *Biometrika*, **37**, 17–23.

Munsell, A. H. (1941). *A color notation*, (9th edn). Munsell Color Company, Baltimore. (Available from Munsell Color Company, 2441 North Calvert Street, Baltimore, MD 21218.)

OFS (Office Fédéral de la Statistique) (1987). *La distribution géographique de la mortalité cancéreuse en Suisse, 1979/81*. OFS, Bern.

Ohno, Y. and Aoki, K. (1981). Cancer deaths by city and county in Japan (1959–1971): A test of significance for geographic clusters of disease. *Social Science and Medicine*, **15**, 251–8.

Rezvani, A., Doyon, F., and Flamant, R. (1985). *Atlas de la mortalité par cancer en France (1971–1978)*. Les Editions INSERM, Paris.

Rogers, D. F. (1985). *Procedural elements for computer graphics*. McGraw-Hill, New York.

RTV (Registro Tumori del Veneto) (1991). *Atlante della Mortalità per Tumori nella Regione Veneto, 1980–86*.

Smans, M. (1989). Analysis of spatial aggregation. In *Recent results in cancer research – cancer mapping*, (ed. P. Boyle, C. S. Muir, and E. Grundmann). Springer Verlag, Berlin.

Stock, P. (1928). *On the evidence for a regional distribution of cancer prevalence in England and Wales*. Report of the International Conference on Cancer, London, July 1928. British Empire Cancer Campaign, London.

Tsutakawa, R. K., Shoop, G. L., and Marienfeld, C. J. (1985). Empirical Bayes estimation of cancer mortality rates. *Statistics in Medicine*, **4**, 201–12.

Walter, S. (1974). On the detection of household aggregation of disease. *Biometrics*, **30**, 525–38.

Zatonski, W. and Becker, N. (1988). *Atlas of cancer mortality in Poland, 1975–1979*. Springer Verlag, Paris.

15. Estimating environmental exposure

G. A. Zapponi

Assessment of environmental exposure to hazardous substances includes measurement of environmental and food concentrations of the substances as a function of time, estimation of inhalation and dermal absorption rates, and assessment of food intake. Other parameters include the bioavailability and absorption of hazardous factors as they are found and distributed within the environment. In this chapter, the main aspects of exposure assessment will be discussed.

Measurement techniques

Basic characteristics of the measurements of environmental parameters

As a rule, determining environmental concentrations of chemical pollutants requires a sampling procedure, preparation of the specimens collected (e.g. purification, extraction), and analytical determination. The sampling procedure is defined in relation to the specific problem and environmental pollutant under study, as well as to established statistical rules. The procedures followed in the treatment and chemical analysis of the specimens depend mainly on the specific substance and the threshold level to be detected. A large number of analytical methods are commonly used in the chemical determination of environmental pollutants, and detailed discussion is beyond the scope of this chapter. These methods include gas chromatography (e.g. for organic chemicals), atomic absorption spectroscopy (e.g. for metals), gravimetric and granulometric analyses (particulate matter), ultraviolet fluorescence (e.g. for sulphur dioxide and hydrogen sulphide), chemiluminescence (e.g. nitrogen oxides), infrared spectroscopy (e.g. for carbon monoxide), ultraviolet spectrophotometry (e.g. ozone), flame ionization (e.g. hydrocarbons), and beta-ray absorption (e.g. dust). The latter methods, which are based on physical principles, are mainly used in routine monitoring of common air pollutants. They are also used in automatic instruments, which routinely collect the sample and provide analytical determination of several parameters. In specific cases, in particular for very low concentrations of some classes of highly toxic contaminants, more refined techniques are employed, such as mass spectrometry (e.g. polychlorodibenzo-*p*-dioxins, polychlorodibenzofurans, etc.) or electronic microscopy for specific studies on dust (e.g. asbestos fibre determination) (Meinke and Taylor 1972; Keith 1979; Schuetzle 1979; Schneider and Skotte 1990).

Determination of the emission rate of a specific hazardous factor at its source

This kind of measurement includes stack emission monitoring as well as the monitoring of pollutant immission into water bodies and on soil. Even if this kind of activity does not directly measure exposure, in many cases it may provide useful data for identifying exposure scenarios, for characterizing the whole pollution process, identifying its sources, and defining mitigation measures. Appropriate models (air and water diffusion models, environmental fate models, environmental partitioning models, etc.) are used for this purpose (Gifford 1981; McCall *et al.* 1983). Many national regulations require that various kinds of emissions be controlled; therefore, data of this type are often available. Generally, the stack emission sampling system is inserted through appropriate holes into the stack at easily accessible sites, where the condition of fluid dynamics is linear. The sampling may take place at random or at specific time periods (e.g. in mean operating and/or maximum rate operating conditions, when the process is started or stopped, etc.), also depending on the statistical variability of the process. In the case of gaseous pollutants, the sample to be analysed is generally collected in phials, flasks, syringes, or bags; or is absorbed in or adsorbed to solutions or solid materials; or is in the form of liquid obtained by condensation at low temperatures. In the case of particulate matter, the sample is generally deposited on appropriate filters. Besides the chemical composition of effluents, it is often necessary to measure the temperature and pressure of the operating conditions; the density, humidity, velocity, and flow rates of emission; as well as the production rate of the specific cycle. There are instruments that operate within the stack itself, based on optic principles, and also remote sensing techniques such as LIDAR and other systems, which are based on the optical properties of plumes emitted from stacks. Water effluent sampling is generally simpler than air effluent sampling, and essentially relies on collecting specific amounts of fluid. There are a number of similar considerations governing the time frequency of sampling, as well as the need to determine not only chemical composition, but also flow rate and other process parameters.

Measurement of environmental levels of specific pollutants in sampling sites within the environment

This category of measurements includes urban or industrial area air quality monitoring, coastal water monitoring, soil quality monitoring, and other environmental monitoring activities. These measurements generally lead to an assessment of environmental concentrations in a specific number of sites (which represent a set of points on a map), but are generally limited for reasons of feasibility and cost. Environmental pollution control generally requires periodic or continuous measurements. The selection of sampling points is often based on specific criteria, rather than purely statistical considerations. As an example, the current EC procedures for urban air quality control are generally aimed at monitoring the most polluted sites; in other examples, sampling sites are chosen in order to assess environmental quality in areas where there is a significant human presence. When using these data for other purposes, it is important to keep in mind the aims of and criteria on which the sampling system is based. In air pollution monitoring, a pump system is generally used to sample a specific volume of air (for high-volume samplers this volume is typically 1–2 m^3/min), and the pollutants are collected in appropriate containers or substrata, substantially analogous to the ones used for stack emission sampling. The duration of sampling depends on the specific purposes of the survey and on the amount of substance to be collected for an efficient chemical determination. It may also be limited by the possibility of losses if there is an excessively long-lasting flow. Monitoring networks, based on automated instruments are generally used in urban air quality control, commonly measuring sulphur dioxide, hydrogen sulphide, nitrogen oxides, carbon monoxide, ozone, the hydrocarbon group, and the amount of particulate matter.

For soil pollutant measurement, the vertical distribution of the pollutant under study is an important parameter, both for achievement of a correct and effective sample and to produce the most useful kind of data for reliable exposure assessment (e.g. in the case of superficial contamination, if an excessively thick layer of soil is sampled, this may dilute the concentration to be detected, providing possibly misleading information).

Drinking water distribution systems are monitored at appropriate points with specific frequencies. This aims to give effective control of the quality of water for human consumption, by examining a wide set of possible contaminants (chemical, microbiological, and physical). On the other hand, the monitoring of recreational coastal waters involves a more limited number of parameters (microbiological, chemical, and physical). The spatial frequency of sampling depends on the type of area under study as well as the mode of recreational use.

Measurement of ambient pollutants in specific spatially limited environments

Techniques that are generally similar to those mentioned above are commonly used to monitor the concentrations of hazardous factors, particularly in the air, in specific spatially limited environments, where they are generally more homogeneous than in the external environment. Typical examples include the monitoring of occupational environments (concerned with the exposure of large social groups, such as factories, offices, schools, etc.) and of indoor domestic environments. This kind of measurement provides information that, generally, can be interpreted fairly easily in terms of exposure. In the case of occupational environments, the selection of the hazardous factors to be monitored is generally based on specific needs. The sampling techniques and analytical methods are similar to those mentioned above; the parameter most frequently measured is the air concentration of hazardous factors. Generally, sampling is also designed to provide information on 'iso-concentration areas', and, therefore, it can be useful to estimate exposure in different sites of the environment under examination. Indoor exposure assessment has to take into account the number of smokers in the house or office, the type of heating system and the fuel used in it, the type of cooking fuel, air conditioning or ventilation, the general characteristics of the neighbourhood, and the volume of local traffic (WHO 1982a).

Personal and portable samplers and monitors

Personal samplers and monitors have recently been developed, which make it possible to monitor directly air pollution concentrations in the exposed individual's breathing area. The main categories of these devices include miniaturized analytical instruments (battery powered, which can directly measure the concentration of specific pollutants), active samplers (which collect and accumulate the pollutant for subsequent analysis), and passive samplers (which utilize a substratum on which the pollutant is absorbed or adsorbed, or with which it may react chemically) (WHO 1982a; Prodi et al. 1988; Vinzents 1988). Miniaturized instruments and active personal samplers contain a pump system, and essentially are a miniaturized version, often of comparable efficiency, of some of the larger instruments discussed above. The sampling duration generally ranges from a fraction of an hour to many hours or a whole day, and further consecutive samplings may be carried out. Passive samplers are simple and inexpensive devices, allowing surveys to be set up to measure the exposure of large numbers of individuals. The response of these devices, however, may be significantly influenced by air turbulence and movement, as well as by the activity of individuals in the study. Therefore, it is advisable to calibrate the measurements that can be obtained with this system, taking into account the possible errors. Passive devices provide good results in radiation exposure monitoring.

Biological monitoring

Exposure to environmentally hazardous factors may also be monitored by measuring the levels of the chemicals of interest or their metabolites in human tissues and fluids, or their binding to DNA or to haemoglobin (Iwasaki 1988; van Sittert 1989; Robinson *et al.* 1990). In the latter two examples the measurement may be considered an indicator of biological effect as well as of exposure. Biological monitoring can provide information which is extremely useful not only for assessing exposure, but also as a means of verifying the capacity of the molecule of interest to reach its target. Monitoring of early biological adverse effects, which are known to be caused by environmental exposure, may also provide important information, even if it may sometimes be difficult to correlate these effects with a specific cause. However, biological monitoring is generally costly, difficult, and time-consuming, and requires an efficient experimental design.

Exposure modelling

The measurements of environmental concentrations of pollutants discussed above do not represent, at least in a strict sense, a measurement of exposure. Rather, they have to be viewed in the light of the parameters and models describing the whole environmental process leading to effective exposure. In the case of air pollution, for instance, more reliable assessment will be possible if the characteristics of the pollutant emission source, as well as the meteorological and wind velocity and intensity parameters are accounted for through appropriate modelling (Gifford 1981). A general model for integrated inhalation exposure assessment should be based on the measurement and/or estimation of concentration values of air pollution originating from multiple sources, on the evaluation of street-level pollution levels induced by traffic (and influenced by the height and characteristics of buildings), on the estimation of indoor–outdoor air pollution relationships, and on the impact of indoor sources, as well as the characterization of population activity patterns. Some models exist for this purpose (WHO 1982*a*). For instance, in the case of indoor exposure, it is assumed that if the outdoor concentration of a non-reactive gas changes, in the absence of internal sources, the indoor concentration will exponentially approach the new outdoor concentration level. The time constant of this process will be directly proportional to the ventilation air-flow rate and inversely proportional to room volume. The presence of an internal source may be considered in the model (WHO 1982*a*).

A simple and effective method for the assessment of integrated inhalation exposure has been proposed, based on the calculation of the 'weighted weekly exposure' (WWE) (WHO 1982*a*). The WWE is simply the weighted average of air pollutant concentrations, as measured or assessed in the various places of exposure. The weight is the duration of single exposures (i.e. the time spent in the various exposure places). Clearly, the WWE may also be measured with portable monitors or samplers; these measurements may also be used for validating WWE theoretical estimations and for defining typical patterns of integrated exposure. This procedure may provide a useful and simple criterion for small-area exposure assessment, based on environmental concentration measurement, human activity, and mobility analysis. Six typical categories have been identified for this purpose: housewives, office workers, industrial workers, outdoor workers, the elderly and infirm, and students (Moschandreas 1981). For each of these subgroups it is possible to define a typical pattern of mobility in various types of places (e.g. home, work-place or school, street at different hours, countryside, etc.). A typical population in an industrial country spends, on average, about 70 per cent of the time inside the home, but this figure varies significantly for the different categories (e.g. elderly people and housewives generally spend much more time at home than students and workers, etc.) (Moschandreas 1981). These considerations may be important in small-area studies based on parameters such as postcode or other equivalent information, in order to assess possible exposure patterns.

Discussion

Some conclusions may be drawn from the above. First, examination of routine environmental data is important to establish whether they represent measurements of the risk factors of interest, simply constitute an indication of general pollution in the environment, or whether they are irrelevant to the specific problem. When the disease under study may be caused by long-term past exposure and the objective data needed for its description are limited or lacking, the use of current or recent environmental monitoring data may be considered, with appropriate 'caveats'. The characterization of the pollution process is particularly important, to verify whether the present conditions may be reliably extrapolated to the past. An inventory of the pollution emission sources existing in the past in the area is essential for this purpose, since emission rates are well characterized for a large number of new and old industrial plants or other sources, and data relevant to past situations may be available (WHO 1982b). The elaboration and modelling of emission data, together with available environmental data, may provide some useful indicators of past and 'historical' exposure patterns. It may be that the particular substance of interest is not included within the set of pollutants considered in routine environmental monitoring, or the monitoring procedure may be too sparse to give useful information in a specific locality. Under such conditions, it is sometimes possible to use available data as predictors of the parameter for which direct information is lacking (often, emission and environmental levels of pollutants emitted by the same source are correlated, and estimates are possible based on such correlation); alternatively, measurements from one site could be used to estimate emissions at another similar site. In this case, a detailed knowledge of the characteristics of the pollution process under study is crucial. Finally, wherever possible, existing data on occupational exposure, indoor and individual exposure data, as well as biological monitoring data, should be integrated with the other information mentioned above. In some cases, the exposure pattern of large groups of the population may be identified; the analysis of these situations may be important in small-area studies. Clearly, this discussion is not exhaustive and the concepts outlined above may be extended to other exposure patterns, including diet, drinking water, and other exposure routes.

References

Gifford, F. A. (1981). Estimating ground-level concentration patterns from isolated air-pollution sources: a brief summary. *Environmental Research*, **25**, 126–38.

Iwasaki, K. (1988). Individual differences in the formation of hemoglobin adducts following exposure to methyl bromide. *Industrial Health*, **26**, 257–62.

Keith, L. H. (1979). *Organic pollutants in water*. Ann Arbor Science. Ann Arbor, Mich. 48106.

McCall, P. J., Laskowski, D. A., Swann, R. L., and Dishburger, H. J. (1983). Estimation of environmental partitioning of organic chemicals in model ecosystems. *Residue Reviews*, **85**, 231–44.

Meinke, W. W. and Taylor, J. K. (ed.) (1972). *Analytical chemistry: key to progress on national problems*, National Bureau of Standards (US), Publication 351, Washington DC.

Moschandreas, D. J. (1981). Exposure to pollutant and daily time budgets of people. *Bulletin of the New York Academy of Medicine*, **57**, 845–59.

Prodi, V., Belosi, F., Mularoni, A., and Lucialli, P. (1988). PERSPEC: a personal sampler with size characterization capabilities. *American Industrial Hygiene Association Journal*, **49**, (2), 75–80.

Robinson, E. P., Mack, G. A., Remmers, J., Levy, R., and Mohadiers, L. (1990). Trends of PCB, hexachlorobenzene, and b-benzene hexachloride levels in the adipose tissue of the U.S. population. *Environmental Research*, **53**, 175–92.

Schneider, T. and Skotte, J. (1990). Fiber exposure reassessed with the new indices. *Environmental Research*, **51**, 108–16.

Schuetzle, D. (ed.) (1979). *Monitoring toxic substances*, ACS Symposium Series 94. American Chemical Society, Washington DC.

van Sittert, N. J. (1989). Individual exposure monitoring from plasma or urinary metabolite determination. *Archives of Toxicology*, Suppl. 13, 91–100.

Vinzents, P. (1988). Personal sampling of total and inhalable dust. *Journal of Aerosol Science*, **19**, (7), 1437–9.

WHO (1982a). *Estimating human exposure to air pollutants*. WHO, Geneva.

WHO (1982b). *Rapid assessment of sources of air, water, and land pollution*, WHO Offset Publ. 92. WHO, Geneva.

16. Mapping environmental exposure

D. J. Briggs

Exposure to environmental pollution needs to be considered in the epidemiology of many diseases, and, at a broader scale, is an important determinant of the quality of life. It is also a strongly geographical phenomenon. Levels of pollutants and other hazards in the environment vary spatially; the degree of human exposure thus differs from one location to another.

The ability to map environmental exposure can help to explore geographical patterns of health outcome and aid in the interpretation of clusters of disease. It can indicate areas of potential future concern. It can provide, also, a broad guide to policy actions and needs; for example, where closer health surveillance may be necessary, where efforts to reduce exposure risk are required, and how effective existing policies have been.

Data on levels of exposure are, however, exceedingly rare. Except in the case of specific monitoring studies (e.g. Akland *et al.* 1985), or where individuals are working in areas of known high exposure risk (e.g. potentially radioactive environments), direct measurements of exposure are not made. For the most part, mapping must consequently rely on indirect approaches, involving the modelling of exposure levels or risk. This paper examines some of the approaches that may be used, and the problems they may encounter.

The geography of exposure

Environmental exposure can be seen as the result of the intersection of two separate geographies: that of the environmental contaminant and that of the recipient individuals or groups (Fig. 16.1). Both of these are highly complex. Many different pollutants occur, including radio-isotopes, chemicals, particulates, vibrations, and organisms. Each may be derived from a wide range of both point and non-point sources; each may be characterized by different properties of mobility and persistence. The environment through which these pollutants move, and in which they are stored and decay, is also exceedingly variable. It can be seen to comprise many different overlaid and overlapping systems (e.g. soil, water, air; urban areas, agricultural land), each of which varies at different scales and in different ways: some, such as the climate, perhaps continuous and regional; others, such as land use, often localized and

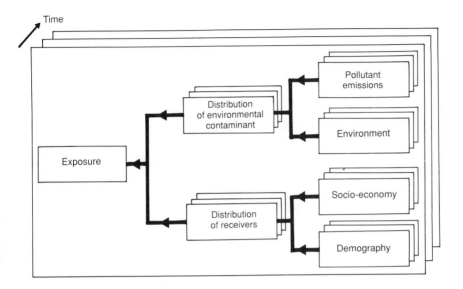

Fig. 16.1   The geographies of environmental exposure.

disjunct. These variations affect the capacity of the environment to absorb, transport, or destroy the pollutants. As a result, different agents may be transferred through the environment by innumerable different pathways, may be stored at different locations for different lengths of time, and may be decomposed by different processes at different rates. Levels of environmental contamination are therefore seen to vary greatly over short distances, and in what may seem like a random manner, while the pattern of one pollutant in the environment cannot necessarily be taken as a guide to the distribution of others.

Nor are these patterns fixed or static. Each varies over a range of temporal scales. Levels of emission may change by the hour or day in response to cycles of industrial or domestic activity. Their rates and directions of transfer may vary equally with day-to-day or seasonal changes in weather: emissions from the Chernobyl explosion, for example, fanned out along four different pathways as wind direction changed during the 4 days after the incident (Gould 1990). In the longer term, over periods of years or decades, technology, land use, vegetation, fauna, soil conditions, climate may all change, and with them the production, dispersal, and distribution of environmental pollutants.

All this, moreover, relates to only one of the two geographies of concern, that of the pollutants themselves. The second geography, that of the recipients, is no less complex. It comprises not merely the distribution of the population *en masse*, as depicted for example by census statistics, but the myriad patterns of movement and rest that lie therein. It is the geography of commuting, social travel, migration; of places of residence, vacation, and work—and of the time spent in each. Like the distribution of the pollutants, it is also a geography which is highly dynamic, changing and shifting by the day, week, season, or year. It is the geography, therefore, of the seemingly random spatial scribblings of each individual accumulated over time.

Approaches to exposure mapping

Faced with this complexity, mapping of exposure is clearly a challenging task. Rarely, as noted, can it be carried out by direct means—simply by plotting the distribution of measured levels of exposure. More commonly, it requires the ability to model the magnitude and distribution of exposure on the basis of other evidence.

The modelling of exposure can be carried out at various levels of abstraction. Four general approaches may be defined:

(1) integrated modelling—the modelling and mapping of actual levels of exposure by intersecting geographical models of pollutant and human distribution (appropriately integrated over time);
(2) concentration mapping—the modelling and mapping of the levels of pollutant in the environment (without regard to human distribution);
(3) dispersion modelling—the modelling and mapping of pollution dispersion from source;
(4) emission mapping—the assessment and mapping of levels of emission or release of pollutants at source.

Clearly this represents a sequence of progressively reduced specificity and power. Which approach is adopted is likely to depend on a number of circumstances, including the degree of knowledge of the processes involved, the scale of analysis, and the availability and quality of data.

Integrated modelling

Ideally, exposure mapping should be based on an integrated modelling approach. To date, however, this has been relatively rarely employed. In part, this reflects the conceptual and computational difficulties involved: it requires the ability to intersect—often with a considerable degree of spatial, analytical, and temporal resolution—data on the distributions of pollutants in the environment with the distributions and/or patterns of movement of recipient individuals or groups. More basically, it reflects the limitations of available data on both environmental conditions and human distributions.

Census data, for example, only provide aggregate statistics on population distribution, at the ward or enumeration district level, and reveal little about detailed patterns of movement through the environment. Similarly, detailed data on the distribution of pollutants are often limited, as outlined below, while the local variations in environmental pollution are typically high—most especially in topographically complex environments such as urban areas (e.g. Simmons and Pocock 1987). Consequently, it is rarely possible to use these data to identify locationally specific exposure, or to model with any precision the patterns of exposure risk for either individuals or tightly defined groups. The best that can normally be achieved is to estimate the percentage of population (or total numbers) living within areas of general exposure risk. Typically, this involves the relatively simple process of overlaying maps of pollutant distribution onto population density maps.

With the development of Geographical Information Systems (GIS), the facility for undertaking such analyses is undoubtedly being improved. The requirement for improved environmental data, however, remains. This approach is therefore only likely to be feasible in the context of local studies, supported by purpose-designed monitoring programmes or surveys.

Concentration mapping

Mapping of environmental concentrations, in contrast, is a well-tried and tested approach. At the national and broad regional levels, there is an abundance of data on a wide variety of agents, derived from routine surveys or monitoring programmes: for example, SO_2 and smoke (e.g. Commission of the European Communities 1989; Warren Springs Laboratory 1990), surface freshwater quality (Commission of the European Communities 1986; Department of the Environment and Welsh Office 1986), bathing water quality (Commission of the European Community 1985; Department of the Environment 1990), and radioactivity (Department of the Environment 1988; Hunt 1989; MAFF 1990). In addition, many more specific, short-term surveys have been carried out (e.g. Campbell 1988).

The quality of these data sources as a basis for exposure mapping is, nevertheless, limited. Few relate explicitly to those agents or sources which are currently of greatest concern, such as carcinogens or mutagens, and the number of stations monitoring the more obscure pollutants is often small (Table 16.1). Sampling and analytical procedures also leave much to be desired. Most of the monitoring networks, for example, are concentrated in specific areas of known high pollution level (e.g. industrial areas in the case of air quality), and the data thus do not provide a wholly representative sample of wider conditions. Although attention is often focused on health outcomes within these high concentration areas, the cumulative population exposure may in fact be higher elsewhere, if large populations are exposed to low concentrations.

As has also been noted, considerable local variability may occur in environmental conditions. Spatial extrapolations from the measured data points must therefore be undertaken with care, and general maps of exposure derived from

Table 16.1 UK air pollution monitoring
stations, 1990 (from Department of the
Environment 1990)

Pollutant	No. of stations
Ozone	17
Carbon monoxide	5
Nitrogen oxides	11
Acid deposition	32
Hydrocarbons	2
Trace gases	1
Atmospheric chemistry	2
Smoke and SO_2	287
Lead	19
Multi-element, incl. lead	5

such data are likely to have limited meaning. Finally, as with all environmental data, there may be significant problems of gaps, errors, or inconsistencies in the data due to problems of conceptualization, sampling, equipment failure, administrative changes, and operator error (see, for example, Briggs and Reeve 1990).

Because of these inadequacies in the available data, many studies must resort to their own surveys. At the local level, this can be highly effective, and countless examples exist (e.g. Beavington 1973, 1977; Lott 1985; Moir and Thornton 1989; Ericson and Mishra 1990; Harrop et al. 1990). The problem, however, is that these tend to be short term, and cannot easily provide data on past conditions. Yet, where exposure is cumulative over time, or where health outcomes are lagged, such data are vital. Moreover, because of the great temporal variability in environmental conditions, surveys of this type may also provide relatively poor estimates of long-term exposure patterns, whereas the spatial variability in the phenomena involved may mean that a very dense network of sites is required. This makes the survey potentially expensive, and cost constraints may, in turn, limit the quality of the results. Problems of vandalism and equipment failure may also dog such surveys (it is not uncommon for 20–30 per cent of installations to be lost), while access to more remote sites may limit opportunities for regular sampling. Numerous relatively low-cost monitoring and survey systems have, however, been devised for environmental monitoring, and these have been used with considerable success. Moss bag collectors, for example, have been widely employed for the analysis of air pollution (e.g. Goodman and Smith 1975; Archibold and Crisp 1983). Corrosion plates have also been applied to assess levels of a range of air pollutants (e.g. Yocum 1962), while solution tablets can be used to assess rainfall acidity (e.g. Jaynes and Cooke 1987).

To acquire data on past, or longer-term, levels of environmental contamination is more difficult. Documentary records may provide some information, but these are notoriously unreliable and difficult to interpret. Potentially more useful in some cases are 'natural monitors'. Lichen, for example, assimilate air pollutants over their lifetime, and may thus yield estimates of the time-integrated average level of contamination (e.g. Nieboer *et al.* 1978; Nyangababo 1987). They are also sensitive to certain air pollutants, and their distribution and species composition may also provide good indicators of average (or possibly extreme) levels of pollution over several years (e.g. Oliver 1968). Reservoir sediments, lake sediments, peat bodies, and ice cores similarly may preserve information on past levels of contaminants in the environment. Few rigorous attempts have been made to use any of these sources as a basis for assessing past environmental exposure of humans, but they have been employed to decipher general historical trends (e.g. Reczynska-Dutka 1986; Pavoni *et al.* 1987; Schintu *et al.* 1989). More ingeniously, Elliott *et al.* (1988) have used museum specimens of birds to assess historical levels of pesticide exposure in wildlife populations (see also Newton 1979).

Dispersion modelling

In the absence of data on pollutant concentrations in the environment, an alternative approach is to derive estimates of their distribution from dispersion models. This approach has been widely used in relation to air pollution, most especially from point sources such as industrial chimneys, and numerous dispersion models have been devised (e.g. Finzi *et al.* 1984; Andresen and Kyaw Tha Paw 1985). Similar models have also been developed for the prediction of pollutant dispersal in streams (e.g. Chytil 1984; Revitt *et al.* 1990), from traffic (e.g. Beiruti and Al-Omishy 1985), in marine environments (e.g. Jeffries and Steele 1989), and the wider environment (van de Meent 1990). Noise dispersal has been modelled in comparable ways (e.g. Briggs and France 1982).

These approaches are especially valuable in relation to exposure to pollutants from clearly defined point or linear sources. They have particular potential, for example, as a basis for defining areas of potential concern around industrial or other installations. They might thus be used to good effect as a means of delimiting optimal search regions for disease clusters associated with nuclear power or reprocessing plants, chemical works, or landfill sites. Their successful application, however, depends upon two requirements: an adequate knowledge of the exposure pathway of the pollutant involved (e.g. whether by air, water, food), and information on levels of emission into that pathway. These requirements are not always met. Lacking the first, different pathways could potentially be explored; lacking the second, recourse can be made to further models of emissions (see below). Either approach, however, is likely to reduce the reliability of the results. Dispersion modelling also becomes excessively complex, and often severely limited by data availability, when applied to dispersed, area sources (e.g. agriculture).

Emission modelling

Data on emission levels are frequently lacking. Often they are not closely or regularly monitored; where monitored, the data may not be available for reasons of commercial confidentiality. In these circumstances, emissions may themselves need to be estimated by modelling processes. Again, many models have been developed, but the majority tend to follow broadly the same form: emissions are estimated on the basis of levels of activity for each specified source, using empirically or theoretically derived emission factors.

These models are widely used at both national and international level to assess and monitor emissions into the environment. Most countries in Europe, for example, calculate emissions of the main atmospheric pollutants (e.g. SO_2, particulates, CO_2, NO_x) from industrial, domestic, energy, and transport sources. The European Commission has also undertaken a project to map emissions of SO_2, NO_x, and volatile organic compounds across Europe, as part of the CORINE Programme (Commission of the European Communities 1990). At a more detailed level, models have also been developed to assess a wide range of other emissions, including road traffic pollution (e.g. Alauzet and Joumard 1989), hazardous chemicals from industrial sites (e.g. Singh 1990), airborne particles (e.g. Simpson 1990), and solid wastes (e.g. Barnard and Olivett 1990).

Such models undoubtedly provide a means of generating estimates of emission levels for a wide range of agents and sources. How reliable the estimates are, however, is open to some debate. Many of the models are at least semi-empirical, and as such depend upon rather limited experimental information which does not fully represent the wide variety of conditions that may be encountered. Technological and other conditions may also change, rendering the models quickly out of date. Estimates of NO_x emissions from road traffic in the UK, for example, were revised upwards by 50 per cent in 1983 when it was discovered that the emission factors being used were significant under estimates (Department of the Environment 1984). More crucially, emission modelling only represents the first stage in estimating environmental exposure. Care must therefore be taken either in using the data thus derived as inputs to further models, or in interpreting patterns of exposure directly from these results.

Spatial modelling

The spatial variability of environmental conditions, and thus of exposure, has already been noted. Environmental data, on the other hand, are often limited.

They typically occur either as detailed measurements for specific sampling or monitoring sites (e.g. air quality, water quality) or as more general classifications for mapped areas (e.g. soil type). Equally, it is apparent that human exposure to environmental pollutants is often local and specific; yet data on human distributions are, in many cases, confined to relatively generalized aggregations (e.g. census statistics). Mapping of environmental exposure for epidemiological or other detailed studies thus depends crucially upon the ability to model spatial distributions. In particular, it relies upon methods of:

(1) spatial interpolation, i.e. the prediction of conditions at unvisited or unmeasured locations from measured data for surrounding locations;

(2) spatial extrapolation, i.e. the estimation of conditions at locations beyond the surveyed area.

Techniques of spatial interpolation are therefore fundamental to exposure mapping: they provide the means to step from generality to detail, and to match broad environmental distributions to specific exposure sites. To undertake spatial interpolation successfully, however, requires a sound knowledge both of the nature of spatial data, and of the nature of spatial variation in the environment.

Spatial data characteristics

Data on both environmental conditions and human distributions take many spatial forms. Many environmental data, for example, refer to point locations: they represent results of routine measurement at specific monitoring sites, analyses and observations at randomly or systematically chosen sample points, or data relating to specific point features (e.g. emissions from chimneys or discharges from sewage outfalls). Similarly, at least at certain levels of generalization, the target individuals or groups may be specified by a point location (e.g. an individual house, the grid reference centroid of a residential area, or a unit postal code).

Many data, also, relate to linear features or networks. Classifications of stream water quality, for example, may have been extrapolated to complete segments or river systems. Data on traffic flow (or the emissions derived therefrom) may be available for the entire road network. Analysis of low frequency electromagnetism may relate to transmission lines. Information on human movements may be expressed in the form of preferred travel pathways or webs. Yet other data are related to areal features. Population data typically are compiled for administrative regions (e.g. enumeration districts or census wards). Data on health outcomes may be aggregated to health district or postcode level. Assessments of pollution may only exist for broad regions or zones (e.g. soil map units, geological regions, vegetation or land use areas). Data derived from dispersion models, or from satellite imagery, may be in raster (i.e. grid-cell) form.

Many data on environmental exposure (or associated phenomena) therefore relate to relatively broad spatial units. As such, they often lack the resolution required for mapping of environmental exposure. To use the data, it is frequently necessary to estimate more local conditions, or more precise distributions by interpolation within the mapped units. Many of the point data available, conversely, refer to very precise locations, and often give limited area coverage. To use these data, there is often the necessity to extrapolate them to wider areas, or to estimate conditions at intermediate sites. Moreover, for many applications, different data sets need to be combined and brought together in a consistent manner. This may require the conversion of the data to a common spatial form. All these processes require the use of advanced methods of spatial modelling. The processes involved are illustrated in Fig. 16.2.

Spatial variation in the environment

Spatial environmental variation can be broken down into two main components: regional trend (or drift), which is essentially predictable, and apparent random or stochastic variation, which for the most part is not. The balance between the two determines the extent to which reliable spatial interpolation is possible.

Regional trends in environmental conditions may take many forms (Fig. 16.3). Some phenomena are distributed in an essentially disjunct fashion, areas of uniformity being bounded by narrow zones of rapid change. Others may vary continuously, along uniclinal, polyclinal, or cyclic gradients. Individual phenomena may show either pattern in different circumstances. Altitude, for example, may be markedly disjunct in areas of tableland or dissected plateaux, yet show more gradual and continuous patterns of variation in areas of rolling or vale-and-scarp terrain. Soils may change abruptly where major geological boundaries occur, or along broad zones of transition associated with subtle topographic or climatic controls. Concentrations of pollutants, likewise, may exhibit sudden variations in complex urban areas, but change only slowly across open country. Over the landscape as a whole, therefore, environmental conditions often show elements of both disjunct and continuous variation (Fig. 16.3).

Superimposed upon this regional pattern, however, is inevitably a degree of more local, and essentially random variation. This is to a large degree a matter of scale; variation which may seem random at a broad scale may be resolved into a recognizable pattern at a more local scale. It is a product, therefore, of the sampling density. This component of the random variation can thus be assumed to be spatially correlated: sites that are close together will be more similar to each other than they will to sites that are farther away. Part of the stochastic element can be considered as residual (i.e. due to sampling or measurement error, temporal variations in conditions at a site, etc). As such, it

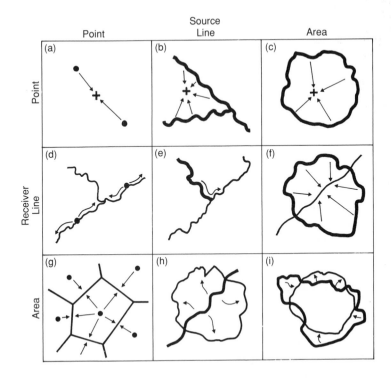

Fig. 16.2 Data types and spatial modelling requirements for exposure mapping. Mapping of environmental exposure often requires that patterns of environmental contamination be predicted on the basis of limited data. This figure illustrates some of the spatial interpolations which may be involved. Note that the arrows do not necessarily indicate flow-lines of the pollutant, but symbolize the process of spatial interpolation. (a) Point-to-point: for example, prediction of levels of air pollution at a location between two monitoring sites; (b) line-to-point: for example, prediction of levels of pollution at a location adjacent to a road network; (c) area-to-point: for example, prediction of levels of pollution at a location within a mapped area of contamination; (d) point-to-line: for example, estimation of the water quality of stream segments on the basis of data from monitoring sites; (e) line-to-line: for example, extrapolation of water quality classes from classified segments to unclassified segments of the stream network; (f) area-to-line: for example, prediction of levels of pollution along a stream or road passing through an area of mapped contamination; (g) point-to-area (tesselation): for example, the mapping of pollution distribution on the basis of data from selected sample locations (e.g. soil sample sites); (h) line-to-area: for example, the mapping of levels of pollution around a linear feature (e.g. roadway); (i) area-to-area: for example, the interpolation of pollution data from one area base (e.g. soil map units) to another (e.g. administrative regions).

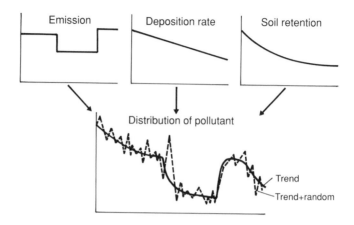

Fig. 16.3   Patterns of environmental variation.

represents spatially uncorrelated variation, or noise. Clearly, the greater the proportion of noise in the data, the less successful will methods of spatial interpolation or extrapolation be.

Spatial modelling techniques

Various methods of spatial interpolation and extrapolation have been developed to cope with these different components of variation. These may be classified broadly into global and local approaches.

Global approaches undertake interpolation on the basis of all the measured data points; probably the most widely used is trend surface analysis. A development of the regression model, this generates smoothed surfaces through the measured points, thereby allowing unmeasured locations to be assessed. It suffers, however, from two major limitations. First, it tends to result in over-smoothing, since it specifically removes outliers. Secondly, it tends to be unstable at the margins of the study area, where control points are sparse, and thus can give inaccurate (or even impossible) extrapolations.

Local models, in contrast, place greatest weight in interpolation on adjacent or surrounding data points, and are thus most appropriate for site-specific estimations, or for deducing detailed (as opposed to generalized) spatial patterns. Many different methods are available, but some of the more common are:

(1) proximal interpolation (e.g. Thiessen polygons);
(2) spline interpolation (e.g. Laplacian-splines);
(3) kriging, in various forms.

Proximal interpolation

Proximal interpolation is based on the assumption of disjunct variation. Each area (or segment in the case of linear features) is considered to be internally uniform, and to be separated from the next by a narrow zone of abrupt change. This, in fact, is the assumption underlying much traditional environmental mapping: soil maps provide a clear example. Map units are delimited by clearly defined boundaries, and each unit is characterized by a named soil type (or association of soil types). Between-unit variation is assumed to be concentrated along the map unit boundary. Internal (i.e. random) variation within the unit occurs both in the form of within-class variation (i.e. the legitimate range of soil conditions recognized in any named soil type) and in the form of inclusions of other soil types, too small to separate. In this context, the best estimate of conditions at any location is therefore provided by the modal value for the map unit in which it lies, adjusted as appropriate to take account of any spatially correlated random variation.

These same principles may also be used in reverse to extrapolate from measured sites to linear segments or areas. In the case of linear features, segment boundaries may be imputed by simply bisecting the line between each pair of sampled points. For point-to-area extrapolation, tesselation procedures are used, for example by constructing Thiessen polygons (e.g. Green and Sibson 1978).

Thiessen tesselation is a standard component of most modern proprietary GIS, and thus is one of the most widely used spatial interpolation techniques. The validity of proximal interpolation is nevertheless limited. Few environmental phenomena are actually distributed in a truly disjunct manner, and the method takes no account of local or random variation in the data. It is also highly sensitive to the distribution of sample points; it is likely to perform especially badly where the samples are unevenly distributed, and also generates unsatisfactory patterns at the edges of sampled areas, where no outlying data points occur. The technique is therefore probably most appropriate with qualitative (i.e. classified) data where the measurable local spatial variability is low.

Spline interpolation

Spline functions have been described as 'mathematical equivalents of the flexible ruler' (Burrough 1986). They provide a means of building locally fitted polynomials to give a continuous surface through spatially distributed data points. Various methods of spline fitting have been developed; the two most extensively used are probably b-splines (in linear, quadratic, or cubic form) and Laplacian-splines.

These methods have been employed for spatial interpolation in a wide range of environmental mapping exercises. Hutchinson and Bischof (1983), for example, computed Laplacian smoothing spline surfaces, using both location and altitude as independent variables, in order to generate rainfall maps across Australia. By also including information on the length of the weather record at each measured site, they were able to weight the data according to their local variance, and thereby incorporate both long- and short-term records without reducing the quality of the whole data set. Similar methods have been used for the modelling of other meteorological variables, including daily solar radiation (Hutchinson *et al.* 1984*a*) and windspeed (Hutchinson *et al.* 1984*b*), and in digital terrain models (Torgersen *et al.* 1983).

Laplacian-spline interpolation has a number of advantages. By taking account of the noise in the available data, it generates surfaces that are sensitive to data quality, and which are normally smooth away from the data points. It also gives a measure of both the estimation error, and the standard deviation of the data; the latter can be used to test the approximate goodness of fit (Hutchinson and Bischof 1983). In addition, the method works well with irregularly scattered data points. On the other hand, like other more sophisticated methods, its computational demands are relatively high, and approximation or reiterative solutions must be used for large data sets (i.e. with more than a few hundred data points).

Kriging

Kriging has become one of the most popular methods of spatial interpolation in recent years. Originally devised primarily for geological prospecting purposes (Matheron 1971), it has since been developed extensively by Webster and his colleagues for agricultural and soil survey applications (e.g. Burrough and Webster 1980; Webster and Burgess 1983; Oliver *et al.* 1989; Webster and Oliver 1989; Oliver and Webster 1990; Oliver 1991). In addition, it has been applied in a range of other fields, including air pollution modelling (e.g. Lajaunie 1984) and groundwater modelling (e.g. Gambolati and Volpi 1979). Thus, it clearly has potential value in the mapping of environmental exposure.

Kriging is, in fact, a suite of spatial interpolation techniques, each designed for different applications or data types (Burrough 1986; Oliver and Webster 1990). It is based upon recognition of the three elements of spatial variation outlined above (i.e. drift, spatially correlated random variation, and noise). At its simplest (i.e. where no drift occurs, or when the effects of drift have been statistically removed), it involves the computation of a measure known as the semivariance. This represents the average difference between all pairs of sites of constant inter-site distance (lag):

$$S(h) = \frac{1}{2n} \sum_{i=1}^{n} (Z_{x,i} - Z_{x+h,i})^2$$

where h = lag;
n = number of sample pairs of lag h;
Z_x = value of variable Z at location x.

Plotting the semivariance against the lag typically produces a curve (the semivariogram) of distinctive form: the semivariance initially rises from some point on the *y* axis, reaches a threshold (the sill) at a certain location, and then levels off (Fig. 16.4). The rising curve of the semiovariogram thus defines the spatially correlated variation in the data. The point of intersection with the *y*

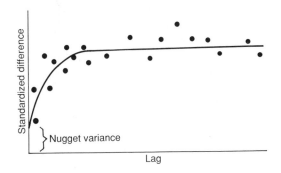

Fig. 16.4 The semiovariogram.

axis is known as the 'nugget variance' and defines the spatially uncorrelated variation, or noise.

So long as the nugget variance is not excessive, such that it swamps the spatial variation in the data, the semivariogram may be used to estimate values at intermediate locations within the survey area. Under these circumstances, kriging seems to provide a powerful interpolation procedure in a wide range of circumstances. It can be applied as an exact interpolator, such that estimated values will exactly equal the measured values at sample sites. No smoothing of the measured surface therefore occurs. This is a major advantage in some circumstances since, in contrast to many other interpolation methods, it means that the most reliable information available (i.e. that at the measured points) is retained.

On the other hand, where the measured values are themselves uncertain, kriging may result in over-fitting of the surface. Like the Laplacian-splines method, it also provides a measure of the estimator error, and thus gives an indication of the quality of the interpolation. Yet, like other methods, it is constrained by a number of circumstances: for example, it cannot provide reliable estimations where the noise in the data (as indicated by the nugget variance) is large. The presence of extreme values may also create instability in the models. In addition, kriging can become computationally impracticable when data sets are large, and may also cease to be conceptually valid when the area covered is inhomogeneous (i.e. when significant disjunct variation occurs). Kriging may also perform rather badly where the sampling network is clustered, since gaps then occur in the semivariogram. Nevertheless, the range

D. J. Briggs

of methods available, and the sequential nature of their operation, enables users to examine the results of the analysis as it proceeds, and to choose subsequent stages in analysis accordingly.

How effective kriging is as a spatial interpolator compared to other methods has been the subject of a number of studies in recent years. Laslett *et al.* (1987), for example, compared several interpolation methods, including kriging and spline interpolation. They concluded that kriging was the only method which performed satisfactorily in all circumstances. On the other hand, van Kuilienburg *et al.* (1982), found little difference in the performance of kriging, inverse-distance weighting, proximal mapping, and conventional choropleth mapping in relation to soil survey. Similarly, Abbass *et al.* (1990), comparing five techniques using geophysical data, concluded that no single method is universally appropriate, although on balance kriging and finite element methods seem to give the most satisfactory performance. The final choice, they suggest, must depend on the distribution of data points, the quality of interpolation needed, and computing power.

Conclusions

The mapping of environmental exposure is clearly an important objective. Reliable and detailed maps of exposure can aid both policy and research. At the broad level, they can help to inform health and environmental policy by indicating regions of potential health risk. At a more detailed scale, they provide vital precursors to local monitoring or experimental studies, by targeting specific areas of concern; likewise, they can help to sharpen the search for discrepancies in health outcome, and to identify their cause.

To date, however, the achievement of this potential has been limited. Most attempts at exposure mapping have amounted to little more than the mapping of pollution levels on the basis of relatively short-term surveys, or their (often intuitive) interpolation from limited monitoring sites. The search for disease clusters, and the testing of health impacts of putative pollution sources, similarly, still tend to rely on somewhat simplistic distance-decay models, which do not necessarily match the dispersion processes involved. With the parallel development of GIS techniques and more advanced methods of spatial interpolation, there is now the opportunity to apply far more rigorous and sensitive techniques. If these can be linked more closely to dynamic models of transfer processes and pathways in the environment, they can give powerful methods for epidemiological research. Yet, even then, they tackle only part of the problem; they still ignore the mechanisms by which humans encounter the pollutants involved. Beyond, therefore, lies an even greater challenge: the intersection of the two geographies—that of the pollutants in the environment and that of human distributions and activity.

References

Abbass, T. El, Jallouli, C., Albouy, Y., and Diament, M. (1990). A comparison of surface fitting alogorithms for geophysical data. *Terra Nova*, **2**, 467–75.

Akland, G. G., Hartwell, T. D., Johnson, T. R., and Whitmore, R. W. (1985). Measuring human exposure to carbon monoxide in Washington, D.C. and Denver, Colorado during the winter of 1982–1983. *Environment, Science and Technology*, **19**, 911–18.

Alauzet, A. and Joumard, R. (1989). Evaluation des emissions de pollutants en France, de 1970 a 2010. In *Man and his ecosystem. Proceedings of the 8th World Clean Air Congress, The Hague, 1989*, Vol. 4, (ed. L. J. Brasser and W. C. Mulder), pp. 423–8. Elsevier, The Hague.

Andresen, J. and Kyaw Tha Paw, U. (1985). Modelling of sulfur dioxide emissions and acidic precipitation at mesoscale distances. *Journal – Air Pollution Control Association*, **35**, 1159–63.

Archibold, O. W. and Crisp, P. T. (1983). The distribution of airborne metals in the Illawara region of New South Wales, Australia. *Applied Geography*, **3**, 331–44.

Barnard, R. and Olivett, G. (1990). Rapid assessment of industrial waste production based on available employment statistics. *Waste Management and Research*, **8**, 139–44.

Beavington, F. (1973). Contamination of soil with zinc, copper, lead and cadmium in the Wollongong city area. *Australian Journal of Soil Research*, **11**, 27–31.

Beavington, F. (1977). Trace elements in rainwater and dry deposition around a smelting complex. *Environmental Pollution*, **13**, 127–31.

Beiruti, A. A. R. and Al-Omishy, H. K. (1985). Traffic atmospheric diffusion model. *Atmospheric Environment*, **19**, 1519–24.

Briggs, D. J. and France, J. (1982). Mapping noise pollution from road traffic for regional environmental planning. *Journal of Environmental Management*, **14**, 173–9.

Briggs, D. J. and Reeve, D. E. (1992). Implications of incorporating environmental data into small area statistical analyses. In *Geographical methods in small area health studies. Proceedings of a meeting held on 22nd June 1990 at the London School of Hygiene and Tropical Medicine*, (ed. A. Westlake), pp. 109–26. Small Area Health Statistics Unit, London School of Hygiene and Tropical Medicine.

Burrough, P. A. (1986). *Principles of geographical information systems for land resources assessment,* Monographs on soil and resources survey, no. 12. Clarendon Press, Oxford.

Burrough, P. A. and Webster, R. (1980). Optimal interpolation and isarithmic mapping of soil properties. I. The semiovariogram and punctual kriging. *Journal of Soil Science*, **31**, 315–32.

Campbell, G. W. (1988). Measurements of nitrogen dioxide concentrations at rural sites in the United Kingdom. *Environmental Pollution*, **55**, 251–70.

Chytil, I. (1984). Dispersion of radioactive pollution in surface waters. *Ecological Modelling*, **26**, 145–53.

Commission of the European Communities (1985). *Quality of bathing water.* Commission of the European Communities, Brussels.

Commission of the European Communities (1986). *Quality of surface fresh water in the Community.* Commission of the European Communities, Brussels.

Commission of the European Communities (1989). *Exchange of information concerning atmospheric pollution by certain sulphur compounds and suspended particulates in the European Community.* Commission of the European Communities, Brussels.

Commission of the European Communities (1990). *CORINE: examples of the use of the results of the 1985–1990 Programme.* Directorate General of Environment, Nuclear Safety and Civil Protection, Brussels.

Department of the Environment (1984). *Digest of environmental protection and water statistics.* HMSO, London.

Department of the Environment (1988). *Monitoring of radioactivity in the UK environment.* HMSO, London.

Department of the Environment (1990). *Digest of environmental protection and water statistics.* HMSO, London.

Department of the Environment and Welsh Office (1986). *River quality in England and Wales, 1985.* HMSO, London.

Elliott, J. E., Norstrom, R. J., and Keith, J. A. (1988). Organochlorines and eggshell thinning in Northern Gannets (*Sula bassanus*) from eastern Canada, 1966–84. *Environmental Pollution,* **52**, 81–102.

Ericson, J. E. and Mishra, S. I. (1990). Soil lead concentrations and prevalence of hyperactive behaviour among school children in Ottawa, Canada. *Environment and Ecology,* **16**, 247–56.

Finzi, G., Bonelli, P., and Bacci, C. (1984). A stochastic model of surface windspeed for air quality control purposes. *Journal of Climate and Applied Meteorology,* **23**, 1354–61.

Gambolati, G. and Volpi, G. (1979). Groundwater contour mapping in Venice by stochastic interpolators. I. Theory. *Water Resources Research,* **15**, 281–92.

Gilbert, O. L. (1968). Bryophytes as indicators of air pollution in the Tyne Valley. *New Phytologist,* **67**, 15–30.

Goodman, G. T. and Smith, S. (1975). Relative burdens of airborne metals in South Wales. In *Report of a collaborative study on certain elements in air, soil, animals and humans in the Swansea–Neath–Port Talbot area together with a report on a moss bag study of atmospheric pollution across South Wales,* pp. 337–61. HMSO, Welsh Office, Cardiff.

Gould, P. R. (1990). Tracing Chernobyl's fallout. *Terra Nova,* **2**, 113–23.

Green, P. J. and Sibson, R. (1978). Computing Dirichlet tesselations in the plane. *Computing Journal,* **21**, 168–73.

Harrop, D. O., Mumby, K., Pepper, B., and Nolan, J. (1990). Heavy metal levels in the near vicinity to roads in a North London Borough. *Science of the Total Environment,* **93**, 543–6.

Hunt, G. J. (1989). *Radioactivity in surface and coastal waters of the British Isles, 1988. Aquatic Environment Monitoring Report.* MAFF, Directorate of Fisheries Research, Lowestoft.

Hutchinson, M. F. and Bischof, R. J. (1983). A new method for estimating the spatial distribution of mean seasonal and annual rainfall applied to the Hunter Valley, New South Wales. *Australian Meteorological Magazine,* **31**, 197–84.

Hutchinson, M. F., Booth, T. H., McMahon, J. P., and Nix, H. A. (1984*a*). Estimating monthly mean values of daily solar radiation for Australia. *Solar Energy,* **32**, 277–90.

Hutchinson, M. F., Kalma, J. D., and Johnson, M. E. (1984*b*). Monthly estimates of windspeed and windrun for Australia. *Journal of Climatology,*

Jaynes, S. M. and Cooke, R. U. (1987). Stone weathering in southeast England. *Atmospheric Environment,* **21**, 1601–22.

Jeffries, D. F. and Steele, A. K. (1989). Observed and predicted concentrations of caesium-137 in seawater of the Irish Sea, 1970–85. *Journal of Environmental Radioactivity,* **10**, 173–89.

Lajaunie, V. C. (1984). A geostatistical approach to air pollution modelling. In *Geostatistics for natural resources characterization*, (ed. G. Verly, M. David, A. G. Journel, and A. Marechal), pp. 877–91. Reidel, Dordrecht.

Laslett, G. M., McBratney, A. B., Pahl, P. J., and Hutchinson, M. F. (1987). Comparison of several prediction methods for soil pH. *Journal of Soil Science*, **38**, 325–70.

Lott, A. (1985). SO$_2$ concentrations near tall stacks. *Atmospheric Environment*, **19**, 1589–99.

MAFF (1990). *Radioactivity in food and agricultural products in England and Wales: Report for 1987*. Terrestrial Radioactivity Monitoring Programme. MAFF, London.

Matheron, G. (1971). *The theory of regionalised variables and its applications*. Les Cahiers du centre de morphologie mathematique de Fontainbleu. Ecole Nationale Superieure des Mines de Paris.

Moir, A. M. and Thornton, I. (1989). Lead and cadmium in urban allotment and garden soils and vegetables in the United Kingdom. *Environmental Geochemistry and Health*, **11**, 113–19.

Newton, I. (1979). *Population ecology of raptors*. T. & A. D. Poysner, Berkhampstead.

Nieboer, E., Richardson, D. H. S., and Tomassini, F. D. (1978). Mineral uptake and release by lichen: an overview. *The Bryologist*, **81**, 226–46.

Nyangababo, J. T. (1987). Lichen as monitors of aerial heavy metal pollution in and around Kampala. *Bulletin of Environmental Contamination and Toxicology*, **38**, 91–5.

Oliver, M. A. (1991). Disjunctive kriging: an aid to making decisions on environmental matters. *Area*, **23**, 19–24.

Oliver, M. A. and Webster, R. (1990). Kriging: a method of interpolation for geographical information systems. *International Journal of Geographical Information Systems*, **4**, 313–32.

Oliver, M. A., Webster, R., and Gerrard, A. J. W. (1989). Geostatistics in physical geography. I. Theory. *Transactions of the Institute of British Geographers N.S.*, **14**, 259–69.

Pavoni, B., Donazzolo, R., Marcomini, A., Degobbia, D., and Orio, A. A. (1987). Historical development of the Venice Lagoon contamination as recorded in radiodated sediment cores. *Marine Pollution Bulletin*, **18**, 18–24.

Reczynska-Dutka, M. (1986). Ecology of some waters in the forest-agricultural basin of the River Brynica near the Upper Silesia industrial region. 4: Atmospheric heavy metal pollution in the bottom sediments. *Acta Hydrobiologica*, **27**, 465–76.

Revitt, D. M., Hamilton, R. S., and Warren, R. S. (1990). The transport of heavy metals within a small urban catchment. *Science of the Total Environment*, **93**, 359–73.

Schintu, M., Sechi, N., Sarritzu, G., and Contu, A. (1989). Reservoir sediments as potential sources of heavy metals in drinking water (Sardinia, Italy). *Water Science and Technology*, **21**, 1891–4.

Simmons, S. A. and Pocock, R. L. (1987). Spatial variation in heavy metal deposition rates in urban areas. *Science of the Total Environment*, **59**, 243–51.

Simpson, R. W. (1990). A model to control emissions which avoid violations of PM10 health standards for both short and long term exposures. *Atmospheric Environment*, **24A**, 917–24.

Singh, M. P. (1990). Vulnerability analysis for airborne release of extremely hazardous substances. *Atmospheric Environment*, **24A**, 769–81.

Torgersen, T., Hutchinson, M. F., Searle, D. E., and Nix, H. A. (1983). General bathymetry of the Gulf of Carpentaria and the Quaternary physiography of Lake Carpentaria. *Palaeogeography, Palaeoclimatology, Palaeoecology*, **41**, 207–25.

van de Meent, D. (1990). Modelling intercompartmental transfers of pollutants: the case of lead. *Science of the Total Environment*, **90**, 41–54.

van Kuilenburg, J., de Gruijter, J. J., Marsman, B., and Bouma, J. (1982). Accuracy of spatial interpolation between point data on moisture supply capacity, compared with estimates from mapping units. *Geoderma*, **27**, 311–25.

Warren Springs Laboratory (1990). *UK smoke and SO₂ monitoring networks: summary tables for 1989*. Warren Springs Laboratory, Stevenage.

Webster, R. and Burgess, T. M. (1983). Spatial variation in soil and the role of kriging. *Agricultural Water Management*, **6**, 111–22.

Webster, R. and Oliver, M. (1989). Disjunctive kriging in agriculture. *Geostatistics*, Vol. 1, (ed. M. Armstrong), pp. 421–32. Reidel, Dordrecht.

Yocum, J. E. (1962). Effects of air pollution on materials. In *Air pollution*, Vol. 1, (ed. A. C. Stern), pp. 199–219. Academic Press, London.

III Statistical methods

Introduction

The chapters in this section deal with the analysis of geographical phenomena which occur on different scales. At the largest scale, questions of ecological bias become paramount and they are discussed by Richardson. At intermediate scales problems of autocorrelation and the need for smoothing are most critical, and these are considered by Richardson, and Clayton and Bernardinelli. At very localized scales, random variation is the dominant problem and the remaining chapters by Bithell, Hills, and Alexander and Cuzick study the questions related to clusters and clustering in a variety of different contexts.

Spatial statistics is currently an active area of methodological research, and several theoretical ideas are being developed. Three main features of spatial problems have stimulated this activity. One is the problem of autocorrelation. Unlike many statistical problems, where a series of independent observations are made, here the spatial structure must be taken into account. For many variables, nearby sampling points are more likely to be similar than distant points and they cannot be regarded as independent samples.

Another important feature is the large amount of replication that is available, especially when disease rates are being mapped, so that the same calculations are performed in several small areas. This leads naturally to the use of Bayesian or empirical Bayes methods, and disease mapping is probably one of the best examples of the utility of the 'shrinkage estimators' first proposed by James and Stein.

These two concepts feature largely in the first two chapters of this section. Richardson discusses methods applicable for studies of large areas, and carefully reviews methods that are appropriate for large-scale correlation studies and spatial regression analyses. A key feature in this work is the use of models that acknowledge, estimate, and adjust for spatial autocorrelation. Problems of ecological bias, which can lead to inaccurate estimates of risk coefficients, and issues of study design, are also discussed. Clayton and Bernardinelli's chapter focuses on the mapping problem, with particular attention directed towards smoothing maps of rates computed for small areas. Because the number of cases in each area is small, these raw rates are very erratic and an unsmoothed map of them exhibits wild variations and is uninformative. Use of the spatial correlation structure, along with Bayesian concepts, suggest ways of smoothing these maps. This chapter reviews the theory of these estimators and applies it to two examples.

A third major area of interest in spatial statistics is the detection of localized clustering of events. Generally this occurs on too small a scale to be detectable by the smoothing methods illustrated in the first two chapters. Another problem is the *post hoc* nature of many cluster investigations. This area still does not have a solid theoretical foundation and several new methods are currently being investigated. Bithell reviews methods for assessing the existence of an increased incidence of disease around a point source, and addresses several important theoretical issues. Hills develops these ideas further and provides an example from a study of multiple point sources, where new questions arise. Alexander and Cuzick take a different approach and focus on the question of the existence of clustering as a general phenomenon without regard to any particular source or individual cluster. A novel problem here is the detection of disease clustering in populations that are known to be unevenly distributed in space, and several new methods for studying this question are reviewed.

17. Statistical methods for geographical correlation studies

S. Richardson

Ecological correlation studies analyse associations between a set of variables defined on aggregated groups of individuals. Within this class, geographical correlation studies are particularly concerned with the joint variation or correlation of variables which represent averages over geographically defined regions.

An example of a geographical correlation study is presented in Chapter 30. Further interesting examples of geographical correlation studies of cancer in relation to major environmental risk factors have been carried out. Several studies have examined water quality. For example, cancer and fluoridation (Chilvers 1983) or type of water (Carpenter and Beresford 1986) has been studied at a large scale and also on a smaller scale. Gastric cancer and leukaemia in relation to dibromochloropropane have been studied at county level (Wong *et al.* 1989), and the influence of chemical toxic waste disposal sites on the surrounding cancer mortality via the pollution of ground water has been studied at a local level (Najem *et al.* 1985). Air pollution studies have mostly been concerned with the link with lung cancer (Buffler *et al.* 1988). Some studies have tried to relate background radiation and cancer mortality, in particular leukaemia (Edling *et al.* 1982). Pesticide use in agriculture and cancer has also been investigated at the geographical level (Stokes and Brace 1988). Finally, industrial exposure has often been correlated with cancer mortality either via the proportion of workers in particular industries (Blot and Fraumeni 1976, 1977) or through the pollution of the surrounding area (Matanoski *et al.* 1981).

When considering results from such studies, it is necessary to be aware of the methodological problems that arise from their design. These problems fall broadly into two categories: statistical problems connected with the spatial structure of the data and problems of interpretation and bias due to the nature of the data.

The statistical methods used in geographical correlation studies are strongly dependent on the scale and the type of geographical variations to be analysed. The testing of geographical association has been classically performed by correlation or regression in studies where measurement errors within each area on the variables of interest are negligible in comparison to the between area variations of the mean of these variables. On the other hand, in small-area studies it is necessary to include a further source of variation corresponding to Poisson fluctuations around the mean within each area. Consequently smoothing methods are needed to study spatial patterns or spatial association, otherwise spurious results might emerge. For instance, positive spatial auto-correlation, resulting solely from the lesser variability of rates in nearby populated town districts versus the greater variability of rates in less populated country districts, would often be detected. The statistical problem of studying association in small-area studies can thus be formulated within the framework of estimation methods for mapping disease rates. For instance, environmental variables can be included as known explanatory variables linked to the mean in the a priori distribution of the rates by regression parameters. Statistical assessment of the regression parameters will then be based on the a posteriori distribution. These methods will be described in detail in the next chapter, and for the remainder of this chapter within-area measurement error will not be considered.

Before investigating the nature of the association between a health indicator and some environmental variable, it is useful to assess as a first step the spatial structure of the health variable alone, which may or may not show a trend or contain outliers, and the type of models that can be used to assess the localized spatial dependence.

Statistical models of spatial variations

Spatial variation can often be thought of as resulting from the superposition of a regular, slowly varying component, analogous to the trend observed in many time-series (referred to as a spatial gradient or a trend surface), and smaller-scale variations around the gradient. As with time-series, this decomposition cannot be specified uniquely and, in practice, the same data might be analysed as stationary with long-range correlations or as having a non-stationary mean and smaller-scale variations. Nevertheless, in epidemiological applications, a gradient structure shared by chronic diseases and exposure indicators alike has been observed at a national level. For example, there is a north-west to south-east gradient for cardiovascular diseases in England which parallels the gradient of a number of socio-economic characteristics or nutritional habits (Pocock et al. 1982); there are also strong north–south contrasts in Italy (Cislaghi et al. 1990), and other examples can be found in Lazar (1982).

Gradients can be represented by linear or polynomial functions of the chosen coordinates for each area, and estimated by regression methods (Cliff and Ord 1981; Ripley 1981; Upton and Fingelton 1985). The fitted trend surface should include all the polynomial terms of a given order to ensure independence from the chosen coordinate scheme. Numerical problems which might occur when fitting high-order surfaces are discussed in Ripley (1981). In particular, it might be desirable to scale the domain to about a square with sides $[-1, +1]$ to avoid extreme values of the polynomial terms. Classical regression methods for fitting gradients are only valid when the residuals have no spatial structure, which is not commonly the case. Autocorrelation tests of the ordinary least squares (OLS) residuals are described in Cliff and Ord (1981) and Ripley (1981). When autocorrelation is present, estimation should proceed by generalized least squares (GLS) or maximum likelihood (ML) with a spatially structured covariance error matrix. These techniques are discussed later in this chapter in the general context of regression with spatially correlated errors.

Alternatively, Cressie (1986) suggested a robust decomposition into gradient-like variations and residuals obtained by overlaying a grid with rows and columns over the area, identifying each district with a particular node of the grid and then using median polish with row and column effects to capture the spatial trend. In an exploratory analysis of sudden infant death syndrome (SIDS) data for the counties of North Carolina, Cressie and Read (1989) carried out weighted median polish on a transformation of the death counts to capture the large-scale variation.

When present in both the exposure and the health indicator rates, gradients complicate interpretation of joint variations since many potential confounder variables may also show the same regular spatial pattern. Hence it is worth investigating the association both before and after the removal of a gradient.

Once the gradient has been identified, it is interesting to investigate whether the residual variations display some spatial pattern indicating the possible influence of exogeneous variables. Of particular interest is the detection of spatial autocorrelation of a variable, which corresponds to the observation throughout the whole spatial domain of similar values in nearby areas. Moran's autocorrelation coefficient, I, has been used to test for spatial auto-correlation in irregular domains. It requires the *a priori* definition of geographical proximity of the areas via a weight matrix $W = \{W_{ij}\}$. The choice of W and the test of I under different null models have been extensively discussed (Cliff and Ord 1981). Some explanatory spatial analysis to detect anomalous spatial values might also be carried out at this stage by inspecting the residuals from a local trend surface or investigating the influence of specific points on the sample autocorrelation function (Cressie and Read 1989; Wartenberg 1990).

Several models have been proposed to characterize further the spatial patterns. Simultaneous autoregressive models (SAR) link the value of the variable in the ith area, Y_i, to a linear function of the values of Y in nearby areas and a random error term without spatial structure (Whittle 1954). For conditional, or Markovian, autoregressive models (CAR), it is the conditional expectation of Y_i with respect to all other values of Y which is defined as a linear function of the values of Y in nearby areas (Besag 1974). Properties of these models have been detailed by many authors and they are briefly summarized here.

A SAR gaussian model for a process with observations Y_i, $1 \leq i \leq N$, at N sites of a domain A is defined by N simultaneous equations:

$$Y_i = \mu_i + \sum_{j=1}^{N} S_{ij} (Y_j - \mu_j) + \epsilon_i, \ 1 \leq i \leq N, \tag{1}$$

where $S_{ii} = 0$ for all i and $\{\epsilon_i, \ 1 \leq i \leq N\}$ are independent gaussian variables with zero mean and variance σ_i^2. Denoting by S the matrix $\{S_{ij}, \ 1 \leq i,j \leq N\}$ and I the identity $N \times N$ matrix, a necessary and sufficient condition for the existence of a set of Y_i satisfying this relation is that $I - S$ is non-singular. Then the distribution of $\mathbf{Y}$ must be multivariate normal $MN(\mu, V_S)$ with $\mu = \{\mu_i, \ 1 \leq i \leq N\}$ and $V_S = (I - S)^{-1} \, \text{diag}(\sigma_1^2, \ldots, \sigma_N^2) \, (I - S^t)^{-1}$.

This model is over parametrized and some simplifying assumptions are needed to be able to estimate it. The simpler SAR model of order 1 expresses the spatial dependence in terms of a known proximity matrix, $W = (W_{ij}, 1 \leq i,j \leq N)$ and an overall parameter a, by imposing the condition: $S_{ij} = a \, W_{ij}$ in Equation (1). Restrictions are also usually made on μ_i and σ_i^2, $1 \leq i \leq N$.

A CAR gaussian model for $\mathbf{Y}$ is defined by the following conditional relationships:

$$\begin{cases} E(Y_i \mid y_j, j \neq i) = \mu_i + \sum_{j=1}^{N} C_{ij} (y_j - \mu_j) \\[2mm] V(Y_i \mid y_j, j \neq i) = \sigma_i^2 \end{cases} \tag{2}$$

and the conditional distribution of Y_i is gaussian, $i = 1, \ldots, N$.

Denoting by C the matrix $\{C_{ij}, \ 1 \leq i,j \leq N\}$, with $C_{ii} = 0$ for all i as previously, a necessary and sufficient condition for existence is that the matrix $\text{diag} (\sigma_1^2, \ldots \sigma_N^2)^{-1} \, (I - C)$ is symmetric and strictly positive definite. Then the distribution of $\mathbf{Y}$ is multivariate normal $MN(\mu, V_C)$ with $V_C = (I - C)^{-1} \, \text{diag} (\sigma_1^2, \ldots \sigma_N^2)$. Note that the symmetry condition implies that $C_{ij} \sigma_j^2 = C_{ji} \sigma_i^2$ for all i,j and positive definiteness implies the existence of $(I - C)^{-1}$. Cressie and Chan (1989) also comment that the coefficients C_{ij} can be interpreted as partial correlation coefficients since $\text{corr} \, (Y_i, Y_j \mid y_k, k \neq i,j)$ $= \text{sign} \, (C_{ij}) \times (C_{ij} C_{ji})^{1/2}$. In the CAR model of order 1, it is assumed that $C_{ij} = a W_{ij}$ in Equation (2) with W satisfying the symmetry condition: $W_{ij} \sigma_j^2 = W_{ji} \sigma_i^2$.

The difference in the simultaneous and conditional formulations implies that for a SAR process, the $\{\epsilon_i, \ 1 \leq i \leq N\}$ are white noise, with ϵ_i correlated with Y_j, $j \neq i$ since $\text{cov}(\mathbf{Y}, \epsilon) = \text{diag} \, (\sigma_1^2, \ldots, \sigma_N^2) \, (I - S^t)^{-1}$; whereas for a CAR process, the innovations $\eta = (I - C) \, (\mathbf{Y} - \mu)$ are correlated, $\text{cov}(\eta) = \text{diag} \, (\sigma_1^2, \ldots, \sigma_N^2) \, (I - C)$ but $\text{cov}(\eta, \mathbf{Y}) = \text{diag}(\sigma_1^2, \ldots, \sigma_N^2)$.

Estimation for CAR and SAR models can be done by maximum likelihood. For autoregressive (AR) processes of order 1, this can be done numerically without too much computational effort once the eigenvalues of W have been computed. Ripley (1988) discusses some numerical problems connected with the maximization of the likelihood. Convenient expressions for the Fisher information and the asymptotic standard errors of $\hat{a}$ in SAR and CAR models are given by Martin (1990b).

Cressie and Chan (1989) fitted a CAR model to the residual variations of the Freeman–Tukey transformed number of SIDS deaths by counties after removal of large-scale variations. They discuss at length the choice of weights. To take into account different population sizes, n_i, of the counties, they defined the conditional variance as inversely proportional to n_i, $(\sigma_i^2 = \sigma^2/n_i)$. Inspecting the variogram, they judged that local dependence did not extend beyond 30 miles and hence they set $C_{ij} = 0$ if $d(i,j)$ is larger than 30 miles, where $d(i,j)$ is the cartesian distance between the seats of the counties i and j. For $d(i,j)$ less than 30 miles, they modelled W_{ij} as proportional to $d(i,j)^{-k}$, where k indicates how fast the spatial dependence decreases. Recalling the symmetry condition for the CAR process, this leads to $C_{ij} = a\,[c(k)d(i,j)^{-k}]\,(n_i/n_j)^{1/2}$, $k = 0, 1, 2$ where $c(k)$ is a constant set to ensure comparability across k. They compared the likelihoods for different values of k, chose $k = 1$ and found weak evidence of a spatial structure when explanatory variables were included in the modelling of the mean.

The spatial structure indicated by a CAR model of order 1 may appear unreasonable for an irregular domain, as the condition $W_{ij}\sigma_j^2 = W_{ji}\sigma_i^2$ with W symmetric does not allow the conditional variances to depend on the number of neighbours of each area. For an SAR process of order 1, the conditional variance given by

$$\mathrm{var}(Y_i \mid y_j, j \neq i) = \sigma^2 (1 + a^2 \sum_j W_{ji}^2),$$

depends in a constrained way both on the parameter a and the weights of neighbours. Extending Künsch's (1987) terminology to irregular domains, Besag (see Besag *et al.* 1991) proposes a generalization of the CAR model, the intrinsic gaussian conditional autoregression (ICAR), where Y_i has an improper multivariate normal distribution. In the particular case where W is the 0–1 contiguity matrix, the conditional mean is assumed to be a perfect local average (no overall non-zero constant mean):

$$E(Y_i \mid y_j, j \neq i) = \frac{1}{W_i^+} \sum_j W_{ij} y_j, \quad W_i^+ = \sum_j W_{ij},$$

the conditional variance to be inversely proportional to the number W_i^+ of neighbours:

$$V(Y_i \mid y_j, j \neq i) = \sigma^2 / W_i^+,$$

and the conditional distributions to be gaussian.

In an ICAR model, the variance–covariance matrix of the $\{Y_i, 1 \leq i \leq N\}$ is not defined since its inverse $\tilde{V}^{-1}$ is equal to $\sigma^{-2}[\mathrm{diag}(W_1^+, \ldots, W_N^+) - W]$ which is only positive semi-definite with a zero eigenvalue. The ICAR model has only one variance parameter, σ^2, which can nevertheless be estimated from the likelihood which involves only $\tilde{V}^{-1}$.

This model assumes a very strong spatial dependence. To accommodate other sources of variations, an additive process can be defined which combines an intrinsic process and additional random errors having no spatial structure (Besag *et al.* 1991). Precisely, **Y** is defined as the sum of a gaussian ICAR process with parameter σ^2 and a vector of independent gaussian variables with mean μ_i and common variance τ^2. The ratio $v = \tau^2/\sigma^2$ measures in some way the strength of the spatial structure, being large if the spatial dependence is weak. The joint distribution of the $\{Y_i, 1 \leq i \leq N\}$ is again an improper multivariate normal distribution with mean μ. The likelihood can be expressed simply in terms of σ^2 and v and hence these parameters can be estimated by maximum likelihood. This is discussed in detail in Mollié (1990) where the Fisher information for the parameters is also given.

SAR and CAR models have been fitted to standardized cancer mortality log transformed data in France both by maximum likelihood and as prior models in an empirical Bayes smoothing of the mortality rates for rare sites (Mollié and Richardson 1991). Table 17.1, extracted from Mollié (1990), gives

Table 17.1 Cancer mortality in 95 French *départements*: maximum likelihood estimation of parameters for different spatial models (from Mollié 1990)

Cancer site	Models						
	CAR		SAR			Additive	
	$\hat{\sigma}^2$	$\hat{a}$	$\hat{\sigma}^2$	$\hat{a}$	$\hat{v}$	$\hat{\sigma}^2$	$\hat{\tau}^2$
Gallbladder (M)	0.078	0.123	0.079	0.072	1.357	0.043	0.058
(SE)	(0.012)	(0.036)	(0.012)	(0.026)	(1.096)	(0.028)	
Multiple myeloma (M)	0.038	0.070	0.038	0.042	∞	0	0.041
(SE)	(0.006)	(0.053)	(0.006)	(0.030)			(0.006)
Gallbladder (F)	0.070	0.168	0.064	0.145	0	0.236	0
(SE)	(0.010)	(0.004)	(0.010)	(0.013)	(0.054)	(0.072)	
Thyroid (F)	0.094	0.166	0.094	0.128	0.214	0.225	0.048
(SE)	(0.014)	(0.008)	(0.014)	(0.017)	(0.177)	(0.093)	

M, male; F, female; SE, standard error.

maximum likelihood estimates for the parameters of first order SAR, CAR, and additive models for four cancer sites over the period 1971–78. The W matrix was defined by binary weights corresponding to contiguity between the 95 French *départements*. The significance levels of the autocorrelation parameters are similar for SAR and CAR. When there is no spatial structure (in the case of multiple myeloma), the additive model gives all the weight to the spatially random component. Note that forcing a SAR or CAR model for this site has led to a slight underestimation of the variance. At the other extreme, for highly autocorrelated sites (female gallbladder and thyroid), the intrinsic component is largely predominant with variance estimate compatible with that of the CAR process (the average number of neighbours is between three and four). For male gallbladder, there is some discrepancy between the additive model and the autoregressive models. The additive model gives similar weight to the two components, but a large standard error for the variance of the intrinsic component which is not significantly different from zero; whereas first-order SAR and CAR models both find significant autocorrelation parameters.

An alternative way to specify a spatial model in the gaussian framework is to choose directly a parametric functional form for the variance–covariance matrix of the multinormal distribution of **Y**, which is linked to the spatial configuration of the sites. This approach is used in kriging and interpolation (Ripley 1981). Direct representation of the variance–covariance error matrix in spatial regression is also commonly used and estimation procedures in this context will be detailed on pp. 190–3.

Adjustment for spatial autocorrelation in correlation or regression

Modified test of correlation coefficients

A first step in the analysis of geographical correlation studies is often the calculation and testing of correlation coefficients between pairs of variables (X, Y) over the N locations of a domain A.

The consequences of neglecting the autocorrelation in the X and Y variables were first pointed out by Bartlett (1935) in the case of stationary time-series. When the autocorrelations are positive, the significance levels of classical tests are overestimated. This phenomenon is more pronounced for spatially auto-correlated variables, with observed significance levels for tests with nominal 5 per cent level increased up to 50 per cent in highly positively autocorrelated cases.

A modified test of the correlation coefficient r_{XY} has been proposed by Clifford *et al.* (1989) for investigating the association between a pair of variables (X, Y). It modifies the degrees of freedom of the classical test of r_{XY}. An effective sample size is calculated based on an estimation of the variance of r_{XY} which takes account of the internal autocorrelations of X and Y. In the case of positive autocorrelation of both variables, this effective sample size, hence the degrees of freedom, will be less than the number of geographical units.

Now suppose that $\mathbf{X}$ and $\mathbf{Y}$ are independent multivariate normal vectors with constant means and $N \times N$ variance–covariance matrices $\Sigma_\mathbf{X}$ and $\Sigma_\mathbf{Y}$, respectively. It can be shown that, to the first order, the variance σ_r^2 of $r_{\mathbf{XY}}$ is given by:

$$\sigma_r^2 \doteq \frac{\mathrm{var}(s_{\mathbf{XY}})}{E(s_\mathbf{X}^2)\,E(s_\mathbf{Y}^2)} \tag{3}$$

where $s_{\mathbf{XY}}$ denotes the empirical covariance between pairs of observations $\mathbf{X}$ and $\mathbf{Y}$ over the N locations, and $s_\mathbf{X}^2$ and $s_\mathbf{Y}^2$ are the empirical variances of $\mathbf{X}$ and $\mathbf{Y}$ respectively.

To estimate $\mathrm{var}(s_{\mathbf{XY}})$ we impose a stratified structure for $\Sigma_\mathbf{X}$ and $\Sigma_\mathbf{Y}$. More precisely, the N^2 locations are divided into K strata $S_0, S_1, S_2, \ldots, S_K$, with $S_0 = \{(\alpha,\alpha),\ \alpha = 1, \ldots N\}$, so that the covariances within strata remain constant, that is $\mathrm{cov}(X_\alpha, X_\beta) = C_\mathbf{X}(k)$, for two locations α and β in stratum S_k. This formulation is flexible enough to allow for non-isotropy or some form of non-stationarity.

An estimate of the variance of $s_{\mathbf{XY}}$ is then given by:

$$\sum_{k=0}^{K} N_k\, \widehat{C}_\mathbf{X}(k)\, \widehat{C}_\mathbf{Y}(k)/N^2, \tag{4}$$

where N_k is the number of pairs of variables in stratum S_k, and $\widehat{C}_\mathbf{X}(k)$ and $\widehat{C}_\mathbf{Y}(k)$ are estimated autocovariances

$$\widehat{C}_\mathbf{X}(k) = \sum_{S_k} (X_\alpha - \overline{X})\,(X_\beta - \overline{X})/N_k,$$

where $\overline{\mathbf{X}}$ is the mean vector over all locations. Thus the estimate takes into account the autocorrelation of both $\mathbf{X}$ and $\mathbf{Y}$. Equations (3) and (4) lead to the following estimate of the variance of $r_{\mathbf{XY}}$:

$$\widehat{\sigma}_r^2 = \frac{\sum N_k\, \widehat{C}_\mathbf{X}(k)\, \widehat{C}_\mathbf{Y}(k)}{N^2\, s_\mathbf{X}^2\, s_\mathbf{Y}^2} \tag{5}$$

In the classical non-autocorrelated case, when either $\Sigma_\mathbf{X}$ or $\Sigma_\mathbf{Y} = I$, it can be shown that the approximation given by Equation (3) is exact and that $(N-2)^{1/2} r_{\mathbf{XY}}/(1 - r^2_{\mathbf{XY}})^{1/2}$ follows a t-distribution with $N-2$ degrees of freedom (df), denoted t_{N-2}. Further, $N = 1 + 1/\widehat{\sigma}_r^2$.

In general, an estimated effective sample size, M is defined by the relationship

$$M = 1 + 1/\sigma_r^2,$$

where $\widehat{\sigma}_r^2$ is given by Equation (5). A modified t-test: t_{M-2} is proposed which rejects the null hypothesis of no association when:

$$\left| \frac{r\sqrt{(\hat{M}-2)}}{\sqrt{(1-r^2)}} \right| > t^{\alpha}{}_{\hat{M}-2} \tag{6}$$

where $t^{\alpha}{}_{\hat{M}-2}$ is the critical value of the t-statistic with $\hat{M}-2$ degrees of freedom.

The modified $t_{\hat{M}-2}$ test can be simply extended to test the partial correlation between two variables $(\mathbf{X}, \mathbf{Y})$ adjusted on variables $\mathbf{Z}_1, \ldots, \mathbf{Z}_p$. We suppose that the vector $(\mathbf{X}, \mathbf{Y}, \mathbf{Z}_1, \ldots, \mathbf{Z}_p)$ follows a multivariate normal distribution. Testing that the partial correlation between $\mathbf{X}$ and $\mathbf{Y}$ conditional on $\mathbf{Z}_1, \ldots, \mathbf{Z}_p$ is zero is equivalent to testing that the correlation between the residuals of the regression of $\mathbf{X}$ on $\mathbf{Z}_1, \ldots, \mathbf{Z}_p$ and of $\mathbf{Y}$ on $\mathbf{Z}_1, \ldots, \mathbf{Z}_p$ is zero. Hence, the modified test can be extended to test the partial correlation by considering the relevant variance–covariances in the conditional distributions of $\mathbf{X}$ and $\mathbf{Y}$ and carrying out the same adjustment of the degrees of freedom. This adjustment will now take into account spatial autocorrelation in the conditional distributions.

In practice, this implies using the modified $t_{\hat{M}-2}$ statistic on the OLS residuals of the linear regression of $\mathbf{X}$ on $\mathbf{Z}_1, \ldots, \mathbf{Z}_p$ and of $\mathbf{Y}$ on $\mathbf{Z}_1, \ldots, \mathbf{Z}_p$, respectively. The following steps are followed:

(1) regress $\mathbf{X}$ on $\mathbf{Z}_1, \ldots \mathbf{Z}_p$ by OLS giving estimated residuals $\hat{\mathbf{U}}$;
(2) regress $\mathbf{Y}$ on $\mathbf{Z}_1, \ldots \mathbf{Z}_p$ by OLS giving estimated residuals $\hat{\mathbf{V}}$;
(3) test the correlation coefficient between $\hat{\mathbf{U}}$ and $\hat{\mathbf{V}}$ using the modified test statistic $t_{\hat{M}-2}$ given in Equation (6) with

$$\hat{M} = (\widehat{\text{var } r_{\hat{U},\hat{V}}})^{-1} + 1. \tag{7}$$

If the residuals $\mathbf{U}$ and $\mathbf{V}$ are not autocorrelated, the variance of the partial correlation coefficient is $1/(N-2)$, hence $\hat{M} = N-1$ as usual.

Monte Carlo studies show that the $t_{\hat{M}-2}$ statistic for testing correlations or partial correlations has indeed a correct significance level (Clifford *et al.* 1989; Richardson 1990*a*). Its power was also shown to be comparable to that of the standard tests of simple or partial correlations, provided that these tests used degrees of freedom compatible with the observed empirical variance of the correlations.

Spatial regression

Testing the association between a dependent variable $\mathbf{Y}$ and a set of independent variables $\mathbf{X}$ can also be tackled by regression techniques. When the variables are spatially distributed it is likely that the assumption of independent errors is violated and that, even after allowing for the spatial structure of the measured variables $\mathbf{X}$, there remains some autocorrelation coming from unidentified or non-measurable spatially distributed variables linked to $\mathbf{Y}$.

The framework is the following: we have a gaussian process $\{Y(\alpha), \alpha \in A\}$ defined on a domain A containing N locations. We have a set of non-random regressors $X = \{\mathbf{X}_1, \ldots \mathbf{X}_p\}$ defined throughout A and we suppose that:

$$\mathbf{Y} = X\beta + \mathbf{U}$$

where β is a $\mathbf{p} \times 1$ vector of parameters and U follows a multinormal distribution $N(\mathbf{0}, \sigma^2 D_U)$.

The log likelihood can be written (up to an additive constant) as:

$$L(\beta, \sigma^2, \mathbf{Y}) = -\frac{1}{2}\log |D_U| - \frac{1}{2}N\log \sigma^2 - \frac{1}{2\sigma^2}(\mathbf{Y} - X\beta)D_U^{-1}(\mathbf{Y} - X\beta).$$

When D_U is known, maximizing over β and σ^2 leads to:

$$\hat{\beta} = (X^t D_U^{-1} X)^{-1} X^t D_U^{-1} \mathbf{Y}.$$

$$\hat{\sigma}^2 = \frac{1}{N}(\mathbf{Y} - X\hat{\beta})^t D_U^{-1}(\mathbf{Y} - X\hat{\beta}).$$

Since the matrix D_U is only rarely known, tests of the regression coefficient β are done conditionally on an estimated structure for D_U. Usually D_U is modelled as $D_U(\theta)$ in terms of a q dimensional vector of parameters θ. In this case the MLE of θ is the value that globally maximizes the profile likelihood:

$$L_p(\theta, \mathbf{Y}) = -\frac{1}{2}\log |D_U(\theta)| - \frac{N}{2}(\log \hat{\sigma}^2)$$

which is only dependent on θ. Maximum likelihood estimation thus involves in the first place the choice of a parametric model for D_U and in a second stage the numerical maximization of the profile likelihood L_p.

The class of spatial autoregressive models (cf. pp. 182–7) has been proposed for modelling $\mathbf{U}$ by analogy to the commonly used time-series method of ARMA modelling of residual errors in regression (Ord 1975). Alternatively, and particularly in the case of non-lattice data, one might specify directly a parametric form for D_U, using what is referred to by Mardia (1990) as direct representation (DR).

Ripley (1981) and Mardia and Watkins (1989) discuss classes of spatial covariance functions that ensure that D_U is always positive definite. For isotropic correlation schemes, the correlation between two points α and β with euclidean distance $d_{\alpha\beta}$ between them is only a function of $d_{\alpha\beta}$. For the disc and spherical models, the correlation between two points is defined as proportional to the intersection area of two discs or two spheres of common radius centred on those points. The corresponding functional form of the correlation can be written as:

$$f_D(r;a) = \begin{cases} \frac{2}{\pi}[\cos^{-1}(\frac{r}{a}) - \frac{r}{a}(1 - \frac{r^2}{a^2})^{1/2}], & 0 \leq r \leq a \\ 0 & r > a \end{cases}$$

for the disc correlation scheme, with radius a, and as:

$$f_S(r;a) = \begin{cases} 1 - \frac{3}{2}(\frac{r}{a}) + \frac{1}{2}(\frac{r^3}{a^3}), \ 0 \le r \le a \\ 0 \qquad\qquad\qquad\quad r > a \end{cases}$$

for the spherical correlation scheme with radius a. These correlation functions both exhibit a fairly linear decrease with increasing distance. A different shape of decrease can be modelled with the help of the two-parameter family of functions. The power correlation scheme defined by:

$$f_P(r;m,a) = \begin{cases} (1 - \frac{r}{a})^m, \ 0 \le r \le a \\ 0 \qquad\quad r > a \end{cases}$$

is such a family, as well as the Bessel correlation scheme, introduced by Whittle (1954), defined by:

$$f_B(r;m,a) = [2^{m-1}\Gamma(m)]^{-1} (ar)^m K_m(ar), \ m > 0, a > 0$$

where K_m are the modified Bessel functions. Setting $m = \frac{1}{2}$ gives an exponential correlation function depending only on one parameter. A more general form of exponential decrease depending on two coefficients can also be defined by:

$$f_E(r;\gamma,\lambda) = \gamma e^{-\lambda r}$$

and was used by Cook and Pocock (1983).

Including the possibility of anisotropy, Vecchia (1988) considered a general form for a rational spectral density function of a two-dimensional process, whose correlation can be expressed in terms of derivatives of the Bessel function $K_0(ar)$. This family of correlation schemes overlaps partially with those introduced by Whittle.

For stationary processes defined on a lattice, a class of separable processes has been considered by Martin (1979) with the property that the correlation function $f(\alpha_1 - \beta_1, \ \alpha_2 - \beta_2)$ between two points in $Z^2 : \alpha = (\alpha_1, \ \alpha_2)$ and $\beta = (\beta_1, \ \beta_2)$, is equal to $f(\alpha_1 - \beta_1, 0) . f(0, \ \alpha_2 - \beta_2)$. Since the two-dimensional correlation structure is simply a product of two one-dimensional correlation structures along rows and columns, many results from time-series modelling can be extended to the class of separable processes. This class of correlation schemes is not isotropic and the effect on the correlation of its rows and columns renders it unsuitable for irregularly spaced data which arise, for example, from aggregation into arbitrary administrative areas.

Mardia and Marshall (1984) have studied the asymptotic properties of the maximum likelihood estimators $(\hat{\beta}, \ \hat{\sigma}^2, \ \hat{\theta})$. Assuming that $\mathbf{Y}$ is a Gaussian process, they give conditions that ensure the consistency and the asymptotic normality of $(\hat{\beta}, \ \hat{\sigma}^2, \ \hat{\theta})$. The information matrix for $(\hat{\beta}, \ \hat{\sigma}^2, \ \hat{\theta})$ is also given. A sufficient condition for continuity of the information is that $f(\cdot\,;\theta)$ is twice differentiable with continuous second derivative. This condition does not hold for the spherical correlation scheme at $r = a$. If θ is known, then there is no bias in the maximum likelihood estimate $\hat{\beta}$. In other cases the bias in $\hat{\beta}$ is in $o(N^{-1})$ (Mardia 1990).

In a study aimed at assessing qualitatively the small-sample properties of the maximum likelihood estimators, Mardia and Marshall simulated 300 replicates of the spherical correlation scheme for sample sizes: $N = 6,8,10$. They note that $\hat{\sigma}^2$ is significantly negatively biased for $N = 6$ and 8. This might imply an underestimation of the standard errors of $\hat{\beta}$, the more so since these standard errors are also estimated conditionally on the estimated $\hat{a}$. Note that for the full Bayes approach considered in the next chapter, uncertainty in the estimation of $\hat{\theta}$ is taken into account in the empirical confidence interval obtained for $\hat{\beta}$ by simulations.

It has been pointed out recently by several authors that maximum likelihood estimation can encounter numerical difficulties even when the number of data points does not prohibit the computation of the maximum likelihood estimate. The profile likelihood can be multimodal and hence some procedures for finding the maximum (e.g. scoring) might only ensure convergence to the nearest local maximum. Examples of bad behaviour are given by Warnes and Ripley (1987). In the case of a CAR model of order 1 with constant overall mean, Ripley (1988) shows unimodality of the profile likelihood as long as $\mathbf{Y}$ is not an eigenvector of W corresponding to the maximal eigenvalue.

Mardia and Watkins (1989) have investigated multimodality in the DR framework. Their study indicates that for small samples, multimodality can be quite frequent for a number of covariance schemes and that for the spherical scheme, this phenomenon is also increased with N, possibly in connection with the lack of a second derivative for the likelihood with respect to the range parameter, a, for this scheme. They recommend that a graphical study of the profile likelihood $L_p(\theta,\mathbf{Y})$. $L_p(\theta,\mathbf{Y})$ can easily be drawn in the cases that they have considered, where the shape of the covariance is modelled in terms of a single parameter; but a study of $L_p(\theta,\mathbf{Y})$ becomes computationally and graphically more involved when there is more than one shape parameter, as in the Bessel and exponential correlation schemes.

When the number of sample points is too large, the maximum likelihood procedure becomes computationally prohibitive, since D_U^{-1} has to be evaluated. For stationary processes defined on a lattice, it is possible to approximate the likelihood (see Whittle 1954; Guyon 1982; and the discussion in Mardia and Marshall 1984). For non-lattice data, the problem was considered recently by Vecchia (1988), who proposed carrying out the estimation with the help of successive partial likelihood functions involving neighbouring observations, which are much easier to handle.

The problem of model choice for the residuals and of its influence on the testing of β has received little attention, particularly when the data is non-lattice. Haining (1987) compares characterizations of D_U in connection with trend surface estimation in the case of regularly spaced aerial survey data. For agricultural field trials, Martin (1990*a*) discusses model selection among the class of separable processes by extending techniques from time-series modelling. The choice of parametrisation of D_U is sometimes made by plotting the variogram of the OLS residuals. Care has to be taken when interpreting the variogram since it is sensitive to the number of pairs of data points used to estimate the empirical covariance at a particular distance. The number of pairs will vary with the distance, in a typical U-shape manner. Ripley (1981) advises the use of cross-validation by successive deletion of data points to assess the fit of the model chosen for the covariance function.

Example

Examples of maximum likelihood estimation with DR for topographic data are given in Ripley (1988), Vecchia (1988), and Mardia (1990). We now present results from a geographical correlation study of the association between male lung cancer mortality and the metal industry in France. These results were partially presented in Richardson (1990*a, b*).

The male lung cancer mortality rate has been standardized over the ages of 35 to 74 and over a two-year period from 1968 to 1969. The data were provided by the French National Institute for Health and Medical Research (INSERM) at the scale of the French *départements*. Cigarette sales were compiled by the French Nationalized Tobacco Company (SEITA). To take into account the time-lag between smoking and the onset of a lung pathology, cigarette sales per head in 1953 were used. Demographic data on the percentages of men employed in the metal industry were taken from the 1962 census (INSEE). After the grouping of the *départements* around Paris into one area and the exclusion of four others with data of poor quality, 82 locations were retained. Coordinates of these locations were recorded in order to be able to adjust a spatial gradient.

Table 17.2 displays regression results obtained using first order CAR or SAR models for U or direct representation for D_U with the disc or exponential correlation schemes. The W matrix for the CAR model was defined with binary 0–1 weights indicating contiguity of the *départements*. For the SAR model, W was further standardized to have row sums equal to 1. Modified $t_{\hat{M}-2}$ tests calculated following Equation (7) are also given. Table 17.2a is concerned with single linear regression between lung cancer mortality and the percentage of workers in the metal industry; Table 17.2b tests this association controlling for cigarette sales; and Table 17.2c further adjusts on a linear spatial trend.

As more explanatory variables are included, the spatial autocorrelation of the residuals decreases so the values of the χ^2 tests of improvement of the like-

Table 17.2 Linear regression between lung cancer mortality rates for men and metal industry workers with different spatial parametrization of the error variance–covariance matrix and comparison with results from the modified t_{M-2} tests

(a) Metal industry (no adjustment)

Model	OLS	CAR	SAR	Disc	Expo.	Modified test
$\beta \times 10^{-2}$	0.291	0.203	0.189	0.132	0.157	$\hat{M} = 16$
t	7.16	5.08	4.34	2.77	3.51	$t_{\hat{M}-2} = 3.00$
(p)	$(<10^{-9})$	(3×10^{-6})	(4×10^{-5})	(7×10^{-3})	(7×10^{-4})	(10^{-2})
χ^2	–	29.8	31.2	11.6	35.0	
(p)	–	(10^{-7})	(10^{-7})	(7×10^{-4})	(10^{-7})	

Simple regression

(b) Metal industry (adjustment for cigarette sales)

Model	OLS	CAR	SAR	Disc	Expo.	Modified test
$\beta \times 10^{-2}$	0.173	0.139	0.126	0.154	0.101	$\hat{M} = 34$
t	5.43	4.22	3.70	4.69	2.90	$t_{\hat{M}-2} = 3.45$
(p)	$(<10^{-6})$	(7×10^{-5})	(4×10^{-4})	(10^{-5})	(5×10^{-3})	(2×10^{-3})
χ^2	–	7	11.4	6.4	14.8	
(p)	–	(9×10^{-3})	(8×10^{-4})	(10^{-2})	(7×10^{-4})	

Multiple regression including cigarettes sales

(c) Metal industry (adjustment for cigarette sales and a linear trend)

Model	OLS	CAR	SAR	Disc	Expo.	Modified test
$\beta \times 10^{-2}$	0.117	0.110	0.102	0.107	0.099	$\hat{M} = 55$
t	3.27	3.04	2.88	2.92	2.70	$t_{\hat{M}-2} = 2.72$
(p)	$(2 \times <10^{-3})$	(4×10^{-3})	(7×10^{-3})	(5×10^{-3})	(9×10^{-3})	(10^{-2})
χ^2	–	0.8	3.84	5.1	5.1	
(p)	–	NS	(5×10^{-2})	(2×10^{-2})	(8×10^{-2})	

Multiple regression including cigarettes sales and a linear gradient lihood between the standard case ($D_U = I$) and the spatial models for D_U are decreased. Similarly the effective sample size $\hat{M}$, which is much reduced from $N = 82$ to $\hat{M} = 16$ in regression (a), is progressively increased when other variables are added. After adjustment for a linear gradient, there is weak evidence of residual spatial structure.

As expected, the difference between the standard (OLS) tests and the spatially adjusted tests, which can be substantial, diminishes with decreasing autocorrelation. When there is evidence of a strong spatial structure in the residuals (Table 17.2a, 17.2b), the influence of the choice of model for D_U on $\hat{\beta}$ is clearly apparent, with estimated slopes varying by about 50 per cent. As the estimated standard errors of $\hat{\beta}$ vary little between models (results not shown), changes in $\hat{\beta}$ are also directly reflected in a 50 per cent variation of the t values between models. Nevertheless, all the models and the modified test agree in the finding of a significant link with the metal industry. The significance levels given by the spatial regressions are smaller than those of the modified tests. This could arise from the noted underestimation of the standard error of $\hat{\beta}$. In Tables 17.2a and 17.2b, it is the disc model which performs the worst in terms of improvement of the likelihood. Further, it is only for this model that we found a bimodal likelihood, with the first peak corresponding to a higher autocorrelation than the second peak. This can be related to the multimodal behaviour of the spherical model found by Mardia and Watkins (1989) in their simulation study. For the disc model in Table 17.2a, it is the first peak that maximizes the likelihood, while in tables 17.2b and 17.2c, the first peak decreases and it is the second peak that, in turn, maximizes the likelihood. The first peak is clearly influenced by the long-range structure of the data.

In conclusion, it is clear that the choice of model for the spatial structure of the residuals can influence notably the estimation and the testing of regression coefficients, even in non-pathological cases where the spatial structure of the data is fairly smooth, as in our example. Other examples, some showing even more discrepancies, are presented in Richardson (1990*b*). The question of strategy for the selection of the residual model deserves further attention.

Ecological bias

The difference between individual and group level estimates of risk measures is often referred to as 'the ecological bias or fallacy'. The issue of ecological bias was first discussed by Robinson (1950), the term ecological fallacy was coined by Selvin (1958), and the original developments concerning this problem were found in the sociological literature (Goodman 1959; Alker 1969; Firebaugh 1978). There have been many publications relating to this topic in epidemiology (Stravasky 1976; Davies and Chilvers 1980; Morgenstern 1982; Richardson *et al.* 1987; Piantadosi *et al.* 1988; Greenland and Morgenstern 1989; Cohen

1990; Richardson and Hémon 1990) and the references quoted are not exhaustive. Several related problems have been discussed under this generic term, leading some authors, sometimes, to argue at cross-purposes. In order to clarify the discussion, we distinguish:

(1) theoretical comparisons between the shape of an individual dose–effect relationship and the relationship obtained by averaging over all individuals in a group;
(2) assuming N groups, decomposition of the total variation and covariation into the average variation within group and the variation of the mean between groups;
(3) assuming linearity of the dose–effect response within each group, comparison between the estimated ecological slope based on N groups and the average of the N within-group slopes.

We adopt the following notation in keeping with Richardson *et al.* (1987). Let X be a risk factor taking values x. Let $f(x) = P(C \mid X = x)$ model the probability of contracting the disease C if an individual is exposed to the risk factor X taking the value x. Let $\mu_G = E(X \mid G)$ be the mean of X inside a group G. When X is dichotomous 0–1, $E(X \mid G)$ represents the prevalence of X in group G, denoted by p_G. Let $E(Y \mid G)$ be the rate of the disease in group G, $E(Y \mid G) = E[P(C \mid X)]$, where the last expectation is taken over all values of X in G.

1. The interest is in comparing the shape, g, of the relationship between $E(Y \mid G)$ and μ_G, $E(Y \mid G) = g(\mu_G)$, to that of the individual dose response, f. Clearly if f is linear: $f(x) = a + bx$, with the same coefficients, a and b, for all individuals of the group G, then

$$g(\mu_G) = E(Y \mid G) = a + b\mu_G = f(\mu_G).$$

Hence f and g are identical. This was first pointed out by Beral *et al.* (1979). In the particular case where X is dichotomous, then b is the individual rate difference and is also the slope relating the group rate of the disease to the prevalence of X in G:

$$E(Y \mid G) = a + bp_G.$$

On the other hand, if f is non-linear, then f and g are no longer identical. For instance, if f is convex, then by Jensen's inequality

$$E(Y \mid G) = g(\mu_G) \geq f(\mu_G).$$

Hence risk measures based on g will, in general, differ from those based on f when f is non-linear (for more details, see Richardson *et al.* 1987).

2. From now on, it is assumed that f is linear. To derive equality of f and g, it was essential to suppose that all individuals of the group G share the *same values* of the intercept a and the slope b (assumption E). Assumption E might be thought less reasonable, if one wants to extend the previous reasoning to estimate ecologically a and b using N groups. Note that assumption E was implicit in all the discussion of Cohen (1990) while, in contrast, departures from it are discussed by Greenland and Morgenstern (1989). Let us consider two ways in which assumption E might break down:

(i) b is identical for all groups but a, the baseline disease rate for the non-exposed, varies between groups;

(ii) both a and b vary between groups.

Case (i) is illustrated in Fig. 17.1. In Fig. 17.1a, the intercepts are the same for all groups and hence the slope of the between-groups variations of $E(X|G)$ and $E(Y|G)$ is equal to that of the within-group variation, so that there is no bias. In Fig. 17.1b or 17.1c, there is an extraneous factor which alters the values of the intercept between groups, resulting in an ecological slope estimate (dashed line) different from the within-group slopes (continuous line).

Much of the discussion on the ecological bias has been centred around a decomposition of the total variation into within- and between-groups components. Assuming that the variables can be considered at two levels, either ungrouped or averaged over groups (symbolized by G), the total variation of a variable (var (X)) can be decomposed into the average variation $A = E[\mathrm{var}(X|G)]$ within each group and the variation $B = \mathrm{var}[E(X|G)]$ of the mean between groups:

$$\mathrm{var}(X) = A + B = E[\mathrm{var}(X|G)] + \mathrm{var}[E(X|G)].$$

Similarly for the covariance:

$$\mathrm{cov}(X,Y) = A' + B' = E[\mathrm{cov}(X,Y|G)] + \mathrm{cov}[E(X|G),E(Y|G)].$$

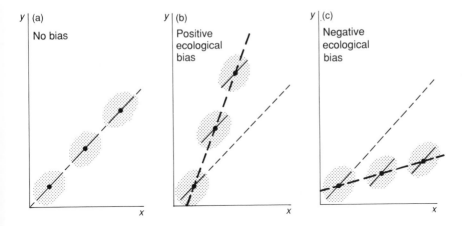

Fig. 17.1 Ecological bias and change in the baseline disease rate between the groups.

The ecological slope estimate is B'/B (referred to as β_e in Piantadosi *et al.* 1988). The slope using the ungrouped data: $(A' + B')/(A + B)$ (referred to as β in Piantadosi *et al.* 1988) is not usually of interest. What is of interest is the average over the groups of the within-group slopes:

$$E\left\{\frac{\mathrm{cov}(X,\,Y|G)}{\mathrm{var}(X|G)}\right\}.$$

If (*i*) holds (i.e. only *a* varies,) the term inside the brackets is independent of *G*, hence this expression is equal to:

$$\frac{E[\text{cov}(X, Y|G)]}{E[\text{var}(X|G)]} = \frac{A'}{A}.$$

When (*i*) does not hold, A'/A does not, in general, equal

$$E\left\{\frac{\text{cov}(X, Y|G)}{\text{var}(X|G)}\right\},$$

and hence referring to A'/A as 'the average within-group regression slope, β_w' as in Piantadosi *et al.* (1988) is somewhat confusing. By simple arithmetic manipulations, $\beta = (A' + B')/(A + B)$ can be decomposed into a weighted average of $\beta_e = B'/B$ and $\beta_w = A'/A$. For instance, by replacing *A*, *A'*, *B*, *B'* by their expressions in the simple equality:

$$\frac{A' + B'}{A + B} = \frac{B}{A + B}\frac{B'}{B} + \frac{A}{A + B}\frac{A'}{A}$$

one obtains:

$$\beta = \frac{\text{var}(E(X|G))}{\text{var}(X)}\beta_e + \frac{E[\text{var}(X|G)]}{\text{var }X}\beta_w$$

which is Equation (4) of Piantadosi *et al.* (1988), originally given by Duncan *et al.* (1961). This last expression is not particularly enlightening. It shows that β always lies between β_e and β_w but cannot say anything on the order of β_e with respect to β_w as is clearly illustrated in Fig. 17.1.

3. Suppose now that we are in case (ii), i.e. that $E(Y|G) = a_G + b_G\mu_G$ with a_G and b_G varying between groups. The ecological slope estimate calculated from the *N* groups:

$$
\begin{aligned}
\beta_e &= \frac{\text{cov}(E(X|G), E(Y|G))}{\text{var}(E(X|G))} \\
&= \frac{\text{cov}(\mu_G, a_G + b_G\mu_G)}{\text{var}(\mu_G)} \\
&= E(b_G) + \frac{\text{cov}(\mu_G, a_G)}{\text{var}(\mu_G)} + \frac{\text{cov}((\mu_G - E(\mu_G))\mu_G, b_G)}{\text{var}(\mu_G)},
\end{aligned}
\tag{8}
$$

using the equality $\text{cov}(XY, X) = E(Y)\text{var}(X) + \text{cov}((X - E(X))X, Y)$.

This derivation follows that given by Greenland and Morgenstern (1989) in the case of a dichotomous 0–1 *X* variable. In this particular case, b_G becomes the rate difference for group *G* and a_G the rate in the unexposed to *X*; μ_G corresponds to p_G, the prevalence of *X* in group *G*.

The ecological rate difference is thus decomposed into three terms. The first term, $E(b_G)$, is the average of the slopes in each group and is the quantity of interest. Of course, the slopes b_G could be influenced by confounding within each group in the usual way. The next two terms are a decomposition of the ecological bias, and it is interesting to discuss necessary conditions for their presence. For the second term to be non-zero, *the intercept* a_G, i.e. the rate in the non-exposed, *must vary between groups*, possibly following the level of another risk factor, a covariate. This covariate is not necessarily a confounder within each group. Hence this second term may be viewed as a bias factor due to *confounding by group* of the variations of disease rates in the non-exposed. For the third term to be non-zero, *the slope* b_G, i.e. the dose response effect or the rate difference for dichotomous exposure, *must vary between groups*. Hence, this third term may be viewed as bias due to groups acting as *effect modifiers*.

For dichotomous risk factors, Greenland and Morgenstern (1989) give artificially constructed examples involving only three groups which show that the bias contribution of the second and third terms of Equation (8) can be made arbitrarily large and may reverse the sign of the within-group association. In their first example, an effect modifier inversely correlated with exposure prevalence is built in. Since the variable creating this effect modification is unidentified, no adjustment can be made.

In their next two examples the risk factor creating the bias is identified. It is thus interesting to investigate whether it is possible to control for the effect of a covariate at a *group level*. It has often been suggested that this could be done by multiple ecological regression on the marginal prevalences of the risk factors (Greenland and Morgenstern 1989; Cohen 1990). It is worth pointing out that for this to be true, the strong assumption of additivity for the joint effect of the two risk factors needs to hold (Richardson and Hémon 1990). Let us model the situation for two dichotomous risk factors as follows.

Let X and Q be two dichotomized risk factors for a disease, with marginal prevalence in a group to be denoted by p_X and p_Q, respectively. Let R_X be the risk ratio corresponding to exposure to X and not to Q and vice versa for R_Q. Let $R_{X,Q}$ be the risk ratio corresponding to simultaneous exposure to X and Q and $p_{X,Q}$ the corresponding joint exposure prevalence in the same group. Then the incidence of the disease in the group is given by:

$$E(Y \mid p_X, p_Q, p_{X,Q}) = a\{1 + p_X(R_X - 1) + p_Q(R_Q - 1) \tag{9}$$
$$+ p_{X,Q}(1 - R_X - R_Q + R_{X,Q})\}$$

where a is the incidence of a group where no individual would be exposed to either X or Q.

If p_X, p_Q, and $p_{X,Q}$ were known for each group, then a correct estimate of $R_{X,Q}$ could be obtained by regression; but this is often unrealistic. Nevertheless, if the joint effect of X and Q is additive, i.e. $R_{X,Q} = R_X + R_Q - 1$, then Equation (9) can be simplified to an expression independent of $p_{X,Q}$:

$$a\{1 + p_X(R_X - 1) + p_Q(R_Q - 1)\}.$$

If, alternatively, the distribution of X and Q in the group are independent, i.e. $p_{X,Q} = p_X \cdot p_Q$ for all groups, then correct estimations of R_X and R_Q require the inclusion of a product term $p_X p_Q$ in the multiple regression. Hence, in the case of additive joint effect or independent joint exposure, estimates of R_X and R_Q could be obtained from an ecological regression, as long as a sufficient number of observations are available and that p_X and p_Q are not too strongly correlated.

The problem of how the departure from these assumptions will affect the estimates of R_X and R_Q is currently under investigation.

Design issues

From the discussion above, it is clear that ecological studies are open to many misconceptions and misinterpretations. We must, nevertheless, point out that geographical studies are the most natural design to study some environmental factors (e.g. water quality or background radiation) where the exposure would be measured with uncontrollably large imprecision by individual epidemiological study designs. In this context, how should we choose a most effective design?

1. The problems of artefacts and errors in the measurement of disease rate in a group, G, having been detailed in other chapters, we only comment on the correct assessment of $E(X|G)$, the mean exposure (or the prevalence) of the risk factor in a group G. This assessment is made more difficult if the *degree of heterogeneity* of exposure is large. Further, if one cannot assume that the individual dose–response relationship is fairly linear in the range investigated, then the whole shape of the distribution of X is influential, the more so if it is widespread.

2. The second aspect of the assessment of mean exposure is that, for chronic diseases, the relevant exposure is not the concurrent exposure of the group G but its past exposure, taking some time-lag between exposure and disease in the group into account. This will be easier to assess for diseases with *shorter latencies and for well-defined groups*. For example, to appraise possible health effects following the Chernobyl accident, a study of geographical comparisons of time trends of childhood leukaemia plotted with respect to date of birth probably provides the most effective design. Here is a case where a point exposure was reasonably assessed, the chosen disease has a short latency, and the critical first trimester prenatal period allows the potentially affected cohort to be identified. The need to include some time-lag in studies of ecological estimates of the relationship between smoking and lung cancer has been illustrated by several authors (Doll and Peto 1981; Decarli and La Vecchia 1986; Richardson *et al.* 1987). They show that unless a delay of 15–20 years between the smoking data and the mortality data is included, no clear relationship emerges. But the interpretation of this time-lag is not straightforward.

3. The problem of considering geographical correlation studies of diseases with long latencies is that it increases the probability of migrations in and out of each geographically defined group. This migration makes it more difficult to carry out correct assessment of exposure for diseases with a long latency. Polissar (1980) provided a detailed discussion of the dilution effect of migrations on ecological relationships when a fraction of the population was wrongly assumed to be exposed. These migration effects are larger in smaller population groups. Hence there is a circular problem, in that studies based on smaller areas will have more homogeneous exposure but more dilution effect due to migrations, particularly if the latency is long. A trade-off between homogeneity and size of the group has to be found.

4. Concerning the possibility to adjust for joint exposures to several risk factors, ecological studies will perform best when the risk factor of interest is overwhelming, so that the biases created by the other risk factors will be small. Such is the case for smoking and lung cancer, where a good correspondance between individual and ecological estimates was found in a study in France (Richardson *et al.* 1987). In other cases, some data on joint exposure, allowing hypotheses to be formulated on the joint exposure distribution in the groups, would be helpful. This is not necessary only in the particular case of additive risk factors. The hypothesis of independence of individual exposures to two risk factors within all groups might be a priori reasonable when one is interested in an environmental risk factor like background radiation exposure, while the confounding factor is at an individual level as, for instance, with smoking. The ecological design will be more appropriate in this case than when the concern is with two individual risk factors (smoking and drinking) which are likely to be interrelated.

The great majority of ecological studies that have been carried out were concerned with hypothesis generation and so were interested in establishing the existence of an association rather than estimating its strength. This is due partly to the many problems outlined in the assessment of group exposure. The next step to improve the design of ecological studies is to concentrate these studies on particular sex- and age-groups and to try to use exposure data relating only to the relevant sex- and age-groups. This may have to be done by combining data on the general population with survey data collected on smaller groups but with adequate stratification. This approach was found to be reasonably successful when relative risks for smoking, lung cancer, and coronary heart disease, estimated either from cohort data or geographically in France, were compared (Richardson *et al.* 1987). It would be interesting to investigate other examples where there is some consensus on the individual dose–effect relationship. Dietary fat and cancer is not an area where such a consensus exists. A strong link between dietary fat and cancer sites such as breast or the colon has been found by international comparisons but has only been weakly reflected, if at all, in individual epidemiological studies. Causes for this discrepancy have been the subject of a lively debate which has brought forward interesting discussions concerning the complementary contributions of individual and ecological studies (Hiller and McMichael 1990; Howe 1990; Prentice and Sheppard 1990; Willett and Stampfer 1990). As many authors point out, the interpretation of a geographical study is strengthened if it is accompanied by a parallel investigation concerning time trends, or there is coherence of the association in different areas, at different time periods or geographical levels, or for diseases with related pathologies (Rosen *et al.* 1985; Prentice and Sheppard 1989).

Acknowledgements

The author gratefully acknowledges A. Mollié's contribution to this chapter and would like to thank her for permission to reproduce Table 17.1 from her Ph.D. thesis. The author wishes to thank C. Guihenneuc and V. Lasserre of the Laboratoire de Statistiques Médicales de l'Université de Paris V for their computing assistance and E. Przybilski for her secretarial assistance. This chapter was written while the author was a Medical Research Council visiting research scientist in the Biostatistics Unit, Cambridge, whose support is gratefully acknowledged.

References

Alker, H. R. (1969). A typology of ecological fallacies. In *Quantitative ecological analysis in the social sciences*, (ed. M. Dogan and S. Rokkan). MIT Press, Cambridge, Mass.

Bartlett, M. S. (1935). Some aspects of the time-correlation problem in regard to tests of significance. *Journal of the Royal Statistical Society*, **98**, 536–43.

Beral, V., Chilvers, C., and Fraser, P. (1979). On the estimation of relative risk from vital statistical data. *Journal of Epidemiology and Community Health*, **33**, 159–62.

Besag, J., Yorke, J., and Mollié, A. (1991). Bayesian image restoration with two applications in spatial statistics. *Annals of the Institute of Statistics and Mathematics*, **43**, 1–59.

Blot, W. J. and Fraumeni, J. F. (1976). Geographic patterns of lung cancer. *American Journal of Epidemiology*, **103**, 539–50.

Blot, W. J. and Fraumeni, J. F. (1977). Geographic patterns of oral cancer in the United States: etiological implications. *Journal of Chronic Diseases*, **30**, 745–57.

Buffler, P., *et al.* (1988). Air pollution and lung cancer mortality in Harris County, Texas, 1979–1981. *American Journal of Epidemiology*, **128**, (4), 683–99.

Carpenter, L. and Beresford, S. (1986). Cancer mortality and type of water source: findings from a study in the U.K. *International Journal of Epidemiology*, **15**, 312–20.

Chilvers, C. (1983). Cancer mortality and fluoridation of water supplies in 35 US cities. *International Journal of Epidemiology*, **12**, 397–404.

Cislaghi, C., Decarli, A., La Vecchia, C., Mezzanotte, G., and Vigotti, M. A. (1990). Trends surface models applied to the analysis of geographical variations in cancer mortality. *Revue d'Epidémiologie et de Santé Publique*, **38**, 57–69.

Cliff, A. D. and Ord, J. K. (1981). *Spatial Processes. Models and Applications*. Pion, London.

Clifford, P., Richardson, S., and Hémon, D. (1989). Assessing the significance of the correlation between two spatial processes. *Biometrics*, **45**, (1), 123–34.

Cohen, B. (1990). Ecological versus case-control studies for testing a linear-no threshold dose–response relationship. *International Journal of Epidemiology*, **19**, 680–4.

Cook, D. G. and Pocock, S. J. (1983). Multiple regression in geographic mortality studies with allowance for spatially correlated errors. *Biometrics*, **39**, 361–71.

Cressie, N. (1986). Kriging nonstationary data. *Journal of the American Statistical Association*, **81**, 625–34.

Cressie, N. and Chan, N. H. (1989). Spatial modeling of regional variables. *Journal of the American Statistical Association*, **84**, 393–401.

Cressie, N. and Read, T. R. C. (1989). Spatial data analysis of regional counts. *Biometrical Journal*, **31**, 699–719.

Davies, J. M. and Chilvers, C. (1980). The study of mortality variations in small administrative areas of England and Wales, with special reference to cancer. *Journal of Epidemiology and Community Health*, **34**, 87–92.

Decarli, A. and La Vecchia, C. (1986). Environmental factors and cancer mortality in Italy: correlational exercise. *Oncology*, **43**, 116–26.

Doll, R. and Peto, P. (1981). The causes of cancer. *Journal of the National Cancer Institute*, **66**, 1191–308.

Duncan, O. D., Cuzzort, R. P., and Duncan, B. (1961). *Statistical geography*. The Free Press, New York.

Edling, C., Comba, P., Axelson, O., and Flodin, U. (1982). Effects of low-dose radiation. A correlation study. *Scandinavian Journal of Work Environment and Health*, **8**, (Suppl. 1), 59–64.

Firebaugh, G. (1978). A rule for inferring individual level relationship from aggregate data. *American Sociological Review*, **43**, 557–72.

Goodman, L. A. (1959). Some alternatives to ecological correlation. *American Journal of Sociology*, **64**, 610–25.

Greenland, S. and Morgenstern, H. (1989). Ecological bias, confounding and effect modification. *International Journal of Epidemiology*, **18**, 269–74.

Guyon, X. (1982). Parametric estimation for a stationary process on d-dimensional lattice. *Biometrika*, **69**, 95–105.

Haining, P. (1987). Trend surface models with regional and local scales of variation with an application to aerial survey data. *Technometrics*, **29**, 461–9.

Hiller, J. E. and McMichael, A. J. (1990). Dietary fat and cancer: a comeback for ecological studies? *Cancer Causes and Control*, **1**, 101–2.

Howe, G. R. (1990). Dietary fat and cancer. *Cancer Causes and Control*, **1**, 99–100.

Künsch, H. R. (1987). Intrinsic autoregressions and related models on the two-dimensional lattice. *Biometrika*, **74**, 517–24.

Lazar, P. (1982). Problems of concurrent trends in etiological research. In *Trends in cancer incidence*, (ed. K. Magnus). Hemisphere Publishing Corporation, Washington.

Mardia, K. V. (1990). Maximum likelihood estimation for spatial model. In *Spatial statistics: past, present, and future*, Institute of Mathematical Geography monograph series, Vol. 12. Ann Arbor.

Mardia, K. V. and Marshall, R. J. (1984). Maximum likelihood estimation of models for residual covariance in spatial regression. *Biometrika*, **71**, 135–46.

Mardia, K. V. and Watkins, A. J. (1989). On multimodality of the likelihood in the spatial linear model. *Biometrika*, **76**, 289–95.

Martin, R. J. (1979). A subclass of lattice processes applied to a problem in planar sampling. *Biometrika*, **66**, 209–17.

Martin, R. J. (1990*a*). The use of time-series models and methods in the analysis of agricultural field trials. *Communications in Statistics – Theory and Methods*, **19**, 55–81.

Martin, R. J. (1990*b*). The role of spatial statistical processes in geographic modelling. In *Spatial statistics: past, present, and future*, Institute of Mathematical Geography monograph series, Vol. 12. Ann Arbor.

Matanoski, G., *et al.* (1981). Cancer mortality in an industrial area of Baltimore. *Environmental Research*, **25**, 8–28.

Mollié, A. (1990). Représentation géographique des taux de mortalité: modélisation spatiale et méthodes bayesiennes. Thèse de doctorat, Université de Paris 6.

Mollié, A. and Richardson, S. (1991). Empirical Bayes estimates of cancer mortality rates using spatial models. *Statistics in Medicine*, **10**, 95–112.

Morgenstern, H. (1982). Uses of ecological analysis in epidemiologic research. *American Journal of Public Health*, **72**, 1336–44.

Najem, G. R., Louria, D. B., Lavenhar, M. A., and Feuerman, M. (1985). Clusters of cancer mortality in New Jersey municipalities, with special reference to chemical toxic waste disposal sites and per capita income. *International Journal of Epidemiology*, **14**, 528–37.

Ord, K. (1975). Estimation methods for models of spatial interaction. *Journal of the American Statistical Association*, **70**, 120–6.

Piantadosi, S., Byar, D. P., and Green, S. B. (1988). The ecological fallacy. *American Journal of Epidemiology*, **127**, (5), 893–904.

Pocock, S. J., Cook, D. G., and Shaper, A. G. (1982). Analysing geographic variation in cardiovascular mortality: methods and results. *Journal of the Royal Statistical Society, Series A*, **145**, 313–41.

Polissar, L. (1980). The effect of migration on comparison of disease rates in geographic studies in the United States. *American Journal of Epidemiology*, **111**, 175–82.

Prentice, R. L. and Sheppard, L. (1989). Validity of international time trend and migrant studies of dietary factors and disease risk. *Preventive Medicine*, **18**, 167–79.

Prentice, R. L. and Sheppard, L. (1990). Dietary fat and cancer: consistency of the epidemiologic data, and disease prevention that may follow from a practical reduction in fat consumption. *Cancer Causes and Control*, **1**, 81–97.

Richardson, S. (1990*a*). A method for testing the significance of geographical correlations with application to industrial lung cancer in France. *Statistics in Medicine*, **9**, 515–28.

Richardson, S. (1990*b*). Some remarks on the testing of association between spatial processes. In *Spatial statistics: past, present, and future*, Institute of Mathematical Geography monograph series, Vol. 12. Ann Arbor.

Richardson, S. and Hémon, D. (1990). Ecological bias and confounding (letter). *International Journal of Epidemiology*, **19**, 764–6.

Richardson, S., Stücker, I., and Hémon, D. (1987). Comparison of relative risks obtained in ecological and individual studies: some methodological considerations. *International Journal of Epidemiology*, **16**, 111–20.

Ripley, B. D. (1981). *Spatial statistics*. Wiley, New York.

Ripley, B. D. (1988). *Statistical inference for spatial processes*. Cambridge University Press, Cambridge.

Robinson, W. S. (1950). Ecological correlations and the behaviour of individuals. *American Sociological Review*, **15**, 351–7.

Rosen, M., Nystrom, L., and Wall, S. (1985). Guidelines for regional mortality analysis: an epidemiological approach to Health Planning. *International Journal of Epidemiology*, **14**, 293–9.

Selvin, H. C. (1958). Durkheim's 'suicide' and problems of empirical research. *American Journal of Sociology*, **63**, 607–19.

Stokes, C. S. and Brace, K. D. (1988). Agricultural chemical use and cancer mortality in selected rural counties in the U.S.A. *Journal of Rural Studies*, **4**, 239–47.

Stravasky, K. M. (1976). The role of ecologic analysis in studies of the etiology of disease: a discussion with reference to large bowel cancer. *Journal of Chronic Diseases*, **29**, 435–44.

Upton, G. and Fingleton, B. (1985). *Spatial data analysis by example*. Wiley, Chichester.

Vecchia, A. V. (1988). Estimation and model identification for continuous spatial processes. *Journal of the Royal Statistical Society, Series B*, **50**, (2), 297–312.

Warnes, J. J. and Ripley, B. D. (1987). Problems with likelihood estimation of covariance functions of spatial Gaussian processes. *Biometrika*, **74**, (3), 640–2.

Wartenberg, D. (1990). Explanatory spatial analyses: outliers, leverage points and influence functions. In *Spatial statistics: past, present, and future*, Institute of Mathematical Geography monograph series, Vol. 12. Ann Arbor.

Whittle, P. (1954). On stationary processes in the plane. *Biometrika*, **41**, 434–49.

Willett, W. C. and Stampfer, M. J. (1990). Dietary fat and cancer: another view. *Cancer Causes and Control*, **1**, 103–9.

Wong, O., Morgan, R. W., Whorton, M. D., Gordon, N., and Kheifets, L. (1989). Ecological analyses and case-control studies of gastric cancer and leukaemia in relation to DBCP in drinking water in Fresno county, California. *British Journal of Industrial Medicine*, **46**, 521–8.

18. Bayesian methods for mapping disease risk

D. Clayton and L. Bernardinelli

The construction of disease maps has been a central part of descriptive epidemiology throughout its history. Until recently, however, statistical methods for mapping disease had changed little. There are two main classes of disease maps—maps of standardized rates, and maps of statistical significance of the difference between disease risk in each area and the overall risk averaged over the entire map.

At first sight the first approach should be preferable since it maps an estimate of the parameter of interest (disease rate), but in recent cancer atlases this has been the less favoured approach. This is due largely to the fact that cancer is relatively uncommon and a map of standardized rates suffers because the rates are overdispersed—their variability only partly reflects genuine geographical heterogeneity, the remaining variance being due to Poisson variability. This leads to several practical problems for the atlas editor, notably that the most extreme rates tend to occur in the areas with the smallest populations—so that the main 'interest' in the map is contributed by the least reliable data—and that rarer cancers seem to vary more than common cancers. Some editors attempt to offset the latter effect by choosing more widely separated category boundaries for rare cancers than for common ones, but a systematic rule is hard to justify. One strategy is to choose category boundaries for each cancer site so that an equal number of areas fall within each category, but this gives an impression that all cancers exhibit approximately equal degrees of geographical variability!

Maps of significance avoid these difficulties but bring different problems. Now the more extreme significance levels tend to be in the areas with the largest populations, even when the size of effect is quite modest, and it is commoner cancers which appear to show more geographical variability than rare cancers. These difficulties stem from a familiar misuse of statistics—the confusion of statistical significance with biological importance!

These considerations led Clayton and Kaldor (1987) to seek a compromise index for mapping purposes. They suggested empirical Bayes estimates of area-specific relative risk which are intermediate between the classical standardized rate ratios and the overall mean for the whole map. When rates are based upon a large number of events the compromise estimate differs little from the standardized rate, but when there is little evidence that it differs from the overall mean the estimate is drawn (or 'shrunk') towards that value. A similar approach to the problem was taken by Manton *et al.* (1989).

Clayton and Kaldor also suggested an important extension of these ideas. They pointed out that, where there is clear evidence of spatial pattern in disease, less reliable estimates should be drawn towards a local rather than a global mean. In generalizing their method to this case they proposed a method very similar to those which had already been investigated in Bayesian approaches to image enhancement (see, for example, Besag 1986). More recent developments have followed the recognition of the connections between the Bayesian theory of image reconstruction and the disease mapping problem. A particularly important development has been the application of modern Monte Carlo algorithms, which allow the uncertainty of estimates to be explored.

Estimation in hierarchical Bayesian models

The Bayesian approach recognizes that two sorts of information are relevant to the estimation of the disease rate in any one area. The first type of information is the observed data on person-time observation and the corresponding count of observed disease events. These data allow the computation of the conventional 'best' estimate of the rate—the observed count divided by the person-time. This is the maximum likelihood estimate under the Poisson assumption. If this were the only information available, it would not be possible to provide any estimate of the rate for an area where the data were missing. However, if the rates for all other areas on the map were known exactly, most people would be prepared to use this information to estimate the missing rate. This is called prior information.

Informally it is clear that some integration of the two types of information is called for. If the cases/person-time data are sparse, then the prior information available from the rest of the map will dominate but, if an adequate number of cases is observed, the local information will be relatively more important. A formal way in which this integration can be achieved is given by the theory of Bayesian inference in hierarchical models. In the present context, Bayes theorem tells us that the posterior distribution for the unknown rate is proportional to the product of the prior distribution, determined by properties of the disease map as a whole, and the likelihood derived from the cases/person-time data. A compromise estimate of disease rate is a measure of the centre of this posterior distribution.

Clayton and Kaldor suggested mapping posterior mean rates. However, since in most cases Bayes theorem does not lead to posterior distributions whose means may be easily calculated, approximations are usually necessary and their adequacy is difficult to assess. In image analysis applications, the posterior mode is often used, since it is easier to compute. This is formally equivalent to the method of maximum penalized likelihood.

Denoting the vector of unknown (log) rates by θ, the likelihood for person-time data by $L(\theta)$, and the prior distribution of log-rates by $\phi(\theta)$, then the posterior distribution is proportional to $L(\theta)\phi(\theta)$. The posterior mode maximizes this and, therefore, also maximizes its logarithm:

$$\log L(\theta) + \log \phi(\theta).$$

The second term may be regarded as a 'penalty' function which handicaps solutions which conflict with the prior model for the map.

The idea of smoothing using 'roughness penalties' goes back to the work of Good and Gaskins (1971). Its use in an explicitly Bayesian context for the estimation of smooth estimates of density distributions and of the intensity function of a time-dependent Poisson process was described by Leonard (1978). In those applications the prior distribution is a stochastic process in one dimension—a random walk, for example. Bayesian image analysis techniques extend this approach to the plane, using spatial processes as prior. Advances in computational algorithms have allowed further extensions of the model to include covariate effects and, by investigating further properties of the posterior distribution for θ, the exploration of the uncertainty associated with the estimation of the map.

Choice of hyperparameter values

The above notation ignores the fact that prior model, $\phi(\ )$, itself needs parameters which specify the overall characteristics of the map to be estimated. The two most important characteristics are

(1) the total variability of underlying rates; and
(2) the tendency for geographically close areas to have similar disease rates.

Parameters which control such characteristics of the prior distribution are often called hyperparameters.

In the simplest case, there is a single hyperparameter which enters as a multiplying factor in the penalty function:

$$\log \phi(\theta;\gamma) = \gamma \log \phi(\theta).$$

Here γ acts as a smoothing parameter—when it is large the penalty function is given relatively more weight, leading to 'smoother' solutions. As we shall see, γ is inversely proportional to the prior estimate of geographical variability.

In the literature on smooth curve fitting, such parameters are usually chosen for optimal prediction of future observations. This is achieved by minimizing a generalized cross-validation criterion. In Bayesian or 'empirical' Bayes approaches, the approach is to obtain a likelihood for γ and use this to estimate γ either by maximum likelihood or by fully Bayesian methods which incorporate a subjective 'hyperprior'. The likelihood for γ captures the information relevant to overall map structure, while the likelihood for θ contains the local information relevant to the rate for each individual area. Bayes theorem provides the mechanism for integrating the overall structural information and the local information.

The likelihood for γ is the probability of all the data in the map given γ and this is given by the integral $\int L(\theta)\phi(\theta;\gamma)d\theta$. This is generally intractable but an approximate likelihood may be obtained using the Laplace integral approximation. We Taylor expand the expression $\log L(\theta) + \log \phi(\theta;\gamma)$ to a quadratic in θ and integrate the resultant multivariate normal error function. Note, however, that when $\phi(\ )$ allows for dependence between the $\{\theta_i\}$, indicating that geographically close areas should have similar rates, the approximation involves the determinant of an $n \times n$ matrix (n being the number of areas).

Similar considerations are involved when investigating the posterior uncertainty for θ. This should be based upon the marginal posterior for θ and this requires integration of the joint posterior for (θ,γ) with respect to γ. While the empirical Bayes idea of substituting an estimate of γ into the conditional posterior distribution for θ, given γ will usually yield acceptable point estimates, the uncertainty associated with these estimates is underestimated if no allowance is made for the uncertainty associated with γ.

Approximation methods, such as the penalized likelihood method, thus suffer from two major disadvantages:

(1) the need for large-scale matrix computations; and
(2) the difficulty of assessing the uncertainties of point estimates of θ.

Both of these problems are avoided by a Monte Carlo approach in which we simulate the joint posterior distribution of θ and γ. Using algorithms, to be described below, we draw a large sample of (θ,γ) values from this distribution (a sample of around 1000 is usually more than enough). When the interest is in γ, we can simply ignore the θ values and concentrate upon the marginal posterior distribution of γ and, more usually, when the interest is in the disease map we ignore the γ values and concentrate upon the marginal distribution of the θ parameters. Point estimates can be obtained by taking the mean of the simulated values, but other aspects of the posterior distribution may also be studied. In particular, we can compute a Bayesian credible interval for the disease rate at each point. We can also compute the proportion of simulated maps which possess some interesting characteristic, thus obtaining a posterior probability that the characteristic is truly present. For these reasons, the Monte Carlo approach is the more attractive. We will return to a more detailed discussion of computational algorithms on pp. 212–13.

Specification of prior models

For simplicity we will first consider the case in which age-standardization of rates is carried out by the 'indirect' method using an external set of age-specific rates. Then the data are the pairs, $(O_i, E_i), i = 1, \ldots, n$ of observed and 'expected' cases in the n localities. It is well known (see, for example, Breslow and Day 1987) that conventional indirect standardization methodology is based upon the assumption that O_i are Poisson variates with expectations $E_i \exp \eta_i$, where the η_i are logarithms of relative risk parameters. The SMRs (standardized mortality ratios) are maximum likelihood estimates of the relative risks, η_i in this model.

Since the standard rates used in the computation of the E_i are derived from some external large population, the SMRs need not be centred around 1.0, and it will be convenient to decompose the model further into an overall mean term, μ, and area effects θ_i:

$$\eta_i = \mu + \theta_i.$$

This is an example of a generalized linear mixed model, or GLMM (Breslow and Clayton 1992), with a Poisson error structure, logarithmic link, one fixed effect (μ), and a set of random effects (θ_i). To complete the model specification it is necessary only to describe the prior distribution of θ given hyperparameter(s) γ.

The simplest prior models, $\phi(\theta; \gamma)$, are models of exchangeability[1] which make no allowance for the locations of areas on the map. These are models for unstructured heterogeneity. Two parametric models have been investigated, a gamma distribution for relative risks, $\exp \theta_i$ and a Gaussian distribution for log relative risks, θ_i. The former leads to the simpler algebraic results, with closed form expressions for the posterior mean, but the latter has considerably greater potential for extension.

A convenient exchangeable Gaussian prior is defined by

$$\phi(\theta; \gamma) \propto \exp \left\{ -\frac{\gamma}{2} \sum_i (\theta_i - \bar{\theta})^2 \right\},$$

where $\bar{\theta}$ is the arithmetic mean of all the log-rates. Note that $\log \phi$ is proportional to the sum of squared deviations of the θ_i from their mean and is readily interpreted as a roughness penalty appropriate for unstructured heterogeneity. It is also important to point out that this function is not a proper distribution, since it does not vary with respect to $\bar{\theta}$. In practice, it will be necessary either to adopt a linear constraint (usually $\bar{\theta} = 0$) or to omit μ. In the latter case, $\bar{\theta}$ will take over the role of μ in the model.

Prior models which allow for more structure in the map incorporate interdependence between the $\{\theta_i\}$, with stronger relationships for areas which are geographically close. The most intensively investigated class of models are the Markov random field (MRF) models in which each θ_i depends upon the others

---

[1] Editorial note: the models called exchangeable here are known as additive models in Chapter 17.

only via its relationship with its immediate neighbours. A particularly convenient class is the gaussian MRF models in which the distribution of θ_i conditional upon the other θs is normal with mean which depends upon the mean of adjacent θ_is.

Clayton and Kaldor (1987) used a Gaussian MRF model in which the conditional variance of each element of θ was assumed to be constant and the conditional expectation was assumed to be a compromise between an overall constant and the (unweighted) mean of neighbouring values. Unfortunately, the model suggested was drawn from work on regular pixel arrays in which the number of neighbours is constant, and is not internally consistent in the case in which the number of neighbours varies. The correct model of this form has density proportional to:

$$\exp \left\{ -\frac{\gamma}{2} \sum_i A_{i+} \theta_i (\theta_i - \bar{\theta}_i) \right\}$$

where $\bar{\theta}_i$ is the mean of the elements adjacent to θ_i weighted with a 'strength of adjacency matrix' A

$$\bar{\theta}_i = \frac{1}{A_{i+}} \sum_j A_{ij} \theta_j$$

where $A_{i+} = \Sigma_j A_{ij}$. The conditional mean and variance relations are:

$$E(\theta_i | \theta_{j \neq i}) = \bar{\theta}_i$$

$$\mathrm{Var}(\theta_i | \theta_{j \neq i}) = \frac{1}{\gamma A_{i+}}$$

In practice it is rather difficult to decide upon a degree of adjacency and the A_{ij} are taken as 1 if areas i and j have a common boundary, and zero otherwise. Such a matrix implies rather strong spatial dependency and may be thought of as a model for local 'clustering'. An alternative model, in the same spirit of that of Clayton and Kaldor, has conditional mean $(1 - \varrho)\bar{\theta} + \varrho\bar{\theta}_i$. In fact this is a special case of the simple adjacency model with $A_{ij} = \varrho$ if the areas are adjacent, and $1 - \varrho$ otherwise. The hyperparameter ϱ, which chooses between unstructured and structured variation of rates (heterogeneity and clustering), may be estimated from the data.

A practical difficulty with this 'compromise' prior is that the likelihood for ϱ may be rather difficult. An alternative, suggested by Besag *et al.* (1991), is to represent θ as the sum of an unstructured heterogeneity component, $\theta^{(1)}$, and a pure clustering component, $\theta^{(2)}$. These two random components have associated hyperparameters $\gamma^{(1)}$ and $\gamma^{(2)}$ which control the strength of each component in the final mixture. This model may also be conveniently represented within the framework of generalized linear mixed models. The model now contains two random sets of random effects—an exchangeable set, and a spatially autocorrelated set.

Although the Gaussian MRF models are convenient, they are not the only possibility. In the more general field of image analysis, there is some experience of discrete MRF models in which the parameter takes on one of a discrete number of 'grey' levels.

The choice of prior model should be determined by empirical considerations, and there is much scope for further work on methods for suggesting and criticizing prior models.

Extensions: covariates and standardization

Invariably it will be necessary to adjust maps for geographical variation in confounding variables. Two types of variable may be distinguished:

(1) those measured for the area as a whole, but not in individuals; and
(2) those, such as age and sex, which are recorded for individuals.

Examples of the former type of covariate include measures of urbanization, climate, and air pollution, and analysis by these is usually termed ecological analysis. The second type of measurement allows tabulation of cases and person-time in strata. Adjustment for confounding variables at this level is sometimes referred to as internal standardization.

The statistical theory and methods outlined here may be extended to allow for either possibility. Clayton and Kaldor showed how the classical indirect standardization algorithm of Mantel and Starke (1968) continues to be applicable in the hierarchical Bayesian modelling framework.

Again these extensions are readily accommodated into the GLMM framework. The extension of the basic model to allow for ecological covariates simply replaces the mean, μ, by a linear regression model:

$$\eta = X\beta + \theta,$$

where, as indicated above, θ itself may be decomposed into a sum of exchangeable and autocorrelated random effects. The probability model for the observed data, given the linear predictor vector η, follows the standard Poisson/log-linear approach to generalized linear modelling of disease rates (Breslow and Day 1987, Chapter 4).

In this model, the length of all covariate vectors and of the random effect vectors is simply n, the number of areas. Extension of the model to allow for covariates measured at subject level necessitates the use of longer vectors to allow for modelling variation between strata (such as age/sex groups) within areas. It is then necessary to introduce a block diagonal matrix Z to ensure that units representing different strata within the same geographical area share the same (random) area effect. Thus, the model then becomes

$$\eta = X\beta + Z\theta,$$

which is the more general form of a GLMM.

For purely descriptive epidemiology, the interest is in θ (or possibly in η), but the methods are equally relevant when the interest is in the ecological coefficients β. In the case where the model allows only unstructured heterogeneity for θ, the model is a regression model with extra-Poisson variation (Breslow 1984).

Of course it is necessary to be aware of the dangers of over-interpretation of ecological analyses. Where, after allowing for the biological effects of a confounding variable, there is a correlation between the residual geographical variability of the disease and the geographical distribution of the confounder, then the ecological analysis will wrongly estimate the confounder effect and, as a result, wrongly estimate the map. This is a manifestation of the 'ecological fallacy'. More formally, the questionable assumption is that the random effects, which represent effects of unmeasured covariates, are uncorrelated with the measured covariates, X. Although it would be perfectly feasible to extend our model to allow for correlated random effects, we have no data for estimation of correlation parameters so that their posterior distributions will be the same as their priors. Nevertheless, it could be argued that such analyses would be quite interesting.

Computational algorithms

Methods for approximate inference in GLMMs have recently been surveyed by Breslow and Clayton (1992). The computational problem lies in the need to integrate over the random effects, θ, to obtain a likelihood for the remaining parameters. Breslow and Clayton discuss two approaches:

(1) the penalized likelihood method, equivalent to approximation of the integration over θ by a Laplace approximation; and

(2) a marginal approach, making use of approximate results for mean and covariance in the marginal distribution of response after summation over the distribution of θ. With these, estimation may proceed using quasi-likelihood ideas.

The latter approach reverts to penalized likelihood for estimation of θ. These are posterior mode estimates based upon the posterior distribution of θ conditional upon estimated values for all other parameters.

The computation of these posterior mode estimates is a problem in non-linear function maximization. The Newton–Raphson method or the equivalent iteratively reweighted least squares (IRLS) algorithm may be used, but requires at each stage the inversion of an $n \times n$ matrix. Besag (1986) has suggested an 'iterated conditional mode' (ICM) algorithm which corresponds to a non-linear Gauss–Seidel or non-linear Jacobi method in different implementations. These latter methods avoid matrix inversion and would appear better suited to large problems. The ICM method bears a close relationship with the 'back-fitting' algorithm of Hastie and Tibshirani (1990). It is well known that such methods may have poor convergence properties and that the convergence may be improved by stepping each parameter by a multiple (>1) of the step size suggested by the Gauss–Seidel approach. This is known as over-relaxation.

The Monte Carlo algorithms mentioned earlier may be regarded as stochastic analogues of these computational methods. The general algorithm is due to Metropolis *et al.* (1953) and arose in applications of statistical thermodynamics. More general applications in statistics were explored by Hastings (1970). A special case, much used in image analysis, is the 'Gibbs sampling' algorithm introduced by Geman and Geman (1984). In this approach, the posterior distribution is simulated by a stochastic version of the ICM algorithm—each unknown rate is replaced by a value drawn from the conditional posterior distribution, conditioning on current values of rates for neighbouring areas. The algorithm may be used, as in Hastings (1970), to obtain posterior moments or, as in Geman and Geman (1984), by incorporating 'annealing' to find posterior modes. The Gibbs sampling approach may be extended to sample the joint posterior distribution of parameters and hyperparameters, thus avoiding the problem of choosing suitable hyperparameter values.

These stochastic algorithms have the property of generating a Markov chain of sample values with equilibrium distribution which may be shown to be equal to the posterior distribution of interest. Thus, samples generated before the attainment of equilibrium must be discarded. In common with the analogous deterministic algorithms, convergence may be slow. Very recently, P. J. Green (personal communication) has incorporated the idea of over-relaxation into the Metropolis algorithm and shown improved convergence as a result.

In all but the smallest problems, the Monte Carlo approach requires less computer time than the approximate methods, and allows exploration of the complete posterior distribution. For these reasons, this is the preferred computational approach.

Examples

In this section we illustrate these methods of spatial analysis using two examples concerning variations in cancer frequency. In the first example, we focus our attention upon covariate relationships, while the second concentrates upon mapping. Most of the calculations reported use the Monte Carlo approach to estimation in the full Bayesian analysis. We have used improper uniform priors for fixed effects, β. However it is well known that Gibbs sampling does not perform well with improper priors for the inverse variance

Table 18.1 Lip cancer incidence and outdoor occupations in Scotland (data from Kemp et al. 1985; Clayton and Kaldor 1987)

Area	Observed	Expected	% employed in AFF	Adjacent areas
0 Caithness	11	3.04	10	1, 53
1 Sutherland	5	1.79	16	0, 2, 55
2 Ross and Cromarty	15	4.26	10	1, 3, 5, 7, 55
3 Skye and Lochalsh	9	1.38	16	2, 4, 5, 55
4 Lochaber	6	1.98	7	3, 5, 6, 15, 30, 55
5 Inverness	9	5.53	7	2, 3, 4, 6, 7
6 Badenoch	2	1.07	10	4, 5, 7, 8, 12, 15
7 Nairn	3	1.08	10	2, 5, 6, 8
8 Moray	26	8.11	10	6, 7, 9, 10, 12
9 Banff–Buchan	39	8.66	16	8, 10
10 Gordon	20	6.63	16	8, 9, 11, 12
11 Aberdeen	31	22.67	16	10, 12
12 Kincardine	9	4.55	16	6, 8, 10, 11, 13, 15
13 Angus	16	10.46	7	12, 14, 15
14 Dundee	6	19.62	1	13, 15, 17
15 Perth and Kinross	16	14.37	10	4, 6, 12, 13, 14, 16, 17, 18, 27, 28, 30
16 Kirkcaldy	19	15.47	1	15, 17, 18
17 NE Fife	17	7.84	7	14, 15, 16
18 Dunfermline	15	12.49	1	15, 16, 27, 29
19 W. Lothian	11	10.20	10	20, 23, 29, 37, 38, 42
20 Edinburgh	19	50.72	1	19, 21, 22, 23
21 Midlothian	7	7.03	10	20, 22, 23, 24
22 E. Lothian	10	8.96	7	20, 21, 24, 26
23 Tweeddale	0	1.76	10	19, 20, 21, 24, 42, 52
24 Ettrick	7	4.18	7	21, 22, 23, 25, 26, 52

25	Roxburgh	7	4.44	10	24, 26, 52
26	Berwickshire	9	2.53	24	22, 24, 25
27	Clackmannan	2	4.32	16	15, 18, 28, 29
28	Stirling	8	8.53	7	15, 27, 29, 30, 31, 33, 34, 35, 36
29	Falkirk	8	15.78	16	18, 19, 27, 28, 36, 37
30	Argyll and Bute	11	8.77	10	4, 15, 28, 31, 44, 45
31	Dumbarton	6	7.20	16	28, 30, 33, 43, 44
32	Glasgow	28	88.66	0	33, 34, 35, 37, 38, 39, 40, 41, 43
33	Clydebank	4	5.27	0	28, 31, 32, 34, 43
34	Bearsden	1	3.62	0	28, 32, 33, 35
35	Strathkelvin	1	7.03	1	28, 32, 34, 36, 37
36	Cumbernauld	1	3.44	1	28, 29, 35, 37
37	Monklands	8	9.35	1	19, 29, 32, 35, 36, 38
38	Motherwell	6	14.63	0	19, 32, 37, 39, 42
39	Hamilton	3	9.34	1	32, 38, 40, 42
40	E. Kilbride	2	5.59	1	32, 39, 41, 42, 46, 48
41	Eastwood	1	5.74	1	32, 40, 43, 46
42	Clydesdale	7	5.62	7	19, 23, 38, 39, 40, 48, 51, 52
43	Renfrew	10	18.76	1	31, 32, 33, 41, 44, 45, 46
44	Inverclyde	9	10.10	0	30, 31, 43, 45
45	Cunninghame	11	12.68	10	30, 43, 44, 46, 47
46	Kilmarnock	3	8.20	7	40, 41, 43, 45, 47, 48
47	Kyle and Carrick	11	12.32	7	45, 46, 48, 49, 50
48	Cumnock-Doon	5	4.75	7	40, 42, 46, 47, 49, 50, 51
49	Wigtown	8	3.31	24	47, 48, 50
50	Stewartry	3	2.88	24	47, 48, 49, 51
51	Nithsdale	7	6.04	7	42, 48, 50, 52
52	Annandale	0	4.16	16	23, 24, 25, 42, 51
53	Orkney	8	2.80	24	0, 54
54	Shetland	7	2.30	7	53
55	W. Isles	13	4.40	7	1, 2, 3, 4

hyperparameters, γ. Instead we have used chi-squared prior distributions with means of 10.0 and 2.0 for exchangeable and autocorrelated effects, respectively. These can be regarded as prior guesses for the γ hyperparameters. The fact that we have little confidence in such guesses is reflected in our choice of only 2 degrees of freedom for these distributions!

Lip cancer in Scotland

Our first example is the data on lip cancer in Scotland discussed by Clayton and Kaldor (1987). The data shown in Table 18.1 take the lip cancer incidence data used by Clayton and Kaldor together with data concerning the percentage of population employed in agriculture, fishing, and forestry (AFF). This was taken from Figure 3.6 of the *Atlas of cancer in Scotland* (Kemp *et al.* 1985), which drew attention to the similarity of the lip cancer map to the AFF map. An association between the two variables is very plausible given the strong role of ultraviolet exposure in lip cancer.

We fitted a GLMM which included a fixed effect regression model for the effect of AFF employment, and both exchangeable and autocorrelated random effects of area. We shall refer to these random terms as modelling 'heterogeneity' and 'clustering' of rates, respectively. Table 18.2 shows parameter

Table 18.2 Employment effect for the lip cancer data

| | AFF employment effect, β | |
Model	Estimate	SD
1 AFF	0.0740	0.006
2 AFF + Heterogeneity	0.0702	0.0147
3 AFF + Clustering	0.0362	0.0124
4 AFF + Het. + Clust.	0.0393	0.0130
2 AFF + Heterogeneity	0.068	0.014
3 AFF + Clustering	0.035	0.012

estimates (posterior means) together with their precision (posterior standard deviation) for the AFF employment effect. For comparison purposes, a simple fixed effects generalized linear model (GLIM) is shown in the first section of the table. The second section shows results obtained from Gibbs sampling (1000 samples), while the third reproduces the approximate analysis of Breslow and Clayton (1992). The Monte Carlo and approximate analysis agree closely where both analyses were successful. However, the approximate method failed in the case of the model with both heterogeneity and clustering terms. This failure occurred because, as in Clayton and Kaldor (1987), the maximum likelihood estimate of the hyperparameters indicates 'pure' clustering, so that estimates of the area effects are drawn entirely towards local means. However, models in which both random components are represented have finite posterior probability and are represented in the Monte Carlo results. The GLIM analysis yields a much smaller standard deviation of the regression coefficient, β. This reflects the fact that this analysis ignores any random influences save the Poisson fluctuation of event counts. Model 2 is an extra-Poisson variation model (Breslow 1934) and gives a similar parameter estimate but with a larger standard deviation. As would be expected from earlier remarks, there is little difference between the results for models 3 and 4. Both of these give a much smaller regression coefficient than we get using models 1 and 2. The reason for this is that the 'clustering' term allows the fitted rates to vary smoothly across the map, and may be thought of as a way of non-parametrically modelling the effect of location. Because AFF employment varies with location in a very similar manner to the variation of disease rates with location, location acts as a confounder. Including it in the model results in a reduction of the coefficient.

How are these results to be interpreted and, in particular, which estimate should we believe? By introducing the clustering term we attempt to control for the confounding effect of location, but location is not itself causally related to disease—it is a surrogate for further unmeasured causal factors. Clearly it is desirable to try to control for such factors, but it is important to remember that a key assumption of the model is that the random effects are unrelated to the covariates, X. If, as seems likely, the other factors which contribute to the location effect are positively correlated with the employment variable, then the model will over-correct and we would obtain an attenuated estimate.

Breast cancer in Sardinia

In our second example we first focus upon estimation of the random location effects, with a view to mapping the incidence of disease. The data (supplied by the Istituto Superiore di Sanità) concern breast cancer mortality in the island of Sardinia during the period 1983–87. There were 805 observed deaths from this cause during this period and we have compared the numbers of observed deaths for each area with expected numbers obtained by applying age-specific rates for the whole of Italy. We have compared analyses for two different scales of data aggregation. The first analysis is for 22 larger areas (Unitá Sanitarie Locali, USLs), while the second analysis concerns a much finer division into 366 communes. Plates 3 and 4 show the results of fitting the model

$$\log Rate = Constant + Heterogeneity + Clustering$$

to the data at the appropriate level. In each figure, map (a) shows the SMRs, while map (b) shows the Bayes estimates. The computations were carried out by Gibbs sampling so that other aspects of the posterior distribution can be explored. Map (c) tabulates the posterior probabilities for each area's relative mortality exceeding the geometric mean of all areas mapped. These are estimated, for example for area i, by the proportion of simulations for which η_i (the linear combination of effects) exceeds the mean, $\bar{\eta}$.

These analyses show that, whereas the SMR is a useful index at the USL level of aggregation, it is too unstable to be useful at the finer level of aggregation. However, the Bayesian estimates continue to be useful on the finer scale. High rates on the north coast and two high pockets in the south of the island can be seen on the map of parameter estimates, and the posterior probability that these areas do indeed have high rates is greater than 90 per cent. There is some suggestion of an unusually low-risk area mid-way up the east coast, but the posterior probability map shows that the evidence is less than convincing.

Table 18.3 (second column) shows the estimates of the hyperparameters, γ, for heterogeneity and clustering effects. The heterogeneity parameter is not

Table 18.3   Hyperparameter estimates for Sardinian data

Random effect term	Hyperparameter γ		SD of effects	
	Estimate	SD(estimate)	Estimate	SD(estimate)
USLs				
Heterogeneity	29.9	14.5	0.17	0.04
Clustering	6.0	2.9	0.21	0.05
Communes				
Heterogeneity	26.0	15.6	0.22	0.06
Clustering	3.8	2.1	0.32	0.07

difficult to interpret since it is the reciprocal of a variance of the random effects. Thus, a value of 25 will generate random effects with a standard deviation of 0.2 (the log-linear model may also be thought of as multiplicative in relative risk so that this figure corresponds to a coefficient of variation of around 20 per cent). The γ hyperparameter for the clustered effects has no such easy interpretation. If the variation of effects is smooth, large variations of θs can take place with little deviation from local means so that the γ hyperparameter is no longer simply interpretable in terms of the standard deviation of the effects it generates. However, in Gibbs sampling the standard deviation of generated effects can be directly computed for each realization of the posterior. The posterior mean and SD of this quantity are shown in the last two columns of Table 18.3. For the heterogeneity effects, these show the expected relationship with the corresponding hyperparameter. This table shows that heterogeneity and clustering effects contribute fairly equally to the estimated spatial variation, the slightly larger contribution arising from the clustering term.

Finally, we suspected that the variation of rates might be attributable to urban/rural differences. Plates 3d and 4d show a classification of areas by degree of urbanization. Preliminary analysis with GLM suggested that a linear relationship with urbanization status coded as 1,2,3 is an adequate model. Table 18.4 shows the estimate we obtained for this fixed covariate

Table 18.4 Effect of urbanization

| Model | Urbanization effect, β | |
	Estimate	SD (estimate)
USLs		
1 Const + Urb	−0.12	0.04
2 Const + Urb + Heterogeneity	−0.11	0.09
3 Const + Urb + Clustering	−0.11	0.12
4 Const + Urb + Het + Clust	−0.11	0.14
Communes		
1 Const + Urb	−0.15	0.04
2 Const + Urb + Heterogeneity	−0.10	0.06
3 Const + Urb + Clustering	−0.13	0.06
4 Const + Urb + Het + Clust	−0.12	0.07

effect using various models. Unlike our previous example, the regression coefficient does not vary greatly with choice of model, indicating that the covariate effect is not seriously confounded by the effect of location. As before, the standard deviation of the estimates is increased by inclusion of random effects. This effect is stronger in the case of the USL analysis. We would speculate that this reflects the lack of degrees of freedom for estimation of variance components with only 22 areas.

References

Besag, J. (1986). On the statistical analysis of dirty pictures. *Journal of the Royal Statistical Society, Series B*, **48**, 259–302.
Besag, J., York, J., and Mollié, A. (1991). Bayesian image restoration with applications in spatial statistics (with discussion). *Annals of the Institute of Statistical Mathematics*, **43**, 1–59.

Breslow, N. E. (1984). Extra-Poisson variation in log-linear models. *Applied Statistics*, **33**, 38–44.

Breslow, N. E. (1984). Extra-Poisson variation in log-linear models. *Applied Statistics*, **33**, 38–44.

Breslow, N. E. and Clayton, D. G. (1992). Approximate inference in generalized linear mixed models. *Journal of the American Statistical Association* (in press).

Clayton, D. and Kaldor, J. (1987). Empirical Bayes estimates of age-standardized relative risks for use in disease mapping. *Biometrics*, **43**, 671–82.

Geman, S. and Geman, D. (1984). Stochastic relaxation, Gibbs distributions and the Bayesian restoration of images. *I.E.E.E. Trans. Pattern Analysis Machine Intelligence*, **6**, 721–41.

Good, I. J. and Gaskins, R. A. (1971). Non-parametric roughness penalties for probability densities. *Biometrika*, **58**, 255–77.

Hastie, T. J. and Tibshirani, R. J. (1990). *Generalized additive models*. Chapman and Hall, London.

Hastings, W. (1970). Monte Carlo sampling methods using Markov chains and their applications. *Biometrika*, **57**, 97–109.

Kemp, I., Boyle, P., Smans, M., and Muir, C. (eds.) (1985). *Atlas of cancer in Scotland, 1975–1980. Incidence and epidemiological perspective (IARC Scientific Publications No. 72)*, International Agency for Research on Cancer, Lyon.

Leonard, T. A. (1978). Density estimation, stochastic processes and prior information. *Journal of the Royal Statistical Society, Series B*, **40**, 113–46.

Mantel, N. and Starke, C. R. (1968). Internal indirect standardization of rates. *Biometrics*, **24**, 997–1005.

Manton, K. G., Woodbury, M. A., Stallard, E., Riggan, W. B., Creason, J. P., and Pellom, A. C. (1989). Empirical Bayes procedures for stabilizing maps of U.S. cancer mortality rates. *Journal of the American Statistical Association*, **84**, 637–50.

Metropolis, N., Rosenbluth, A. W., Rosenbluth, M. N., Teller, A. H., and Teller, E. (1953). Equations of state calculations by fast computing machines. *Journal of Chemical Physics*, **21**, 1087–92.

19. Statistical methods for analysing point-source exposures

J. F. Bithell

This chapter discusses methods available for the analysis of clusters or aggregations of cases of disease in the situation where a suspect source of risk is known or specified a priori. In practice, clusters are often noticed first and then related *post hoc* to some previously unsuspected source. Although it is tempting to use point source methods in this situation, it must be continually borne in mind that the inferential value of the resulting tests is weakened by the selection problem, i.e. the difficulty that we do not know how many similar clusters might have arisen by chance but did not. Thus, in the famous case of the excess of childhood leukaemia found near the nuclear reprocessing plant at Sellafield, UK, for example, the initial finding was reported by a Yorkshire Television programme (Yorkshire Television 1983). The interest presumably arose in part as a result of anecdotal evidence and it would certainly not be possible to determine how many other populations or medical comparisons might have been liable to be reported in a similar fashion. This dramatic excess, giving a relative risk in Seascale of around 10, was in fact so impressive that it was responsible for initiating a government inquiry (Black 1984) and considerable further research. Although the methods of this chapter will use this example to illustrate methodological points, the selection problem must be continually borne in mind when interpreting the results.

Geographical data can clearly be represented by points in two dimensions and, in the first instance, we use the spatially homogeneous cartesian coordinate system to do so. The effect of specifying a point source of some kind, say S, is to impose an origin on the coordinate system and this makes it natural to consider an origin-specific system such as polar coordinates. At the same time, it is one of the objects of statistical analysis to achieve a reduction of the dimensionality of data and thus it is inevitable that we should sooner or later consider *distance*, or some monotonic transform of it, despite the protests of some geographers that it inadequately describes geographically significant information. Indeed, it may well be more appropriate to consider angular bearing or to measure distance from a geographical object other than a point, such as a coastline, for example. As far as the methods described in this chapter are concerned, however, the important thing is that we agree to consider a single, one-dimensional quantity which is supposed to be related to

risk. The essential unsuitability of untransformed distance means that we will
be well advised to consider an inverse measure of 'closeness'; it may well also
be advantageous to use methods invariant under monotonic transformations,
which is equivalent to using the rank order of the distances.

The chapter will, in fact, consider methods based on ranks as well as on a
metric and will further make a distinction between case-control methods and
methods suitable for when population denominators are known. First, more
traditional methods of analysis and their drawbacks will be considered briefly.

Traditional methods

Traditional methods of analysing geographical data usually involve calculating
incidence rates in different regions. Thus, in a systematic analysis of childhood
leukaemia in the north of England, for example, Craft *et al.* (1984) calculated
the incidence rates in the 675 electoral wards in the region and displayed them
on a map. The recent availability of small-area population data in the UK
made it possible to do this for units small enough to be relevant to localized
effects, but the interpretation of such rates is made more difficult by sampling
error and the variation of unit size. Some authors have attempted to get round
these difficulties by reporting significance levels for excesses, instead of rates,
i.e. calculating the probabilities of the observed or greater numbers of cases
under the null hypothesis. This practice, however, has its own drawbacks: it
will emphasize chance excesses in small subregions and give little weight to
moderate increases in risk in larger subregions. (See Chapter 18 for further
discussion.) Furthermore, a display of regions on a map, though informative
from an exploratory point of view, invites a subjective assessment rather than
an objective statistical analysis; the latter requires a method of relating disease
incidence to a specific location, i.e. as argued above, to distance in the first
instance. Other disadvantages of the traditional approach are discussed by
Bithell and Stone (1989).

Population-based tests of no association with distance

Once we think in terms of testing the null hypothesis that there is no association
between disease risk and distance, a large number of tests suggest themselves.
Suppose that we have population data, i.e. the expected numbers of cases
under the null hypothesis, $e_1, e_2, \ldots, e_N$, in each of N subregions which, for
convenience, we can assume to be ranked in order of increasing distance from
our point source S, say. We will also have observed counts of the numbers,
$r_1, r_2, \ldots, r_N$, of cases in these subregions, which it will often be reasonable to

assume are Poisson distributed. Conditionally on their total $n = \Sigma r_i$, the $\{r_i\}$ will have a multinomial distribution and will comprise sufficient statistics for the relative risks ϱ_i in the subregions. The best test of the null hypothesis H_0: $\varrho_1 = \varrho_2 = , \ldots , = \varrho_N$ will clearly depend on the alternative hypothesis, H_1, determined by the ϱs, but it can be shown (Bithell 1991) that the most powerful test is that based on the average score over all cases when the subregions are scored by values proportional to the $\log(\varrho_i)$ assumed under H_1. This tells us the best test to use if we have a good idea of the alternative we should be considering.

It is, however, in the nature of investigative epidemiology that we can rarely be sure what this should be. It would be preferable not to have to make parametric assumptions dependent on the effect of distance, but even if we use ranks the alternative would still require us to specify how the relative risk changes as we move further from S. One possibility might be to use a maximum likelihood ratio (MLR) test, which would proceed by obtaining estimates of the ϱs and using their logarithms as the scores. This would provide a procedure which would be asymptotically most powerful against a completely general alternative. However, because we have not provided any information about the alternative, such a test is effectively a test of heterogeneity and would not necessarily be at all powerful against a single specific alternative. The essential difficulty, which cannot be avoided, is that the best test depends on the alternative hypothesis and specifying this presupposes more knowledge than will generally be available.

A partial remedy to this problem is provided by a class of tests introduced by Stone (1988) which are constructed by reference to alternatives in which we assume only that the risk does not increase with increasing distance. Specifically, we consider the general alternative hypothesis H_M: $\varrho_1 \geq \varrho_2 \geq , \ldots , \geq \varrho_N$. Now the maximum likelihood estimators (MLEs) for the ϱs can be obtained by solving a problem in constrained optimization which is analogous to the problem of isotonic regression; this in turn permits us to use the likelihood ratio test as before, but with the likelihood now maximized subject to the order restriction on the ϱs. Stone also proposed a 'Poisson maximum' test based on the MLE $\hat{\varrho}_1$ of ϱ_1, which turns out to be the largest cumulative relative risk in the region as a whole. Stone conjectured that in some circumstances this may provide a test almost as powerful as that based on the MLR, but it now seems clear that, in general, this is unlikely to be so and, given the availability of cheap computing power, it may well be preferable to carry out a Monte Carlo test using the MLR statistic. (See also Chapter 20.)

An example

These tests are illustrated by data on childhood leukaemia and lymphoma occurring in the years 1966–83 within 50 km of the plant at Sellafield. The data were provided by the Childhood Cancer Research Group (Stiller *et al.* 1991) and the population expectations for 91 electoral wards are calculated from OPCS population data, using national tumour registration rates and adjusting for age in five-year groups. Altogether, 51 cases were recorded, of which five were in the nearest ward, Seascale, which had an expectation of only 0.389. Various tests were carried out on the data, as follows:

(1) Stone's test, based on the order-restricted maximum likelihood ratio;
(2) the Poisson maximum test, based on the estimate of $\hat{\varrho}_1$ only;
(3) a closeness score test with scores given by the reciprocals of the ward ranks;
(4) as above, but with scores given by the reciprocals of the ward distances in km.

In each case the null distribution was estimated by simulating 9999 replications having the same form as the data set, each time sampling the observed number of cases, 51, from the multinomial distribution with probabilities proportional to the expectations calculated from the population data. The resulting estimates of the significance levels achieved are reported in Table 19.1.

Table 19.1 Estimated significance levels based on 9999 simulations for tests of risk in relation to point sources defined as (a) the centre of the Sellafield installation and (b) the grid reference attaching to the postcode

| | | | Closeness scores | |
Point source location	Stone's test	Poisson maximum	1/Rank	1/Distance
(a) Centre of Sellafield	0.0040	0.0002	0.0001	0.0004
(b) Postcode location	0.0559	0.0140	0.0434	0.0026

The top row relates to data in which the ranks and distances were calculated by reference to a point, S_1, in the centre of the Sellafield site, OS reference (30250, 50350). This location for S is that used in previous studies (Bithell and Stone 1989).

However, in a more comprehensive study currently in progress, different nuclear installations in England and Wales were located in the first instance by using the grid references associated with their postcodes. This procedure locates S at a point, S_2, with grid reference (30290, 50430), i.e. a point approximately 90 m NNW of S_1. This in turn demotes Seascale to the second nearest ward, with a dramatic effect on the rank-based statistics, as shown by the second row of Table 19.1. We exhibit this comparison not for scientific reasons, but to demonstrate the sensitivity of the rank-based tests to small changes in the data.

Properties of the tests

The results of the tests reported in Table 19.1 are specific to this particular data set, of course, and to investigate the properties of the tests in general we need to investigate the operating characteristics of the tests, such as the power. Following Stone (1986), the approach used here was to estimate the expected significance level (ESL), first introduced by Dempster and Schatzoff (1965). As its name implies, the ESL is the average significance level that would be returned by a given test if the alternative were always true. A major advantage is that it is not specific to a particular Type I error, α, and indeed it can be interpreted as the power averaged over all values of α.

Table 19.2 summarizes the results of a simulation experiment in which the performances of five test statistics were compared under an alternative hypothesis specifying that the relative risk (RR) declines like

$$\varrho_i = 1 + 9 \times \exp(-d_i/5)$$

where d_i is the distance of ward i from S in km. This is similar to the pattern of relative risk observed near Sellafield (see Fig. 19.1). The simulated data were

Table 19.2 Estimates of the expected significance levels based on 5000 simulations for five tests of closeness applied to 51 cases distributed in the 91 wards according to the relative risk function $1 + 9 \times \exp(-\text{distance}/5)$

		Closeness scores		
Stone's test	Poisson maximum	1/Rank	1/Distance	Most powerful
0.0398	0.0788	0.0220	0.0158	0.0142

constructed by applying this pattern of RR to the actual expectations in the wards around Sellafield and sampling 51 cases, the number actually observed.

The test statistics considered were:

(1)–(4) as in the actual Monte Carlo tests reported above;
(5) a closeness score test as in (3) and (4), but with closeness score in ward i given by:

$$\log(1 + 9 \times \exp(-d_i/5))$$

These latter scores were chosen to give the most powerful test against the alternative under consideration, so we would expect the ESL to be smallest for this statistic. That this is indeed the case can be seen from Table 19.2, which shows estimates of the five ESLs based on 5000 simulations. Stone's MLR test appears to be distinctly less powerful in this example, although we must, of course, bear in mind that the information required to construct the most powerful test is never available in practice. The Poisson maximum is even less powerful than the likelihood ratio test against this alternative, despite the fact that the latter associates the highest risk with the first ward. Considering that the closeness scores based on the reciprocals of rank and distance are somewhat arbitrary, they have performed rather well, suggesting that the closeness score tests are fairly robust to departure from the optimum scores.

The results of this simulation study are part of a more comprehensive investigation currently being conducted, whose results will be reported elsewhere (Bithell 1991). Whether Stone's MLR test will perform acceptably well in a wide range of circumstances remains to be seen; in the light of this limited investigation, it certainly seems likely that it will, at any rate, be consistently better than the Poisson maximum test.

Case-control methods

If the locations of the cases are known exactly, it may be preferable to use a sample of controls and to compare the distributions of case and control distances from S. In particular, this has the following potential advantages:

(1) For small-scale effects it may be important to determine the locations of individual cases and controls more precisely than is possible from population data.

(2) Population data inevitably have an element of inaccuracy, especially between censuses, which results mostly from migration effects.

(3) In principle, the case-control approach permits analyses which control for confounding factors not available for census data.

The natural analogue of the closeness score test applied to Poisson data would consist of adding such a score for the cases and determining the null conditional distribution of the resulting statistic under random permutations of the cases and controls. The analogue of Stone's test—which was also proposed but not applied by Stone—effectively tests the hypothesis of uniformity of the probability that an individual is a case rather than a control. The 'Bernoulli maximum', which is analogous to the Poisson maximum, is ineffective for normal case-control studies, since the observed significance level cannot be less than the fairly high probability under the null hypothesis that the first individual is a case. The MLR test, however, is feasible.

Example continued

The case-control tests have been exemplified by applying them to the 50 cases whose actual postcoded addresses were within 50 km of the centre of the Sellafield site, S_1. A sample of controls was obtained for an earlier investigation

(Bithell 1990) by sampling addresses from the telephone directory and, though this might be an unacceptable sampling frame for a serious epidemiological investigation, it will suffice for the purposes of illustration. Of the original sample of addresses, some 65 were within 50 km of S_1. The first row of Table 19.3 shows the results of applying Stone's MLR test as well as score tests based on the reciprocals of the ranks and the distances. As in the Poisson case, the data show a great concentration of risk near S_1: the first five individuals in the data set are cases. It will be seen that Stone's test gives a less significant result than the closeness score tests. This is in spite of the fact that the scores were chosen quite arbitrarily: a non-linear transformation of distance, for example, would lead to a different result for the third test shown.

Table 19.3   Estimated significance levels based on 999 simulations for tests of risk in relation to Sellafield, based on 50 cases and 65 controls: (a) genuine data and (b) data set modified by transposing the first case with the first control

	Stone's test	Closeness scores	
		1/Rank	1/Distance
(a) Actual data	0.017	0.004	0.003
(b) Modified 'data'	0.052	0.259	0.013

It is instructive to examine the effect on the test statistics of modifying the data set somewhat: specifically, the second row of Table 19.3 shows the effect of transposing the first case with the first control. It will be seen that the closeness test based on ranks shows a much larger reduction in significance than the test defined in terms of distance.

Clearly the results of tests on one data set can provide only a pointer to the properties of tests in general. The theory of case-control tests is a little less straightforward than for the Poisson case, but further studies are in progress and may be expected to indicate the extent to which Stone's test provides a reliable general-purpose method in situations where we have no information about likely alternatives.

Estimation

It is perhaps unfortunate that preoccupation with clusters has encouraged epidemiologists to concentrate on hypothesis testing almost to the exclusion of estimation. In the case of data related to a point source, there are methods available for estimating and displaying the relationship between risk and distance.

For example, thinking in terms of the case and control distributions of distance described above, we can construct density estimates of the underlying probability distributions and take the ratio of these. It turns out that this estimates a 'relative risk function' which measures the risk at a point (or distance from S in this case) relative to the average risk over the whole population contributing to the sample. Relative risk functions in two dimensions are described by Bithell (1990) and used to depict risk over the whole of a region, but a one-dimensional version is not materially different. Thus we may estimate the risk relative to the mean as a function of distance x as

$$\hat{\varrho}(x) = \frac{\hat{f}_{\text{cases}}(x)}{\hat{f}_{\text{controls}}(x)}$$

where, for both cases and controls, $\hat{f}(x)$ is an estimate of the density of distances constructed, for example, using normal kernels:

$$\hat{f}(x) = \frac{1}{\sqrt{(2\pi)}nh} \sum_i \exp \left\{ -\frac{1}{2} \left(\frac{x - X_i}{h} \right)^2 \right\}$$

where $\{X_i\}$ are the respective data values and h is the 'bandwidth' or smoothing parameter. Figure 19.1 depicts the relative risk of childhood leukaemia as it varies by distance from Sellafield, constructed in this manner from the cases and controls described previously. Because the resulting function depends on

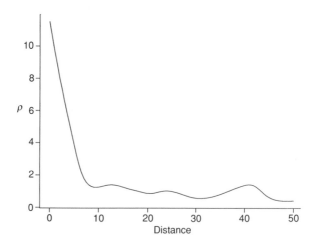

Fig. 19.1   A function estimating the relative risk at different distances from the Sellafield plant constructed from samples of 50 cases and 65 controls using kernel density estimates with a bandwidth of 10 km.

the bandwidth, the method may at present be best regarded as an exploratory one, although there certainly are objective methods available for choosing *h* (Silverman 1986). In principle, the same sort of analysis could be constructed using smoothed population data instead of the control sample.

A semi-parametric method, recently introduced by Diggle (1990), effectively fits a functional form, for example a negative exponential function, to the relative risk, while using a density estimate in the denominator to estimate the distribution of distance for the controls. This permits estimation of specific parameters, of course, though their interpretation obviously depends on the validity of the parametric model.

Discussion

In discussing statistical procedures for analysing the existence or extent of geographical clusters of disease, it is important to distinguish between the cases where there is or is not a pre-specified focus of putative risk. If there is not, we are seeking an arbitrary pattern over some geographical domain. Many methods of doing this have been advanced in the literature, including tests based on cases and controls (Smith and Pike 1974; Cuzick and Edwards 1990). Locating an individual cluster can be regarded as a problem in estimation and may be achieved by constructing an estimate of a (relative) risk function and looking for its peak (Bithell 1990).

This chapter, however, has been concerned with the complementary problem relating to a pre-specified source. Fewer papers have been published on this topic, partly perhaps because of the reluctance to use distance explicitly, and perhaps also because any notion that we are comparing a distribution of distances for cases with either a population distribution or a control distribution runs into difficulty unless we concentrate on tests that are sensitive primarily to differences in the tail of the distribution. The methods discussed in this chapter offer possibilities for dealing with this situation. In epidemiological applications, however, we must remember the caveat in the introduction to this chapter and resist the temptation to identify sources of risk after inspecting our data.

Acknowledgements

The data reported in this chapter were kindly provided by Dr G. J. Draper, Director of the Childhood Cancer Research Group and his staff. The calculations were effected with the assistance of Mrs S. J. Dutton, who was supported by a grant from Nuclear Electric plc.

References

Bithell, J. F. (1990). An application of density estimation to geographical epidemiology. *Statistics in Medicine*, **9**, 691–701.

Bithell, J. F. (1992). The comparative characteristics of tests for risk in relation to point sources. Technical Report, in preparation.

Bithell, J. F. and Stone, R. A. (1989). On statistical methods for analysing the geographical distribution of cancer cases near nuclear installations. *Journal of Epidemiology and Community Health*, **43**, 79–85.

Black, D. (1984). *Investigation of the possible increased incidence of cancer in West Cumbria*. HMSO, London.

Craft, A. W., Openshaw, S., and Birch, J. M. (1984). Apparent clusters of childhood lymphoid malignancy in Northern England. *Lancet*, **i**, 96–7.

Cuzick, J. and Edwards, R. (1990). Spatial clustering for inhomogeneous populations. *Journal of the Royal Statistical Society, Series B*, **52**, (1), 73–104.

Dempster, A. P. and Schatzoff, M. (1965). Expected significance level as a sensitivity index for test statistics. *Journal of the American Statistical Association*, **60**, 420–36.

Diggle, P. J. (1990). A point process modelling approach to raised incidence of a rare phenomenon in the vicinity of a pre-specified point. *Journal of the Royal Statistical Society, Series A*, **153**, 349–62.

Silverman, B. W. (1986). *Density estimation for statistics and data analysis*. Chapman and Hall, London.

Smith, P. G. and Pike, M. C. (1974). A note on a 'close-pairs' test for space clustering. *British Journal of Preventive and Social Medicine*, **28**, 63–4.

Stiller, C. A., O'Connor, C. M., Vincent, T. J., and Draper, G. J. (1991). The National Registry of Childhood Tumours and the leukaemia/lymphoma data for 1966–83. In *The geographical epidemiology of childhood leukaemia and non-Hodgkin lymphomas in Great Britain 1966–83*, (ed. G. J. Draper), OPCS Studies in Medical and Population Subjects. HMSO, London.

Stone, R. A. (1986). Statistical methodology and causal inference in studies of the health effects of radiation. Unpublished D.Phil. thesis. University of Oxford.

Stone, R. A. (1988). Investigations of excess environmental risks around putative sources: statistical problems and a proposed test. *Statistics in Medicine*, **7**, 649–60.

Yorkshire Television (1983). *Windscale: the nuclear laundry*. Documentary programme, 1 November.

20. Some comments on methods for investigating disease risk around a point source

M. Hills

A fundamental problem when assessing risk around a point source is the difficulty of specifying, in advance, the size of the area for which the risk is to be assessed. To see why this is a problem, suppose the increased risk is largely confined within an area B, centred on the point source P, and suppose an area A is chosen for study. If A is much smaller than B, the study may lack power because the number of cases is small; if A is much larger than B, the study may fail to detect any increased risk because the true rate ratio for A is lower than for B.

Stone (1988) and Bithell and Stone (1989) have presented methods for testing for an increased risk which do not require a single area to be specified in advance. Instead a number of small areas $A_1, \ldots, A_k$, which together more than cover any area likely to be of interest, are studied. Let these areas be arranged in order according to their distance from the point source P, and let the number of cases expected in these areas from standard age-specific rates be $E_1, \ldots, E_k$ with observed numbers $O_1, \ldots, O_k$. Then O_i may be taken to be an observation from the Poisson distribution with mean $\lambda_i E_i$. The hypothesis which corresponds to there being no increased risk in any of the areas, compared to standard rates, is

$$H_0: \quad \lambda_1 = \lambda_2 = \ldots = \lambda_k = 1.$$

Stone and Bithell suggest testing H_0, against isotonic alternatives

$$H_1: \quad \lambda_1 \geq \lambda_2 \geq \ldots \geq \lambda_k.$$

They argue that an elevated risk around a point source, regardless of how far it extends, will result in an isotonic trend with distance of this kind.

The maximum likelihood estimates of the λ_i subject to the isotonic restraint are easily found using the algorithm described in Barlow *et al.* p. 72 (1972). These estimates are then used for the likelihood ratio test of H_0 versus the best isotonic alternative. The sampling distribution of the likelihood ratio is obtained by repeatedly simulating observations from Poisson distributions with mean E_i, which are then used to obtain estimates of λ_i subject to the isotonic restraint, and the likelihood ratio. As a way of avoiding simulation,

Stone (1988) suggested using the largest value of O/E when areas are merged in order of increasing distance as an approximation to the likelihood ratio test. Exact p-values may be calculated for this test but the computation is heavy.

If H_0 is judged untenable compared to isotonic alternatives, this could be due to a trend in risk with distance, but it could also be due to a level of risk for the total area which is different from that implied by the standard rates, without there being any trend with distance. In practice it is important to know whether there is any evidence for trend independently of the level of risk for the total area, and this may be judged by testing the weaker hypothesis

$$H_0': \quad \lambda_1 = \lambda_2 = \ldots = \lambda_k = \lambda_0$$

in which λ_0 is unknown. This allows for the possibility that the total area may have a risk which is different from that implied by the standard rates. Under H_0' the distribution of the number of cases in the ith area is Poisson with mean $\lambda_0 E_i$, which depends on an unknown parameter, thus precluding direct simulation. Conditional simulation, in which the number of simulated cases is kept the same as the total number actually observed, eliminates the unknown parameter and may be used to carry out the test. A test of H_0' may also be based on the circle with largest value of O/E, but the p-value must be obtained by simulation rather than by direct calculation.

Implementation

In the Small Areas Health Statistics Unit (SAHSU) at the London School of Hygiene and Tropical Medicine, we have started to investigate point sources by obtaining observed and expected numbers of cases for a range of circles centred on the point source. Expected numbers are obtained from age-specific rates for the disease concerned, based on both Great Britain and the region in which the point source is located. The areas $A_1, \ldots, A_k$, ranked by distance from the source, are the bands between successive circles; the first band is the first circle, the second band is the area between the second and first circle, and so on.

The main parameters for the family of circles are the radius of the smallest, the radius of the largest, and the number of circles. Some rule for interpolating between the smallest and largest is also required. As smallest we use 0.5 km. This is very small (sometimes including no population) but it offers the chance to pick out extremely localized clusters. As the largest we use, say, 10 or 20 km, depending on the situation. Purely as a matter of convenience, 10 circles in all are used, giving, for example, radii:

0.5, 1.0, 2.0, 3.0, 4.9, 6.3, 7.4, 8.3, 9.2, 10.0.

Here the first four are chosen to concentrate on local clustering, while the rest produce roughly equal increments in area up to 10 km. The first two circles typically produce no cases if the disease is uncommon.

Examples

Table 20.1 shows three examples from a study of cancer of the larynx around several possible point sources: Column (1) refers to the radii of the circles; the distance of each band from the point source is taken to be the radius of the outer circle defining the band. Columns (2) and (3) refer to the observed and

Table 20.1   Three examples of observed and expected values for cancer of the larynx (incidence) in circles of increasing size. Expected numbers are based on rates for standard administrative regions

	(1) d	(2) O	(3) E	(4) CO	(5) CE	(6) O/E	(7) CO/CE	(8) λ
Example 1	0.5	0.00	0.27	0.00	0.27	0.00	0.00	1.40
	1.0	0.00	1.03	0.00	1.30	0.00	0.00	1.40
	2.0	10.00	7.38	10.00	8.68	1.36	1.15	1.40
	3.0	10.00	6.93	20.00	15.61	1.44	1.28	1.40
	4.9	24.00	15.90	44.00	31.51	1.51	1.40	1.40
	6.3	12.00	10.41	56.00	41.92	1.15	1.34	1.17
	7.4	9.00	8.28	65.00	50.20	1.09	1.29	1.17
	8.3	11.00	8.58	76.00	58.78	1.28	1.29	1.17
	9.2	8.00	9.97	84.00	68.75	0.80	1.22	0.80
	10.0	6.00	8.58	90.00	77.33	0.70	1.16	0.70
Example 2	0.5	0.00	0.11	0.00	0.11	0.00	0.00	1.31
	1.0	0.00	0.81	0.00	0.92	0.00	0.00	1.31
	2.0	3.00	3.02	3.00	3.94	0.99	0.76	1.31
	3.0	5.00	5.58	8.00	9.52	0.90	0.84	1.31
	4.9	18.00	15.85	26.00	25.37	1.14	1.02	1.31
	6.3	29.00	20.42	55.00	45.79	1.42	1.20	1.31
	7.4	29.00	18.27	84.00	64.06	1.59	1.31	1.31
	8.3	12.00	14.48	96.00	78.54	0.83	1.22	0.98
	9.2	12.00	14.96	108.00	93.50	0.80	1.16	0.98
	10.0	18.00	13.51	126.00	107.01	1.33	1.18	0.98
Example 3	0.5	1.00	0.02	1.00	0.02	50.00	50.00	50.00
	1.0	0.00	0.15	1.00	0.17	0.00	5.88	1.80
	2.0	0.00	0.53	1.00	0.70	0.00	1.43	1.80
	3.0	2.00	0.98	3.00	1.68	2.04	1.79	1.80
	4.9	6.00	2.79	9.00	4.47	2.15	2.01	1.80
	6.3	5.00	3.60	14.00	8.07	1.39	1.73	1.73
	7.4	5.00	3.16	19.00	11.23	1.58	1.69	1.73
	8.3	6.00	2.50	25.00	13.73	2.40	1.82	1.73
	9.2	1.00	2.60	26.00	16.33	0.38	1.59	0.80
	10.0	3.00	2.38	29.00	18.71	1.26	1.55	0.80

expected values in the bands. Columns (4) and (5) refer to the observed and expected values for the circles and are the cumulative sums of the numbers in the bands. Columns (6) and (7) refer to the O/E ratios for the bands and circles respectively, and the estimated values of the λ_i under a decreasing monotonic restriction are given in column (8). Plots of O/E for the bands versus the distance of the band from P are shown in Fig. 20.1. The p-values for a variety of tests, using these examples, are shown in Table 20.2.

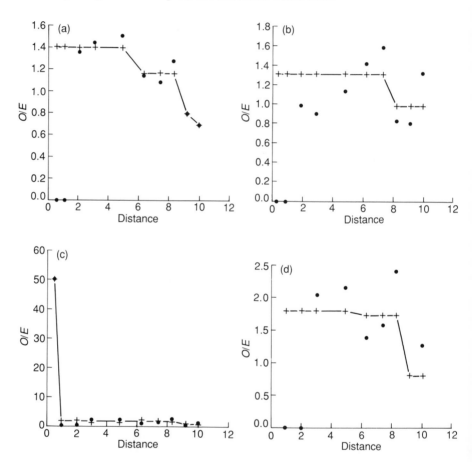

Fig. 20.1 Plots of O/E for the bands versus the distance of the band from P. (a) Example 1; (b) Example 2; (c) Example 3; (d) Example 3, omitting the first band. ●, Raw data; +, smoothed data, using an isotonic restraint.

These three examples, selected from a total of 10 sites, are chosen solely to illustrate some of the problems that arise when trying to interpret the results of the significance tests described on pp. 231–2. No conclusions about the risk of cancer of the larynx should be drawn from these three examples in isolation.

Table 20.2 *p*-values for tests of H_0 and H_0' for the three examples and for the pooled data from these examples

			p-value	
	Ex.1	Ex.2	Ex.3	Pooled
Unconditional simulation (H_0)				
Circle with largest *O/E*	0.499	0.446	0.018	0.339
Likelihood ratio (H_0)	0.128	0.183	0.007	0.007
Conditional simulation (H_0')				
Circle with largest *O/E*	0.627	0.651	0.030	0.185
Likelihood ratio (H_0')	0.161	0.364	0.054	0.074

Example 1

There is a slight suggestion of a downward trend with distance, largely due to the last two bands. The likelihood ratio test of H_0 gives a *p*-value of 0.128. In this situation we would expect the likelihood ratio test for trend alone (H_0') to give a similar result, and indeed the *p*-value is 0.161.

The largest value of *O/E* in the circles is 1.40, based on 24 cases where only 15.9 were expected. The nominal *p*-value for this result is 0.035. Adjusting for selection, the probability of observing an *O/E* ratio greater than or equal to 1.40 in all 10 circles is 0.499. The reason for this very large change from nominal to adjusted is due to the appreciable probability of one case in the first circle (giving *O/E* = 3.7) and two cases in the second circle (giving *O/E* = 1.53).

Example 2

There appears to be a slight drop in risk after about 7 km, but the two likelihood ratio tests show no significant departures from either H_0 or H_0'. Looked at separately, the circle with radius 7.4 km has the value 1.31 for *O/E* with nominal *p*-value 0.0123 but, on adjustment for selection, this becomes 0.446. This is an example of how using the nominal *p*-value for the largest *O/E* can be very misleading.

Example 3

This kind of situation arises whenever there is a single case in the first circle, where the expected value is low. Apart from the first circle there appears to be little trend with distance. The largest *O/E* ratio is 50.0 with nominal *p*-value

0.020. This barely changes when adjusted for selection because almost the only way of achieving an *O/E* ratio larger than 50.0 is with one case in the first circle. Because of the difficulty of simulating low *p*-values with high precision, the adjusted value shown in Table 20.2 is actually lower than the nominal value, due to random error in the simulated value. The likelihood ratio tests give *p*-values of 0.007 for H_0 and 0.054 for H_0'.

In our limited experience with using these methods, the test based on the circle with largest value of *O/E* is best avoided. There is a high chance that the largest value will arise from a single case in the smallest circle, and such a result is more a comment on the discrete nature of the Poisson distribution than evidence of a raised risk near the source. The likelihood ratio test of H_0 is more useful, but to distinguish the situation where there is an increased risk, but no trend, from the situation where there is a trend, it is best to test H_0' as well.

Aggregating over sites

In view of the rarity of the diseases we are commonly interested in and the possibility that the original site was selected because of an apparent excess of cases, it is essential to be able to widen an enquiry to other sites and to aggregate the evidence obtained, including the evidence from the original site.

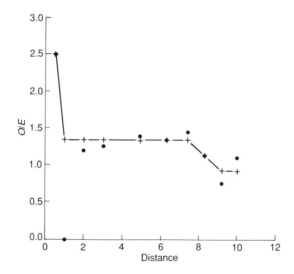

Fig. 20.2   The result of aggregating the observed and expected values for each band over the three sites represented in the three examples. •, Raw data; +, smoothed data, using an isotonic restraint.

Using the same range of circles for each site offers the possibility of simply aggregating the observed and expected values for each band over the sites. Figure 20.2 shows the result of aggregating over the three sites represented in the three examples. There appears to be little evidence for trend, apart from that supplied by the case in the first circle and the decline in risk after about 7 km. Table 20.2 shows that the likelihood ratio test rejects H_0. Unfortunately the test for H_0', which we should like to carry out to see whether there is a trend with distance as well as with values of λ which differ from 1, cannot be carried out using the pooled data alone because each site may have its own (different) value of λ_0. An alternative approach is to combine the three separate p-values for testing H_0'; these are 0.161, 0.364, and 0.054, and combining these in the standard way, using $-2 \Sigma \log p$ gives the value 11.511. Looking this up as chi-squared on $2 \times 3 = 6$ degrees of freedom gives a combined p-value of 0.074.

Discussion

Because of the role of the expected values in these methods, the choice of standard rates is critical. A common technique in epidemiology is to compare the number of cases among a group of people, characterized by some factor, with the number expected for subjects without the factor, living in the same area. The difficulty we meet in studies of point sources is that the factor of interest *is* residence in the area, so we must choose some other group for comparison. In SAHSU we are currently dividing England, Wales, and Scotland into socio-economic strata based on census characteristics, and then estimating age- and sex-specific rates for each stratum. The circles are similarly divided into strata and the rates appropriate to each stratum are applied to find the expected numbers. In this way the areas under study are compared with socio-economically similar areas, as well as areas from the same region (see Chapter 11 for further discussion).

References

Barlow, R. E., Bartholomew, D. J., Bremner, J. M., and Brunk, H. D. (1972). *Statistical inference under order restrictions*. J. Wiley and Sons, New York.

Bithell, J. F. and Stone, R. A. (1989). On statistical methods for analysing the geographical distribution of cancer cases near nuclear installations. *Journal of Epidemiology and Community Health*, **43**, 79–85.

Stone, R. A. (1988). Investigations of excess environmental risks around putative sources: statistical problems and a proposed test. *Statistics in Medicine*, **7**, 649–60.

21. Methods for the assessment of disease clusters

F. E. Alexander and J. Cuzick

Clusters and clustering

Clustering is a poorly defined concept in the medical literature. This is not surprising since an adequate definition is extraordinarily difficult (Elliott 1989). An important distinction to make is the notion of an individual cluster, corresponding to an excess number of cases in one small area or around a particular point source, and the concept of a general tendency for clustering, by which is meant a more heterogeneous 'clumped' distribution of disease cases than would be expected from the variation in population density and chance fluctuations.

From a modelling point of view, one can give a precise mathematical formulation of these concepts, but such models are generally too inflexible to encompass the full range of possibilities seen in practice. Thus another important distinction to recognize is the difference between a cluster or clustering in a mathematical model and in an empirical set of data. It is the latter which is addressed in the medical literature and necessarily any definition will take the rather less precise form indicated in the preceding paragraph. For example, Knox (1989) has given the following definition: 'a cluster is a geographically bounded group of occurrences of sufficient size and concentration to be unlikely to have occurred by chance.'

Figure 21.1 shows an example of a point pattern arising in a uniform underlying population. The random pattern arises from a Poisson process and contains a number of aggregations or clusters, including the one highlighted, but these are entirely due to chance variation. The problem of *post hoc* cluster identification is illustrated by the Texas sharpshooter who positions his target in precisely this position *after* shots have been fired to the target. Eyeballing patterns for evidence of clustering becomes virtually impossible when the underlying population is heterogeneous (Fig. 21.2). Apparent clusters are now merely pointers to areas of high population density.

Null hypothesis: no clustering

We begin by considering what we mean by the null situation of 'no clustering'. The geographical distribution of disease will normally display structure at a

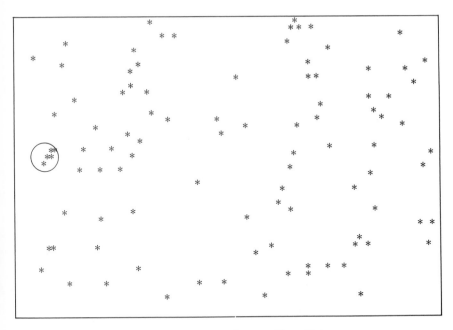

Fig. 21.1   Sample point pattern for a uniform Poisson process.

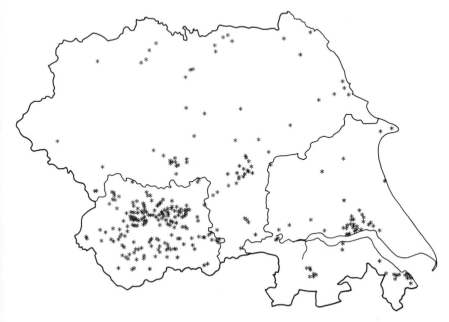

Fig. 21.2   Sample point pattern for a non-uniform Poisson process arising from an uneven population density.

variety of scales; there will be regional trends, large-scale heterogeneity (e.g. by UK county or French *département*), and also variations in incidence due to geographical change of known risk factors. All of these are important but not relevant to the issue of detecting localized clustering. Note, however, that the choice of known risk factors for which to make adjustment represents a decision on 'uninteresting clustering' (Cuzick and Edwards 1990) which needs to be explicit and which will depend on the context. In general, we shall wish to adjust for large-scale variations in risk (Hills and Alexander 1989) when studying localized clustering.

We suppose that the study area, A, is partitioned into a large number of small areas $\{A_j\}$ and that stratum (age, sex, risk-factor) specific reference incidence rates $\{r_i\}$ are available, together with counts $\{n_{ij}\}$ of the population at risk in each A_j. Let Θ be the relative risk of some *large* area containing A_j. This factor is included to accommodate the large-scale trends and heterogeneity mentioned above. Then an appropriate null hypothesis (H_0) is that the number D_j of cases in A_j has Poisson distribution with mean equal to the 'expected number'

$$E_j = \Theta \Sigma r_i n_{ij}. \tag{1}$$

Spatial clustering may be defined as any departure from H_0 in which the variability of the $\{D_j\}$ is *increased*.

If this happens, then cases will tend to group together in some areas and these will be *clusters*. Note that in the absence of a predetermined putative risk we are taking 'clustering' as the primary concept and 'cluster' as derived from it. We return to this point later.

The distribution of cases under this null hypothesis is closely related to an underlying Poisson process. Indeed, if the partition $\{A_j\}$ is allowed to be arbitrary, then under H_0 the case locations are a realization of a Poisson process which is, technically, non-homogeneous but whose intensity at $\mathbf{x}$,

$$\lambda_0(\mathbf{x}), \tag{2}$$

depends only on the population distribution (by stratum) at x and large-scale geographical factors (via Θ). For the present purposes λ_0, θ, r_i, n_{ij}, are all assumed to be known, although in practice Θ will usually have to be estimated. In the sequel we shall not always distinguish between situations which do, and do not, condition on the total observed number of cases, $D+$.

Models for clustering

Two particular mechanisms of clustering are worth distinguishing. The first, called *true contagion* (Cliff and Ord 1981) occurs when some of the events are not independent of each other. One parametrization of this takes parent locations (or events) generated by a Poisson process and the number of daughter events located at each parent determined by a generalizing distribution. For the second, which we shall call *localized heterogeneity*, the number in each small area follows a Poisson distribution with mean $\lambda_i E_i$, but each λ_i is independently selected from a suitable distribution.

If, for either of these models, the study area were decomposed into small areas of equal size, then the number of events in a random small area would follow a composite distribution. In several special cases the same distribution arises from true contagion and localized heterogeneity. If, for example, the generalizing distribution were logarithmic, the composite distribution is negative binomial and this also occurs for localized heterogeneity if the local intensity is sampled from a gamma distribution.

These situations may be relaxed slightly by allowing the clusters arising in the true contagion model to be dispersed around the parents and the intensity varying continuously in the local heterogeneity model. The composite models are then known as the *Poisson cluster process* and the *doubly stochastic Poisson process*, respectively.

Broadly, these two correspond to the two biological models which are appropriate: transmission of an infectious agent and local excesses of environmental risk. We have hinted at the mathematical duality of the two which is, in fact, total (Bartlett 1953). The biological distinction also becomes rather blurred in chronic disease epidemiology because of the inclusion of healthy carriers and long, variable latent periods.

Methods

There is a large body of theoretical work on the analysis of spatial point patterns (e.g. Cliff and Ord 1981; Diggle 1983). Most methods are based on either cell counts or distances (event-event or point-event). A special problem in the analysis of disease clustering is the heterogeneity of the human population. Other difficulties are the relative sparseness of the data and, often, the desire of both the general public and the scientific investigator to detect quite small, subtle, and unspecified variations from the null hypothesis.

Cell count methods

The requirement that accurate counts of human populations at risk be available has traditionally led to the use of census units as basic cells.

Potthoff and Whittinghill (1966a,b) have shown that the locally most powerful test of Equation (1) with estimated mean against the compound gamma-poisson alternative gives rise to the test statistic

$$S = \sum_i \frac{D_i(D_i-1)}{E_i} \, . \tag{3}$$

S has an asymptotically normal distribution, with mean

$$\mu = \frac{D_+ (D_+ - 1)}{E_+} \text{ and variance } \frac{2(N-1)\mu}{E_+} . \tag{4}$$

One disadvantage of this is that the investigator has no control over the scale of the clustering that he is studying. An alternative method, due to Urquhart and Black (COMARE 1988), uses an algorithm to amalgamate the smallest UK census districts (enumeration districts, or EDs) into areas with expected number of cases (E_i) approximately equal to a pre-specified constant size E. They then applied Pearson's chi-square goodness-of-fit test to investigate departures from Poisson variability. Calculations on a uniform population and negative binomial alternative hypothesis (Hills and Alexander 1989) suggest that this method may lack power and, since we are concerned with excess variability, theoretical considerations suggest that the dispersion test using

$$\sum_i \frac{(D_i - E_i)^2}{E_i} \tag{5}$$

is likely to be preferable. When all the E_is are exactly equal to E and the total number of cases is taken as fixed then this is equivalent to the Potthoff–Whittinghill test. In general, they are not the same and their relative power for various alternatives requires further investigation.

Distance methods

All these methods consider circles defined by geographical distance, population density, population count, number of cases, or a combination of these. Usually either the number of cases or the population size is fixed and the other is the random variable. Two general points arise. First, the size of the circles may differ depending on the local population density. Secondly, since population counts are known only for pre-defined census areas, the circles are either exact circles with estimates of their population or approximations to circles composed of appropriate amalgamations of, for example, EDs. In the latter situation the populations are known exactly. We shall refer to both as 'circles'.

Distance methods using control locations

Two distance methods (Cuzick and Edwards 1990; Diggle 1990) use control locations to explicitly (or implicitly) specify the nuisance function λ_0 which measures the local population density (see Equation (2)). There are then two sequences of points, $(x_1, \ldots, x_n)$ (cases) and $(x_{m+1}, \ldots, x_{m+n})$ (controls), and the null hypothesis is the *random labelling hypothesis* that $(x_1, \ldots, x_n)$ is a random sample from $(x_1, \ldots, x_{n+m})$. No particular distributional form is assumed for either cases or controls. Cuzick and Edwards identify the k nearest neighbours to each point (for some suitable small integer(s) k) and use as test statistic

$$T_k = \sum_{i=1}^{n} \sum_{j=1}^{n} \delta_{ij} , \tag{6}$$

where $\delta_{ij} = 1$ if $i \neq j$ and x_j is one of the k nearest neighbours of x_i. The distribution of T_k is asymptotically normal with mean

$$\frac{n(n-1)k}{(m+n-1)}$$

and variance depending on the particular configuration. The covariance structure is also available, so that testing for a combination of T_ks (with, for example, $k = 1, 2, 4, 8$) is straightforward. The test for single k can be seen as a special case of a join-count statistic with T_k represented by a Geary–Moran statistic (Moran 1948).

The method of Diggle uses the second moment properties of the process; specifically $K_{11}(s) = \lambda_0^{-1} \times$ mean (number of cases within distance s of an arbitrary case) and K_{22}, is defined analogously in terms of the control series. Departures from the null hypothesis are identified by positive values of estimates of

$$D(s) = K_{11}(s) - K_{22}(s). \tag{7}$$

λ_0 can be estimated using kernel density, or other appropriate methods.

The particular strength of this method is that it focuses on estimation of the scale of the clustering; however, the usefulness of this may be limited, since 'scale' is determined by geographical rather than population measures. Formal significance testing uses Monte Carlo methods.

The choice of suitable controls is critical for both methods. In certain situations (e.g. in the analysis of data from a matched case-control study) they may well be available at the same time as the case locations, in which event they are a natural way of specifying all the 'nuisance' heterogeneity included as matching criteria. In other situations considerable care (and possible expense) will be required in their selection.

Distance methods using population counts

The geographical analysis machine (GAM; Openshaw *et al.* 1988) was originally aimed at detecting individual clusters. It was highly visual and clusters were revealed by an abundant overlay of drawn circles. These are (potentially) centred on any one of a large number of grid locations and can have any one of a large number of radii, or can have size specified by population or case counts. A circle is plotted if it satisfies a local significance criterion based on Poisson probabilities. Global statistical testing is now available using Monte Carlo methods with the number of drawn circles as test statistic. This is essentially a point-event distance method.

A second method due originally to Besag (1989) (see also Besag and Newell 1991) as a modification of the GAM for detecting individual *clusters*, which aimed to minimize its Type I errors and other theoretical drawbacks, considers circles centred only on case locations and tests for significance the 'distance' to the kth nearest case. Because of the heterogeneity of the population, distance is replaced by the expected number of cases, E, arising among the population, P_c, within an appropriate circle around a case c. The circle is built from discrete EDs. The probability that E is less than the observed value λ is

$$p = 1 - \sum_{j=0}^{k-1} \exp(-\lambda)(\lambda)^j/j! \tag{8}$$

If p is less than a specified value, a circle is drawn around the case.

This idea is the basis of another test of *clustering* (the NNA test; Alexander *et al.* 1989, 1991a) in which the same idea is applied to large data sets and attention focused upon the percentage of cases with $p < 0.05$ (called 'clustered' cases). Technical differences between the two include the use of two values of k (the particular choice depending on the frequency of disease) and the use of actual locations instead of EDs, with a local estimate of λ around each case, being derived by smoothing ED populations. Monte Carlo testing is used.

This test uses as its statistic the sum over all cases of transform of the P_cs. Corresponding work for homogeneous populations summarized in Cliff and Ord (1981) indicates that a statistic of this type is likely to be appropriate but gives little guidance on the particular form. Our own work indicates that the simple sum ΣP_c is unduly influenced by cases which are not within clusters and, in consequence, lacks power. Testing by Monte Carlo simulation will always be necessary.

A variant of the Cuzick–Edwards test, the 'one-sample limit' is similar to the NNA test but takes as its statistic

$$\Sigma Q_c$$

where Q_c is the number of cases arising in the circle centred as c and having a fixed pre-defined expected number of cases within it. Thus the circles now have their denominators fixed rather than their numerators. An advantage of this method is that formulae for the mean and variance are available and asymptotic normality can be established. Preliminary results suggest that the power of this test is similar to that of the NNA test.

General comments

For most of these methods (Potthoff–Whittinghill, Urquhart–Black, Cuzick–Edwards, NNA) the *primary* aim is to provide a global statistical test of clustering. Estimation is not straightforward since no specific parametric form is assumed for the alternative process. However, estimating the geographical scale of clustering is a specific aim of the Diggle method. The other methods all share a degree of arbitrariness in the size (however determined) of circles or cells considered; inspection of the effect on the results of change of size will provide some guidance on the scale of clustering by geographical distance (GAM), population size (GAM, Cuzick–Edwards), number of cases (GAM, Besag, NNA), but this is a very informal data analytic procedure. Similarly, the proportion of clustered cases (NNA, Besag) provides some indication of the extent of clustering (i.e. how many cases arise under the influence of the aetiology that causes clustering).

Comparative performance

Little guidance is available on the comparative performance of the methods. A simulation study (Cartwright *et al.* 1990) has compared the power of three of the methods against five alternatives. In general, the Potthoff–Whittinghill and NNA methods had similar power and the Cuzick–Edwards rather lower. When the one-sample limit variant of the Cuzick–Edwards test was used, comparable power to the Potthoff–Whittinghill and NNA methods was observed. Knowledge of the power of tests and their sensitivity to particular alternatives is an essential prerequisite to interpretation of their results (Wartenberg and Greenberg 1990).

A collaborative study using artificial data is currently in progress to explore this question further. No large-scale patterns were used in the generation of the data but one important conclusion has been that the consequences of 'clustering' may be manifested as larger-scale heterogeneity. Thus care is required in the decisions to adjust for large-scale structure. All methods showed reasonable success in identifying clustering and in giving (approximate) locations to clusters, but all yielded false positive results. We conclude that the methods can safely be applied to identify areas for further research, but that extreme caution is necessary before results are disseminated.

Interpretation and application

It is important to recognize that the investigation of clustering and clusters will be motivated by diverse aims. They will, in general, include monitoring community health, allaying public concern, and providing aetiological clues (Rothman 1987). Rothman has stressed that useful clues from cluster investigations are relatively rare (see also Warner and Aldrich 1988). The 'payoff for clustering research comes from the specific hypotheses which emerge to explain the observed pattern' (Rothman 1990). We would add that confirmation and refinements of existing hypotheses should also be included among the payoffs. Always, however, the interpretation is tentative and will require confirmation from in-depth analytical studies. In any event, the likelihood of useful aetiological clues is enormously increased if the cases have been ascertained using a fixed protocol (rather than in some *ad hoc* way), and their numbers are large. Inferences are much stronger if clustering involves several clusters. Any interpretation involving a causal role for a source with a single *post hoc* cluster must be extremely tentative. Investigation of a cluster of this type may involve enormous expenditure of professional time and public money (see example 4 below). With hindsight, this will have been justified from a scientific point of view only if it leads to identification of an aetiological factor which is either

(1) a substantial cause of the total burden of the particular disease in society; or
(2) an overwhelming cause of disease in a particular area, though rarely causative elsewhere (example 3 below).

In general, we believe that it is not normally appropriate to justify the expenditure of public resources on an isolated cluster not supported by a test of generalized clustering. Exceptions will occur as a result of interaction between the magnitude of the excess and the availability of reasonable explanatory hypotheses. Testing a hypothesis for replication in comparable areas (if it remains an environmental hypothesis), or using alternative study designs (if a biological model is postulated), will be essential.

Some examples will illustrate these points:

1. Cluster investigations that have identified important aetiological factors:

(a) dental caries, enamel discolouration, and fluoridization (Black and McKay 1916; McKay 1929, 1933; Dean 1938);
(b) soya beans and asthma attacks (Antó *et al.* 1989; Sunyer *et al.* 1989; see also Chapter 27).

In both instances a long and painstaking research programme led, in succession, to the generation then testing of a hypothesis, to intervention, and finally to the reduction of disease.

2. Hodgkin's disease in young adults. There has been a long history of anecdotal reports of clustering, of inconsistent results of tests for generalized tendency to exhibit space–time clustering (reviewed by Smith 1978; Alexander 1990), and a collection of epidemiological evidence supportive of a specific infectious aetiology model (the 'late host-response model') (Gutensohn and Cole 1981). Now tests of spatial clustering have shown consistently positive results (Alexander *et al.* 1989; Urquhart 1989; Glaser 1990) and, more recently, have suggested that such clustering occurs more commonly in isolated areas, although the overall incidence rate there is lower (Alexander *et al.* 1991b). This has been contemporaneous with laboratory findings of the Epstein–Barr viral genome in approximately 30 per cent of tumour samples (Staal *et al.* 1989; Weiss *et al.* 1987, 1989). The two independent areas of research support each other and offer hope for further aetiological insight.

3. Mesothelioma in Turkey. A *post hoc* observation of high rates of malignant pleural mesothelioma in a small village (Karain, with a population of 500–800) in Turkey (Baris *et al.* 1975) was confirmed by a subsequent survey (Baris *et al.* 1978). The 'cluster'

persisted in time with this rare disease (normal incidence is of the order of 1–2 per million person-years) representing 86 per cent (108) of the deaths due to cancer from 1970 to 1987. Detailed epidemiological study, which included analyses of rock and dust samples, has identified exposure to naturally occurring erionite fibres as the cause (Baris *et al.* 1987). This is of overwhelming local importance, but is not of aetiological relevance to cases of mesothelioma arising elsewhere, where the exposure is absent. (See Chapter 26.)

4. The Sellafield cluster. This is one paradigm of an isolated *post hoc* cluster report which has led to an enormous volume of research. To date, seven years on from the original media report, two government committees have reported (Black 1984; COMARE 1986), and two cohort studies (Gardner *et al.* 1987*a,b*) and one case-control study (Gardner *et al.* 1990) have been published. Other studies are in progress. The localized excess has been confirmed and the perspective has shifted from a putative environmental risk to a hypothesis involving occupational exposure of men before their child's conception. (See Chapter 25.) Despite considerable controversy over the plausibility of the biological mechanisms involved (Evans 1990), it is conceivable (Greaves 1990; Peto 1990) that the eventual outcome will be confirmation of the hypothesis and a real increase in knowledge of the aetiology of childhood leukaemia.

Conclusion

We have chosen to focus on the idea of clustering as opposed to specific clusters and have defined it in purely statistical terms. Statistical methods can then (with some error) determine whether it is present. They cannot tell whether it is 'real' in the sense of an extension of Knox's definition (1989):

'– the cases are related to each other through some social or biological mechanism or have a common relationship to some other event or circumstance.'

Cluster investigations represent one of many tools for hypothesis generation and refinement, but new putative causes will always require further, more specific, studies before the results become secure.

References

Alexander, F. E. (1990). Clustering and Hodgkin's disease. Guest editorial. *British Journal of Cancer*, **62**, 708–11.

Alexander, F. E., Williams, J., McKinney, P. A., Cartwright, R. A., and Ricketts, T. J. (1989). A specialist leukaemia/lymphoma registry in the UK. Part 2: clustering of Hodgkin's disease. *British Journal of Cancer*, **60**, 948–52.

Alexander, F. E., McKinney, P. A., Cartwright, R. A., and Ricketts, T. J. (1991*a*). Methods of mapping and identifying small clusters of disease with applications to geographical epidemiology. *Geographical Analysis*, **23**, (2), 156–73.

Alexander, F. E., Ricketts, T. J., McKinney, P. A., and Cartwright, R. A. (1991*b*). Community lifestyle characteristics and risk of Hodgkin's disease in young people. *International Journal of Cancer*, **48**, 10–14.

Antó, J. M., Sunyer, J., Rodriguez-Roisin, R., Suarez-Cervera, M., and Vazquez, L. (1989). Community outbreaks of asthma with inhalation of soybean dust. *New England Journal of Medicine*, **320**, 1097–102.

Baris, Y. I., *et al.* (1975). An outbreak of pleural mesothelioma in the village of Karain/ Urgup. *Anatolia: Kanser*, **5**, 1–4.

Baris, Y. I., *et al.* (1978). An outbreak of pleural mesothelioma and chronic fibrosing pleurisy in the village of Karain/Urgup in Anatolia. *Thorax*, **33**, 181–92.

Baris, Y. I., *et al.* (1987). Epidemiological and environmental evidence of the health effects of exposure to erionite fibres: a four-year study in the Cappadocian region of Turkey. *International Journal of Cancer*, **39**, 10–17.

Bartlett, M. S. (1953). Spectral analysis of two-dimensional point processes. *Biometrika*, **51**, 299–311.

Besag, J. (1989). Contribution to the discussion at the RSS meeting on cancer near nuclear installations. *Journal of the Royal Statistical Society, Series A*, **152**, 367–8.

Besag, J. and Newell, J. (1991). The detection of clusters in rare diseases. *Journal of the Royal Statistical Society, Series A*, **154**, 143–55.

Black, D. (1984). *Investigation of the possible increased incidence of cancer in West Cumbria*. Report of independent advisory group. HMSO, London.

Black, G. V. and McKay, F. S. (1916). Mottled teeth: an endemic developmental imperfection of the enamel of the teeth heretofore unknown in the literature of dentistry. *Dental Cosmos*, **58**, 129–56.

Cartwright, R. A., Alexander, F. E., McKinney, P. A., Ricketts, T. J., Hayhoe, F., and Clayton, D. G. C. (1990). *Leukaemia and lymphoma. An atlas of distribution within areas of England and Wales 1984–1988*. Leukaemia Research Fund, London.

Cliff, A. D. and Ord, J. K. (1981). Spatial processes: models and applications. Pion, London.

COMARE (1986). *First report. The implications of the new data on the releases from Sellafield in the 1950s for the conclusions of the report on the investigation on the possible increased incidence of cancer in West Cumbria*. HMSO, London.

COMARE (1988). *Second report. Investigation of the possible increased incidence of leukaemia in young people near the Dounreay Nuclear Establishment, Caithness, Scotland*. HMSO, London.

Cuzick, J. and Edwards, R. (1990). Tests for spatial clustering in heterogeneous populations. *Journal of the Royal Statistical Society, Series B*, **52**, 73–104.

Dean, H. T. (1938). Endemic fluorosis and its relation to dental caries. *Public Health Reports*, **53**, 1443–52.

Diggle, P. J. (1983). *Statistical analysis of spatial point patterns*. Academic Press, London.

Diggle, P. J. (1990). *Second-order analysis of spatial clustering in inhomogeneous populations*. Technical Report MA90/35 Lancaster University.

Elliott, P. (ed.) (1989). *Methodology of enquiries into disease clustering*. Small Area Health Statistics Unit, London.

Evans, H. J. (1990). Leukaemia and radiation. *Nature*, **345**, 16–17.

Gardner, M. J., Hall, M. J., Downes, S., and Terrell, J. D. (1987*a*). Follow up study of children born to mothers resident in Seascale, West Cumbria (birth cohort). *British Medical Journal*, **295**, 822–7.

Gardner, M. J., Hall, A. J., Downes, S., and Terrell, J. D. (1987*b*). Follow up study of children born elsewhere but attending schools in Seascale, West Cumbria (schools cohort). *British Medical Journal*, **295**, 819–22.

Gardner, M. J., Snee, M. P., Hall, A. J., Powell, C. A., Downes, S., and Terrell, J. D. (1990). Results of case-control study of leukaemia and lymphoma among young people near Sellafield nuclear plant in West Cumbria. *British Medical Journal*, **300**, 423–9.

Glaser, S. L. (1990). Spatial clustering of Hodgkin's disease in the San Francisco bay area. *American Journal of Epidemiology Supplement 1*, **132**, S167–S177.

Greaves, M. F. (1990). The Sellafield childhood leukaemia cluster: are germline mutations responsible? *Leukaemia*, **6**, 391–6.

Gutensohn, N. and Cole, P. (1977). Epidemiology of Hodgkin's disease in the young. *International Journal of Cancer*, **19**, 595–604.

Gutensohn, N. and Cole, P. (1981). Childhood social environment and Hodgkin's disease. *New England Journal of Medicine*, **304**, 135–40.

Hills, M. and Alexander, F. E. (1989). Statistical methods used in assessing the risk of disease near a source of possible environmental pollution: a review. *Journal of the Royal Statistical Society, Series A*, **152**, 353–63.

Knox, E. G. (1989). Detection of clusters. In *Methodology of enquiries into disease clustering*, (ed. P. Elliott). Small Area Health Statistics Unit, London.

McKay, F. S. (1929). The establishment of a definite relation between enamel that is defective in its structure, as mottled enamel, and the liability to decay. *Dental Cosmos*, **71**, 747–55.

McKay, F. S. (1933). Mottled enamel: the prevention of its further production through a change of the water supply at Oakley, Idatis. *Journal of the American Dental Association*, **20**, 1137–49.

Moran, P. A. P. (1948). The interpretation of statistical maps. *Journal of the Royal Statistical Society, Series B*, **10**, 243–51.

Openshaw, S., Craft, A. W., Charlton, H., and Birch, J. M. (1988). Investigation of leukaemia clusters by use of a geographical analysis machine. *Lancet*, i, 272–3.

Peto, J. (1990). Radon and the risks of cancer. *Nature*, **345**, 389–90.

Potthoff, R. F. and Whittinghill, M. (1966a). Testing for homogeneity: I. The binomial and multinomial distributions. *Biometrika*, **53**, 167–82.

Potthoff, R. F. and Whittinghill, M. (1966b). Testing for homogeneity: II. The Poisson distribution. *Biometrika*, **53**, 183–90.

Rothman, K. J. (1987). Clustering of disease (editorial). *American Journal of Public Health*, **7**, 13–15.

Rothman, K. J. (1990). A sobering start for the cluster busters conference. *American Journal of Epidemiology*, **132**, 6–13.

Smith, P. G. (1978). Current assessment of 'case-clustering' of lymphomas and leukaemias. *Cancer*, **42**, 1026–34.

Staal, S. P., Abinder, R., Beschorner, W. E., Hayward, G. S., and Mann, R. (1989). A survey of Epstein–Barr Virus DNA in lymphoid tissue. *American Journal of Clinical Pathology*, **91**, 1–5.

Sunyer, J., Antó, J. M., Rodrigo, M., and Morell, F. (1989). Case-control study of serum immunoglobulin-E antibodies reactive with soybean in epidemic asthma. *Lancet*, i, 179–82.

Urquhart, J., Black, R., and Buist, E. (1989). Exploring small area methods. In *Methodology of enquiries into disease clustering*, (ed. P. Elliott). Small Area Health Statistics Unit, London.

Warner, S. C. and Aldrich, T. E. (1988). The status of cancer cluster investigations undertaken by state health departments. *American Journal of Public Health*, **78**, 306–7.

Wartenberg, D. and Greenberg, M. (1990). Detecting disease clusters: the importance of statistical power. *American Journal of Epidemiology*, **132**, S156–S166.

Weiss, L. M., Stickler, J. G., Warnke, R. A., Putilo, D. T., and Sklar, J. (1987). Epstein–Barr viral DNA in tissues of Hodgkin's diseases. *American Journal of Pathology*, **129**, 86–91.

Weiss, L .M., Movahed, L., Warnke, R. A., and Sklar, J. (1989). Detection of Epstein–Barr viral genomes in Reed–Sternberg cells of Hodgkin's disease. *New England Journal of Medicine*, **320**, 502–6.

IV   Studies of health and the environment

22. Environmental epidemiology: a historical perspective

B. Terracini

Since Hippocrates, it has been recognized that human health is largely determined by the environment, i.e. by 'the conditions under which any person or thing lives or is developed; the sum-total of influences which modify and determine the development of life or character' (*Oxford English Dictionary* 1989). Untoward effects (in humans, as well as in animals and plants) may derive from:

(1) chemical, physical, and biological agents artificially (and often involuntarily) introduced into air, water, and/or soil in the course of, or as a consequence of, productive and other human activities, i.e. man-made pollution;

(2) exposures deriving from personal behaviour, including diet, tobacco smoke, alcohol intake, sexual habits, etc.;

(3) naturally occurring hazards.

The latter hazards may take a variety of forms: some examples are food contamination by toxins produced by fungi (such as aflatoxins), excesses or deficiencies of macro- or micronutrients in diet, inadequate concentration of elements in air or drinking water, background radioactivity, etc.

Only problems related to man-made pollution are mentioned under the heading 'environment' in the latest supplements to the British Encyclopedia (*Britannica Book of the Year* 1985–90). This is not surprising: policy decisions aimed at the control of involuntary exposures (ranging from herbicides in drinking water to passive tobacco smoke) are more complex than those required for the control of conscious and voluntary exposure to well-known hazards, such as active tobacco smoke (nevertheless, the existence, in several countries, of a state tobacco monopoly, substantially contributing to state revenues, is a major political problem).

Differences in disease occurrence among genetically similar populations are likely to reflect environmental influences, but simple geographical comparisons cannot discriminate between the contribution of man-made pollution, personal behaviour, and naturally occurring hazards. For instance, the estimate, based on geographical comparisons, that over 70 per cent of all cancers are determined by the environment relates to the sum of all factors that accompany cultural differences and not exclusively to exposure to pollutants (International Agency for Research on Cancer 1990).

Hazard and risk are two different concepts. The former means the inherent potential of an agent (chemical, physical, etc.) to produce a health-related effect within an exposed population, whereas risk corresponds to the probability of the occurrence of an effect.

Environmental epidemiology

In the past, this term has been used to describe the use of conventional epidemiological techniques in order to hypothesize about, study, and interpret associations between disease and environmental agents (as opposed, for instance, to genetic epidemiology).

A broader approach is currently envisaged, which is primarily focused on exposure circumstances, and which considers as dependent variables all possible health effects of environmental agents to which populations are exposed (Buffler 1988; Goldsmith 1988). The identification of previously unrecognized hazards due to exogenous exposures is still central to environmental epidemiology, but it is apparent that other scientific activities have become equally important in deciding on further studies or matters of policy. Such activities include:

(1) the identification of previously unrecognized environmental exposures to agents known to be hazardous and, when required, the quantification a posteriori of the ensuing risks (either absolute, relative, or attributable);
(2) the estimate of individual exposures to environmental hazards;
(3) risk assessment;
(4) the evaluation of either the need for, or the effectiveness of, preventive measures.

There are several reasons for the shift from disease- to exposure-centred environmental epidemiology. First, particularly in developed countries, degenerative, chronic diseases (such as cancer, lung emphysema, etc.) have become the prevailing pathology: the aetiology of many of these conditions is multifactorial, i.e. no specific hazard can be considered as a necessary cause. To further complicate the picture, many environmental hazards (e.g. excess dietary fat, asbestos, etc.) are causally associated with more than one disease.

Secondly, most environment-induced ill-effects are dose-related. For a given hazard, there may well be exposures either low enough, or of short enough duration, as to be negligible in terms of risk. It has also become obvious that ill-effects are frequently the result of interaction (addition, synergism, antagonism, etc.) between different hazards. For the same exposure to a given hazard, the risk may differ according to which other hazards are present or not.

Thirdly, analytical techniques for measuring pollutants in the environment have been used more and more, and their sensitivity has increased by several orders of magnitude. Consequently, there has been a dramatic increase in hazard-specific environmental data requiring risk evaluation.

Finally, health authorities, public opinion, and the scientific community have become increasingly concerned by the number of environmental contaminants for which potentially deleterious effects are unknown or poorly understood.

In evaluating the potential impact of a hazard, the severity of known ill-effects is just one of the items to be considered. Others include the frequency of the condition, the prevalence of exposed persons, and the nature and properties of the environmental agent. The domain of environmental epidemiology also covers markers of exposure and reversible effects, as long as they are relevant to prevention or to risk assessment.

Risk assessment is the process of estimating indirectly (for the purpose of policy decisions) the potential health consequences of exposure to a hazard, based on the information that is available at a given time. When data on the effects on humans are insufficient, assessment can be attempted from estimates of intake by humans and knowledge of the effects of the agent in experimental systems.

The workplace is an important source of pollutants for the general environment and the same hazards often affect both the workers and the general population. Away from the workplace, individual exposures (and risks) are usually many times lower and can be estimated less accurately. Thus, the statistical power of epidemiological studies on exposures in the general environment tends to be low. Risks, however, can be estimated indirectly, through extrapolation (based on some assumptions) from the results of occupational studies.

A short history of environmental hazard identification

Before the advent (or use) of modern epidemiological methods

Historically, only physicians and surgeons were in a position to point out the possible damaging effects of environmental exposure. The observer had to be well motivated in order to watch properly, describe, infer about, and report what he saw. Sometimes, he had to face the reluctancy of the conventional medical milieu to accept facts which did not conform with current ideas (Semmelweiss' observations on the cause of puerperal fever is a case in point). Obviously, such a system only picked up associations between diseases and/or exposures which were so unusual that comparisons with controls were unnecessary and inference required very little arithmetic, if any. The observations of a clinician have been compared to those of somebody looking out of the window at a bird table (Acheson 1979). He will hardly notice a doubling of the usual number of sparrows, but if he sees a couple of cockatoos, it is immediately apparent that something extraordinary is happening. Such a cockatoo were the scrotal cancers in chimney sweepers first described by Sir Percival Pott in 1775. Pott did not report the number of chimney sweepers with cancer he observed, but he expanded in detail on the brutal conditions of their short lives, as a contributing factor to their unhappy fate (Clayson 1962).

Throughout the nineteenth and the first part of the twentieth century, clinicians identified a number of cockatoos, particularly in the workplace. This is not surprising. The industrial revolution led to the introduction of a huge number of new chemical and physical agents in the workplace at relatively high concentrations, and for many decades not much consideration was given to the possibility of controlling and reducing workers' exposure. Although causality was often demonstrated only at a later stage, through formal epidemiological studies, in some instances the evidence from clinical reports was so overwhelming that (at least in some countries) some form of prevention-oriented policy was introduced.

In 1921, for instance, published reports on the occurrence of bladder cancer in workers employed in dyestuff production were so numerous and consistent as to induce the International Labour Organization to declare that occupational exposure to aromatic amines in this kind of industry entailed a carcinogenic risk and that most likely the chemical agents were 2-naphthylamine and benzidine. This was confirmed by R. Case some 30 years later, in cohort studies on chemical workers in Britain (International Agency for Research on Cancer 1987).

Occasionally, not only causes but also mechanisms of disease have been profitably investigated in large (and unbiased) series of cases, in the absence of formal epidemiological studies. In Britain, occupational skin cancer was made compulsorily notifiable early in the twentieth century. In 1947, Henry analysed clinical data and the occupational histories of over 3700 cases notified between 1920 and 1945. He found that the cancer site was largely governed by the manner in which the carcinogenic materials were handled (for instance, 71 per cent of skin cancers in patent fuel workers occurred on the head and neck v. 40 per cent in pitch loaders). In addition, the average latent period was 40–60 years for cancers caused by oils v. 20–30 years for those caused by tar and pitch (Clayson 1962).

Nowadays, clinical observations of an unusual association provide a hunch but not proof of causality, the elucidation of which is left to more refined epidemiological methods (the implementation of the relevant studies, nevertheless, may take some time). Not long ago, however, several human teratogens were recognized in the absence of formal (i.e. controlled) epidemiological studies. They include maternal alcohol abuse (which produces a typical fetal alcohol syndrome), Kanechlor ('Yusho' syndrome), and methylmercury (microcephaly) (Hemminki and Vineis 1985).

There are other examples of degenerative diseases, monofactorial in aetiology, that were first recognized as distinct conditions only when and where the necessary cause was present in the environment. The 'Spanish toxic oil syndrome' is a new, well-defined disease, unreported before 1981, which killed over 300 people in Spain and was caused by adulterated rapeseed oil illegally introduced onto the food market (Tabuenca 1981). The exercise of identifying 'new', previously unclassified diseases is a part of environmental epidemiology—the burden is on clinicians and veterinarians.

The advent of modern epidemiology

John Snow's analyses of the cholera outbreak in London in 1854 (Snow 1855) represent the beginning of modern epidemiology because of his skill in organizing observations in order to verify a hypothesis, i.e. that sewage in water causes cholera. From descriptive data at the level of London districts, Snow first recognized an association between the source of the water supply and the disease. Then he collected information for subdistricts and found that the association was stronger at this level. Finally, he showed that the association persisted when the population in the same neighbourhood was classified according to the company supplying water to their houses. This allowed him to rule out the alternative hypothesis, that differences in disease between subdistricts were confounded by social class.

Snow's epidemiology was more than mere arithmetic. As much as Percival Pott had been 80 years before, he was impressed by, and described, the miserable conditions of life of those affected. He asserted that overcrowding and lack of hygiene were additional risk factors for cholera, and hypothesized that the disease was caused by a transmissible agent. Two further features of Snow's field investigation are that he personally walked from house to house in order to collect the required information on the water supply and that he submitted his report within weeks of the onset of the epidemic.

During the second part of the nineteenth century, aetiological studies were mainly concerned with infectious diseases, with much reliance on laboratory investigation and little attention to study design. The supremacy of the deterministic concept of causality was typically reflected in the postulates of Henle-Koch (MacMahon and Pugh 1970): a micro-organism should be considered as causally related to a disease when it is present in all subjects affected by 'the disease in question' (i.e. necessary cause) and when it is absent, or found as a fortuitous parasite, in other diseases (i.e. sufficient cause). In addition, the agent should be isolated in the laboratory and should reproduce the disease if inoculated in an experimental animal.

The weakness of the deterministic approach soon became obvious, even for infectious diseases. A complex web of causation for cholera, which included social factors, had already been implicated by Snow. In fact, Henle-Koch's first postulate implies circular reasoning, since the '(infectious) disease in question' cannot be defined until a particular agent has been arbitrarily selected as the necessary cause (MacMahon and Pugh 1970). The need for new models of aetiology became apparent later, when degenerative diseases started to dominate the scene.

After Lind's pioneering work on scurvy, and before recent trials on the chemoprevention of cancer, aetiology-oriented experimental studies were uncommon and limited to non-fatal conditions, such as dental diseases. Early in the twentieth century, two series of trials demonstrated that mottled teeth and caries are causally associated, respectively, to excessive and insufficient fluorine concentration in the drinking water (Murray 1989). The study on mottled teeth (McKay 1933), in Oakley, Idaho, was perhaps the first occasion on which problems typical of intervention studies were rationally faced:

1. When it started, in 1925, there was a clear hypothesis, which originally alluded to springs and not specifically to fluorine. The hypotheses came from the observation that almost all children living in town had mottled teeth v. 0/4 children served by another spring located out of town (fluorine concentrations in the two springs were measured during the study, under conditions of double blindness between clinicians and chemists).

2. The trial was not randomized but the choice of controls was reasonable: the prevalence of mottling was compared between children born before the adoption of the new spring and those born afterwards.

3. At the beginning of the study, the citizens of Oakley were invited to express their opinion on the trial (and to vote on a proposal calling for a bond issue to finance a new water supply).

Until now, however, the major contribution to environmental epidemiology has come not from experimental studies but from observational, hypothesis-testing studies, relating disease to exposure at the individual level. For most human carcinogens evaluated as such by IARC, demonstration of the hazardous properties of the agent was obtained in either case-control or cohort studies (International Agency for Research on Cancer 1987).

The first reported case-control study, published by Lane Claypon in 1926, concerned the role of reproductive experience in the aetiology of breast cancer (Cole 1979). The case-control design was also used in the very first investigations into cancer and tobacco smoke, carried out before the Second World War (US Department of Health, Education and Welfare 1964). However, the value of case-control studies became clearly apparent following the seminal studies on smoking and lung cancer carried out by Wynder and Graham and Doll and Hill in the early 1950s. This decade ended with the publication of a methodological review (Mantel and Haenszel 1959), which a few years ago still ranked among the 10 most cited papers ever published in the *Journal of the National Cancer Institute* (Cole 1979).

Discussion of the process by which new aetiological hypotheses are formed is beyond the scope of this book. Nevertheless, it is clear that, in the past, concerns about the carcinogenicity (International Agency for Research on

Cancer 1987) or teratogenicity (Hemminki and Vineis 1985) of specific chemicals often originated from unusual observations reported by alert clinicians. Nowadays, it would be inappropriate to rely excessively on clinicians' hunches to detect hazards entailing low relative risks for common diseases. Moreover, as discussed in Chapter 1, only weak evidence is obtained from geographical correlation studies, because of the problems of making inferences about individuals from grouped data (i.e. the ecological fallacy). For example, even for aflatoxin B1, the epidemiological evidence for carcinogenicity was described as 'limited' when data from correlation studies only were available (International Agency for Research on Cancer 1982). Exploratory case-control studies may be helpful but are expensive. For chemical hazards, knowledge of structure–activity relationships as well as other toxicological data may provide useful insights: environmental epidemiologists need to have access to and be able to interpret this type of information.

A new discipline

After the Second World War, there was an increasing awareness of the need for a rational, systematic, explicit, and reproducible approach to the evaluation of causality of associations. It was apparent that the causal significance of an association was a matter of judgement which went beyond a statement of statistical probability. Hill (1965) elaborated a set of criteria for causality, but with emphasis that they should be used flexibly and that none of them gave incontrovertible evidence for or against causality. Hill's approach largely overlaps with that used during the preparation of the first US report on the effects of tobacco (US Department of Health Education and Welfare 1964). Hill's criteria included:

(1) the strength of the association;
(2) the consistency of findings in different studies;
(3) the specificity of the association;
(4) the relationship in time;
(5) the existence of a dose–response gradient between exposure and disease occurrence;
(6) biological plausibility;
(7) coherence of the evidence with the natural history of the disease;
(8) experimental (or *quasi*-experimental) evidence; and
(9) reasoning by analogy.

Hill's criteria have been used and expanded upon in the exercise conducted by IARC over the past 20 years in assessing causality from the epidemiological evidence for carcinogenicity of environmental agents; these expanded criteria have also been applied to teratogens (Hemminki and Vineis 1985). Compared to Hill's original formulation, IARC has been more explicit about the importance of study design and the control of confounding variables.

A frequent shortcoming is the poor definition of the exposures under evaluation, thus blurring the distinction between *source* and *cause*, well known in the epidemiology of infectious diseases. For example, among exposures recognized by IARC (1990) as causally associated with human cancer, furniture and cabinet making is a *source* of hazard (the actual carcinogen has not yet been identified) whereas 2-naphthylamine is a *cause* of cancer. For chemicals, at best, 'exposure' in epidemiological studies corresponds to technical or commercial products, whose impurities may vary between periods and places. Causal inference concerning the pure compound requires additional information, such as the demonstration of carcinogenicity of the pure compound in laboratory animals or knowledge of the interaction between the chemical and its cellular targets (both criteria exist in the case of 2-naphthylamine).

It is not surprising, therefore, that of the 55 exposures listed by IARC as *carcinogenic to humans*, 12 are described as industrial processes, nine as mixtures, 19 as pharmaceutical drugs or groups of drugs, and only 15 as chemicals or groups of chemicals other than drugs (not all of which unequivocally correspond to a Chemical Abstract Service code number).

Inaccurate definition of exposure may weaken both causal inference and risk assessment. Consistency with past knowledge requires reasonable confidence that any new knowledge alludes to the same agent. This is not the case, for instance, of the 'rubber industry' as a process entailing exposures that are carcinogenic to humans, since chemicals to which rubber workers have been exposed have varied greatly over time and in different places.

Beyond associations between exposure and disease

Biochemical or molecular epidemiology (Perera 1987; Hulka and Wilcosky 1988) is the application of epidemiological methods to studies investigating internal exposures (i.e. the contact of the body tissue with a chemical) and/or biochemical outcomes. Relevant biological variables include markers of:

(1) internal dose (in tissues, blood, or secretions);
(2) physiological response (i.e. effects other than overt disease);
(3) asymptomatic disease (e.g. tumour-specific antigens); and
(4) susceptibility (e.g. α-antitrypsin in lung emphysema).

Markers of internal dose may describe either absorption (e.g. urinary concentration of cotinine, a major metabolite of nicotine) or the dose reaching a tissue or cellular target (biologically effective dose markers, e.g. DNA adducts with an electrophilic compound).

In aetiological studies, biochemical markers are often more accurate estimates of the actual dose reaching the target than commonly used surrogates (such as job description or number of cigarettes), thus leading to increased statistical power. For late outcomes, a major problem is the limited persistence of the markers, so that they provide little information on previous exposure. Exceptions are foreign compounds persisting in the human body (such as lead, arsenic and other metals, DDT, polychlorinated biphenyls, etc.), the toxicology of which is sufficiently known to estimate past intake from current concentrations in human tissues. For mutagens and carcinogens, identification of permanent changes in DNA is another promising lead.

Biochemical epidemiology is relevant to environmental epidemiology in other respects also. For some pollutants, monitoring markers of exposure in the general population has become a common practice over the years (e.g. *ad hoc* surveys on blood lead concentration in children). The novelty derives from the increased availability of methods (particularly for exposure to carcinogens) and the range of new questions raised by their application. For instance (Vineis *et al.* 1990): what is the source of aromatic amines forming adducts to haemoglobin in non-smokers and non-occupationally exposed? To what extent are inherited susceptibility factors, such as metabolic phenotypes, determinants of bronchial cancer in smokers?

Finally, when risk assessment requires extrapolation from animal to man (which is not uncommon), the procedure is likely to be more accurate if it takes into account both the dose reaching the target and interspecies differences in biotransformation.

Markers of physiological response are effects detectable early after exposure to an environmental hazard, not necessarily related to or predictive of overt disease, e.g. increased chromosomal aberrations in circulating lymphocytes in cigarette smokers. Often, a major limitation to the use of 'early effects' as outcome measures for epidemiological studies is the uncertainty over their biological significance.

At the end of the twentieth century

Currently, the tendency is towards progressively larger hypothesis-based studies, to increase statistical power and the sensitivity to detect causal associations. Assessment of causality has taken advantage of the proper use of multivariate analysis in studies measuring a relatively large number of potential confounders.

It is obvious, however, that simply increasing the size of a study and the number of exposure-related variables will not, in themselves, overcome the limitations of inadequate definitions of exposure and surrogate estimates (e.g. total body intake, at best) of the dose actually reaching the target organ or cells.

Biochemical epidemiology might contribute to circumvent, at least in part, these shortcomings. Nevertheless, there are at least two reasons for considering it unrealistic that epidemiological methods will be able to recognize more than a limited number of the ill-effects associated with environmental agents. First, the number of environmental agents that could be investigated is enormous. Secondly, for effects occurring after a long latent period, awaiting their demonstration before implementing preventive measures would be unethical.

Currently, environmentally related (potential) health problems often need to be faced in the absence of observations in man. Under these circumstances, a proper use of toxicological data and knowledge of the mechanisms of injury may greatly contribute to the goals required of environmental epidemiology.

Acknowledgement

I am grateful to Paolo Vineis for his criticism of this manuscript.

References

Acheson, E. D. (1979). Clinical practice and epidemiology: two worlds or one? *British Medical Journal*, 1, 723–6.

Britannica Book of the Year (1985–90). Britannica Inc.

Buffler, P. A. (1988). Epidemiology needs and perspectives in environmental epidemiology. *Archives of Environmental Health*, 43, 130–2.

Clayson, D. B. (1962). *Chemical carcinogenesis*. J. & A. Churchill, London.

Cole, P. (1979). The evolving case-control study. *Journal of Chronic Diseases*, 32, 15–27.

Goldsmith, J. R. (1988). Keynote address: Improving the prospects for environmental epidemiology. *Archives of Environmental Health*, 43, 69–74.

Hemminki, K. and Vineis, P. (1985). Extrapolation of the evidence on teratogenicity of chemicals between humans and experimental animals: chemicals other than drugs. *Teratogenesis, Carcinogenesis and Mutagenesis*, 5, 251–318.

Hill, A. B. (1965). The environment and disease: association or causation? *Proceedings of the Royal Society of Medicine*, 58, 295–300.

Hulka, B. S. and Wilcosky, T. (1988). Biological markers in epidemiologic research. *Archives of Environmental Health*, 43, 83–9.

International Agency for Research on Cancer (1982). *IARC monographs on the evaluation of carcinogenic risk of chemicals to humans, supplement 4. Chemicals, industrial processes and industries associated with cancer in humans*, IARC Monographs vols 1–29. Lyon.

International Agency for Research on Cancer (1987). *IARC monographs on the evaluation of carcinogenic risk to humans, Supplement 7. Overall evaluations of carcinogenicity*, An updating of IARC Monographs vols 1–42. Lyon.

International Agency for Research on Cancer (1990). *Cancer: causes, occurrence and control*, (ed. L. Tomatis). IARC Scientific Publications, No. 100. Lyon.

McKay, F. S. (1933). Mottled enamel: the prevention of its further production through a change of the water supply at Oakley, Ida. *Journal of the American Dental Association*, 20, 1137–49.

MacMahon, B. and Pugh, T. F. (1970). *Epidemiology, principles and methods*. Little, Brown and Co., Boston.

Mantel, N. and Haenszel, W. (1959). Statistical aspects of data from retrospective studies of disease. *Journal of the National Cancer Institute*, **22**, 719–48.

Murray, J. J. (1989). *The prevention of dental disease*, (2nd edn). Oxford University Press, Oxford.

Oxford English Dictionary (1989). (2nd edn). Clarendon Press, Oxford.

Perera, F. P. (1987). Molecular cancer epidemiology. A new tool in cancer prevention. *Journal of the National Cancer Institute*, **78**, 887–98.

Snow, J. (1855). *On the mode of communication of cholera*, (2nd edn). Churchill, London. Reproduced in *Snow on cholera*, Commonwealth Fund, New York (1936); reprinted by Hafner, New York (1965).

Tabuenca, J. M. (1981). Toxic allergic syndrome caused by ingestion of rapeseed oil denatured with aniline. *Lancet*, **2**, 567–8.

US Department of Health, Education and Welfare, Public Health Service (1964). *Smoking and health: Report of the Advisory Committee to the Surgeon General of the Public Health Service*, Public Health Service Publication, No. 1103, Washington DC.

Vineis, P., Faggiano, F., and Terracini, B. (1990). Biochemical epidemiology: uses in the study of human carcinogenesis. *Teratogenesis, Carcinogenesis and Mutagenesis*, **10**, 231–7.

23. Guidelines for the investigation of clusters of adverse health events

R. B. Rothenberg and S. B. Thacker

The foregoing sections provide a detailed discussion of the statistical and epidemiological aspects of studies of the occurrence of disease in small areas. This chapter will consider a more pragmatic issue—the response of health authorities to the report of a 'cluster' of health events. As defined previously (Chapter 21), clusters have a specific statistical meaning. In common parlance (and in the day-to-day responsibilities of the public health worker), a 'cluster' is usually a report of a perceived health problem from a concerned citizen or group. The report can vary greatly in the quality of its information, the clarity of its purpose, and in the motivation which generated it. Such reports pose a number of pragmatic epidemiological, statistical, and social issues for which health workers, until recently, have had little practical guidance.

In July 1990, the Centers for Disease Control in the United States issued a set of guidelines for evaluating clusters (CDC 1990). Though not sufficiently specific to cover the entire range of problems that may arise, they none the less provide a reasonable framework for day-to-day action. Use of this framework should reduce unproductive effort but assure recognition of issues worth pursuing.

The guidelines were developed on the basis of a number of important assumptions (discussed in detail in preceding chapters). First, in many reports of cluster investigations, a geographical or temporal excess in the number of cases cannot be demonstrated. Secondly, when an excess is confirmed, the likelihood of establishing a definitive cause-and-effect relationship between the health event and an exposure is slight. Thirdly, a cluster may be useful for hypothesis generation, but is not likely to be useful for hypothesis testing. Frequently, the issues raised by a cluster cannot be definitively answered by the investigation *per se* and require an alternative epidemiological approach. Finally, from the public health perspective, the perception of a cluster in a community may be as, or more, important than the reality of its existence.

In the following sections, based in large measure on the CDC guidelines, we describe a systematic approach to cluster evaluation.

Managing the investigation of clusters: skills and knowledge required

The investigation of a perceived cluster of adverse health effects is not simply an isolated epidemiological or statistical exercise. Appropriate response by health authorities requires specific skills, including a sensitivity to the social and cultural issues of the situation, understanding of the principles of risk perception, understanding of the functions of public media, and awareness of potential legal ramifications of the investigation.

Scientific tools

Managing clusters is a form of public health surveillance (i.e. the ongoing collection, analysis, and dissemination of information important to public health practice) (see Thacker and Berkleman 1988). Cluster investigation is not necessarily a primary mechanism for investigating aetiological relationships. Thus, the investigator may be looking more at patterns (spatial, temporal, or both) in data than searching for specific associations between agent and disease. As described in previous chapters, a variety of statistical techniques is available to detect and characterize such patterns. None is the universal technique of choice. The investigator should select the particular epidemiological or statistical approach in accordance with the circumstnaces under study—the nature of the condition, the type of data available on the cases, the availability of comparison/denominator data, and so forth. The investigator will need to know the assumptions and limitations of the method, as well as its sensitivity and specificity. Finally, the investigator must be able to determine the power of any planned study to detect a clustering of events.

Once the presence of a cluster or excess of disease or injury is confirmed, comprehensive investigation may require a capacity to conduct environmental sampling. Such a capacity includes: the knowledge and equipment necessary to design an appropriate sampling scheme and to collect specimens; access to laboratories with adequate facilities and experienced staff to analyse these specimens quickly and accurately, with appropriate attention to quality control/assurance procedures; and the ability to interpret the results appropriately. Similarly, the capacity must exist to collect, analyse, and interpret biological monitoring specimens (whether used as measures of exposure or adverse health effects). A reported cluster of disease may, in fact, represent a cluster of incorrectly performed laboratory tests (CDC 1987).

Psychological factors

Cluster investigators must possess a working understanding of the various ways in which individuals respond to stressful situations and react to uncertainties (Rothenberg *et al.* 1990). Investigators should be able to recognize the source of community suspicions (e.g. of deliberate delay and cover-ups on the part of health authorities) and seemingly unrealistic (to the investigators) demands for allocation of resources, schedules, etc. Investigators must respond to these without hostility and be familiar with appropriate techniques to respond. Finally, investigators should realize that the perception of a problem must be dealt with responsibly and sympathetically, even if there is no demonstrable underlying community health problem or cluster of disease.

Risk communication

Once the investigator has established an estimate of the degree of risk inherent in the situation under study, this estimate must be communicated to the community in a comprehensible manner. Simply presenting the numbers will not suffice. The risk must be put in perspective through comparison with risks associated with more familiar activities, such as driving a car or taking an aeroplane (Thacker and Berkleman 1988). Particular care must be exercised to ensure that this is done in a sensitive, non-condescending manner.

In addition, the 'risk' perceived by community members does not necessarily parallel the estimates of risk that are produced by mathematical or scientific assessments of the situation (Slovik 1987). Public health agencies must recognize this fact and be prepared to address it. This difference in perceptions is more than just a failure to communicate adequately the 'true' risk or a failure of the community to understand. Public perception of risk is influenced by the extent to which the source of the risk is voluntary or imposed, the degree of control the individual or community has over the source of the risk, the degree to which the source of the risk is familiar and easily comprehended (or visualized), and the potential adverse social and economic ramifications (Slovik 1987).

Public media

Public health agencies must be aware of media 'imperatives', the factors that influence the various media (print, television, etc.) in their selection and presentation of stories (e.g. the desire for a pictorial/visual component, the presence of conflict or controversy, the presence of strong emotive content, and the availability of a target for blame). This point has been elaborated by Greenberg and Wartenberg (1990). Because the media tend to simplify complex, technical explanations, with the concomitant loss of subtle distinctions or qualifications, investigators must distil messages that they wish to convey and present them in the way that they are most likely to be transmitted without confusion or distortion. The investigator must use simple presentations (whether oral or written) that stress a few key points; provide any background necessary to allow understanding; and be straightforward regarding what is fact, what is speculation, and what is not known at all. Most of all, investigators must remain co-operative and responsive and must be prepared to provide all of the above rapidly, before distortion and discord have been introduced into the public exchanges.

Legal ramifications

Many of the situations that prompt requests for investigation ultimately involve government intervention or litigation (ongoing or contemplated litigation may, in fact, stimulate the request for the investigation). Since the investigation report is likely to be used in that litigation or to justify that intervention, members of public health agencies must have a basic understanding of the principles of tort law that relate to legal proof of causality and responsibility— and must understand how these differ from the (sometimes stricter) requirements of scientific proof. Such principles include: the concept of negligence (which entails the breach of duty that caused or substantially contributed to harm or damage); the concept of breach of warranty (the understanding that an action or situation is safe); the concept of strict liability (which focuses on the product rather than on the conduct); and the concept of failure to warn (Black 1990). To establish legally a cause and effect relationship, it is necessary to convince those deciding the issue that a preponderance of the evidence indicates the association. This is interpreted (Black 1990) as meaning that the probability that the outcome was due to exposure is at least 50 per cent (i.e. the attributable risk in the exposed is 50 per cent or greater).

Organizational requirements

A citizen who reports an apparent cluster wants assurance that the most appropriate and responsible person is quickly informed and then acts accordingly. Health agencies should develop a reporting process that is quick, traceable, and reaches the appropriate person regardless of chosen entry point for the concerned citizen. The response process should be triage-oriented, so that it proceeds smoothly from one level of action to the next, and terminates effectively when resolution is reached. The health agency should develop a feedback and notification process that educates and enlightens with efficiency and courtesy, and a referral process that assures timely and competent field investigation and public health response.

In order to assure smooth and timely public health responses, four organizational components are recommended:

1. A locus of responsibility and control. The health agency should designate an individual with stature in the agency to serve as the identifiable point of responsibility (the Programme Director). Agencies may vary considerably in this choice (e.g. Director of Environmental Health, State Epidemiologist, Director of Cancer Control Activities,

Chronic Disease Director, or County Health Officer). The specific appellation or designee will be a function of local circumstances and priorities. The choice is less important than the estbalishment of a locus.

2. A process for involving concerned groups and individuals. The health agency should consider the establishment of an Advisory Committee (or group with similar title) to oversee the decision-making process for cluster evaluation. Such a committee might include representatives from the health agency, from other government agencies, from the private and voluntary sectors, from concerned citizens' groups, and from the media, as well as including selected individuals. (Again, the exact composition will be a function of local circumstances.) This committee should be asked to provide oversight, guidance, and advice to the Programme Director. The duties should be carefully specified a priori and agreed to by the committee members. Since the committee is likely to be composed of persons with diverse backgrounds, oversight rather than technical decision-making should probably be the major focus.

3. A set of operating procedures. The health agency should establish a written protocol for cluster evaluations. The protocol should include mechanisms for reaching responsible persons and a detailed enumeration of the triage process (guidelines for such a protocol are suggested below). This protocol should be disseminated to appropriate persons in the health agency to assure proper handling of the report, whatever the point of entry.

4. Dedicated resources. For those health agencies with a recurrent need for cluster evaluations, some dedication of staff and support resources is required. The Programme Director will probably not be able to perform the required day-to-day tasks and may not be the appropriate person for primary contact. Cluster activities will frequently be a part of the responsibility of a number of staff members, but the duties and responsibilities should be clearly designated.

Just as there is no perfect statistical test for evaluating all clusters, there is no perfect organizational structure for all health agencies. The specifics of organization are a function of local circumstances.

Guidelines for a systematic approach

This section, taken from the Centers for Disease Control guidelines, outlines a four-stage approach to the evaluation of a reported cluster (CDC 1990). It does not speak directly to the particular outcome of concern (e.g. cancer or birth defects), to the types of data available (mortality, hospital discharge, or disease registries), or to the specific analytical techniques. Usually, these particulars will be a function of local resources and circumstances. Rather, these guidelines focus on a set of stages for the management of a reported cluster, from original contact to final disposition. These stages may be viewed as a series of filters which provide responses appropriate to the reported problem. The diagrammatic summary (Fig. 23.1) highlights the need for a feasibility assessment prior to performing an actual study, and the need for separating the issue of increased frequency of occurrence from that of potential aetiologies.

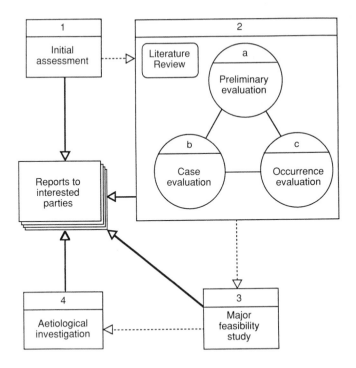

Fig. 23.1 Stages in a cluster investigation.

Several caveats should be borne in mind. The boundaries between the stages are not fixed. Often, the health agency will choose to follow a different order, to combine steps, or to pursue a problem on several fronts. Considerable local judgment and discretion are required. In addition, the cluster investigation can be resolved at a number of points along the path by a report to those invested in the process. Termination of the enquiry implies, as well, the generation of an internal report for the health agency and its advisory groups. Such reports are useful communication tools, particularly if regularly scheduled and available to an established, but flexible, list of recipients.

Finally, although there are some tacit assumptions about the internal organization of the health agency (e.g. presence of a public affairs office and establishment of a cluster advisory committee), it is well recognized that there is considerable variability in health agency structure and function. The guidelines are meant to be tailored to local circumstances. It is assumed that if the health agencies choose to establish an Advisory Committee, consultation will take place at critical decision points.

Stage 1   Initial contact

The purpose at this stage is to collect information from the person(s) or group(s) first reporting a perceived cluster (hereafter referred to as the caller).

The initial contact is critical. The caller must be referred quickly to the responsible health agency unit, and the problem should never be dismissed summarily. The majority of potential cluster reports can be brought to successful closure at the time of initial contact, and the first encounter is often one of the best opportunities for communication with the caller about the nature of clusters.

Procedures

1. Gather identifying information on the caller, unless anonymity is requested: name, address, telephone number, organization affiliation, if any. If anonymity is requested, advise the caller that the inability to follow up may hinder further investigation.

2. Gather initial data on the potential cluster: suspected health event(s), suspected exposure(s), number of cases, geographical area of concern, time period of concern, and how the caller learned about the cluster.

3. Obtain identifying information on cases: name, sex, age (or birth date, age at diagnosis, age at death), race, diagnosis, date of diagnosis, date of death, address (or approximate geographical location), telephone number, length of residence at site of interest, contact person (family, friend) and method for contact, and physician contact. In the initial encounter much of this may be approximate, and in some instances the health department official may choose not to collect identifying information right away. This type of information may, in practice, be gathered over the course of several contacts.

4. Discuss initial impressions with the caller. There are a number of points which frequently arise:
   (a) A variety of diagnoses speaks against a common origin.
   (b) Cancer is a common illness (with a 1 in 3 lifetime probability). The risk increases with age, and cases among older persons are less likely to be true clusters.
   (c) Major birth defects are less common than cancer, but still occur in 1–2 per cent of live births.
   (d) Length of residence must be substantial to implicate a plausible environmental carcinogen, because of the long period of latency required for most known carcinogens.
   (e) Cases that have occurred in people now deceased may not be helpful in tying exposure to disease, because of the limited ability to obtain good information on exposure and possible confounding factors.
   (f) Rare diseases may occasionally 'cluster' in a way that is statistically significant, but this, in itself, may be a statistical phenomenon not related to exposure.

5. Request further information on cases, more complete enumeration, and plan a follow-up telephone contact, as needed.

6. Assure the caller that he or she will receive a written response to the report of the cluster. (Often, this will simply confirm in writing what has already been communicated by telephone.)

7. Maintain a log of initial contacts, whether written, by telephone, or in person. The log should include the day, date, time, caller identification, health event, exposure, and geographical area. Follow-up contacts should be logged in as well, with a brief note as to purpose and result. If possible, the log should be cross-referenced and computerized so that all those at the health agency who deal with the problem have the same information.

8. Notify the health agency public affairs office (or equivalent) about the contact. In many agencies, this is analogous to notification of the commissioner's office of a press contact.

There is often considerable pressure, early in a cluster investigation, to collect new environmental data or to use existing measurements, although specific area assessments are unlikely to exist. It is advisable to avoid premature environmental measurement, since it is unfocused and often uninterpretable.

Outcome

1. If the initial contact suggests that further evaluation is needed (e.g. single and rare disease entity, plausible exposure, or plausible clustering), proceed to Stage 2, preliminary evaluation.

2. If the initial contact permits satisfactory closure, prepare a summary report for the caller and for the Advisory Committee (or other supervisory group).

Stage 2   Assessment

Once the decision has been made at Stage 1 to proceed further with an assessment, it is important to separate two concurrent issues: whether an excess number of cases has actually occurred, and whether the excess can be tied aetiologically to some exposure. The first usually has precedence, and may or may not lead to the second. This stage initiates a mechanism for evaluating whether an excess has occurred. Three separate elements are identified:

(1) a preliminary evaluation (Stage 2a) to assess quickly from the available data whether an excess may have occurred;

(2) confirmation of cases (Stage 2b) to assure that there is a biological basis for further work; and

(3) an occurrence investigation (Stage 2c) whose purpose is a more detailed description of the cluster through case-finding, interaction with the community, and descriptive epidemiology.

In addition, the investigators may wish to do a literature review and seek consultation with other investigators during the course of this stage (see Fig. 23.1). These activities are often interrelated and may occur in parallel. The health agency is encouraged to exercise flexibility in conducting this portion of the investigation, and to recognize that a linear approach is often not possible.

Stage 2a   Preliminary evaluation

Data from the initial contact, possibly with augmentation from other sources, are used to perform an in-house calculation of observed versus expected occurrence.

Purpose: to provide a quick, rough estimate of the likelihood that an important excess has occurred.

Procedures

1. Determine the appropriate geographical area and time period in which to study the cluster.
2. Determine which cases will be included in the analysis. This stage does not involve case verification, so all cases will be assumed to be real. However, some cases may need to be excluded from the analyses because they occurred outside the geographical area or time period decided on, or because the health event for the case differs from that of other cases. It may be helpful to tabulate frequencies of health events and look at related descriptive statistics.
3. Determine an appropriate reference population. Occurrence rates (or other statistics) calculated for the cluster must be compared to those for a reference population in order to assess whether there is an excess number of cases. (Choice of the reference population must be made carefully.)
4. If the number of cases is sufficient, and if a denominator is available (e.g. population of a community, number of children in school, or number of employees in a workplace), calculate occurrence rates, standardized morbidity/mortality ratios, or proportional mortality ratios. Compare the calculated statistic with that for the reference population to assess significance.
5. If the number of cases is not large enough to obtain meaningful rates, or denominator data are unavailable, consider using one of the statistical tests specifically developed to assess space, time, or space–time clustering. These are described elsewhere (CDC 1990).

Outcome

1. If this preliminary evaluation suggests an excess number of cases, proceed to case evaluation.
2. If preliminary evaluation suggests no excess, then prepare a response to the caller indicating findings and advising that no further investigation is needed.
3. If preliminary evaluation shows no excess, but the data are suggestive of a question of biological and public health importance, further assessment may still be warranted. It must be stressed that a decision to proceed further at this point should not be based solely on an arbitrary criterion for statistical significance.

Stage 2b   Case evaluation

Purpose: to verify the diagnosis.

Some health agencies may choose to verify diagnoses before calculating preliminary rates (Stage 2a). Because verification may be costly, however, agencies may often (or usually) do rate calculations first.

Procedures

1. Obtain verification of the diagnosis through contact with the responsible physicians or from the appropriate health event registry. Verification is often a multi-step process, involving initial contact with the patient, family, or friends, subsequent referral to the responsible physicians, and permission to examine the records.
2. Whenever possible, obtain pathology verification and copies of relevant pathology reports or medical examiner's report.
3. In some instances, histological re-evaluation may be required. Often, however, confirmation and re-evaluation are difficult to obtain.

Outcome

1. If cases are verified, and an excess is confirmed (Stage 2a), proceed to Stage 2c, the occurrence investigation. (As noted, however, this may be ongoing already.)
2. If some (or all) of the cases are not verified, and an excess is not substantiated, prepare a response to the caller outlining findings and advising that further evaluation is not warranted.
3. If some of the cases are not verified, but biological plausibility persists and the data are suggestive, consider initiating or continuing the occurrence investigation.

Stage 2c   Occurrence evaluation

Purpose: to design and perform a thorough investigation to determine if an excess has occurred and to describe the epidemiological characteristics.

The occurrence evaluation is meant to define the characteristics of the cluster in depth and often requires field investigation. It begins with a written protocol which outlines the costs and utility of data collection, the methods to be used, and the plan of analysis. The major product should be a detailed description of the cluster. Up to an including this stage, resource allocation is still relatively small.

Procedures

1. Determine the most appropriate geographical (community) and temporal boundaries.
2. Ascertain all potential cases within the defined space–time boundaries.
3. Identify the appropriate data-bases for both numerator and denominator and their availability.
4. Identify statistical and epidemiological procedures to be used in describing and analysing the data.
5. Perform an in-depth review of the literature and consider the epidemiological and biological plausibility of the purported association.
6. Assess the likelihood of being able to establish a relationship between exposure and the event under consideration.
7. Assess community perceptions, reactions, and needs.
8. Complete the proposed descriptive investigation.

Although an Advisory Committee can be most helpful at any point in the process, and it is usually warranted to involve such a committee early, the

committee may be of particular importance at this point. The occurrence
evaluation may vary considerably in size and content; consensus on the
appropriate level of effort will facilitate acceptance of the results.

Outcome

1. If an excess is confirmed, and the epidemiological and biological plausibility is
   compelling, proceed to Stage 3, the major feasibility study.
2. If an excess is confirmed, but there is no apparent relationship to an exposure,
   terminate the investigation with particular emphasis on the risk communication
   aspects of the issue.
3. If an excess is not confirmed, terminate the investigation and report findings to the
   caller.

Stage 3   Major feasibility study

Purpose: to determine the feasibility of performing an epidemiological study
linking the health event and a putative exposure.

The major feasibility study examines the potential for relating the cluster to
some exposure. It should consider all the options for geographical and
temporal analysis, including the use of cases that are from a different geographical locale or time period and not part of the original cluster. In some
instances, the feasibility study itself may provide answers to the question under
study (Bender *et al.* 1988).

Procedures

1. Reread the detailed literature review, paying particular attention to known and
   putative causes of the outcome(s) of concern.
2. Consider the appropriate study design, with attendant costs and expected outcomes
   of the available alternatives. This includes a consideration of sample size, the
   appropriateness of using previously identified cases, the appropriate geographical
   area and time period, and the selection of controls.
3. Determine the data needed on cases and controls, including physical and laboratory
   measurements.
4. Determine the nature, extent, frequency, and methodology for environmental
   measurements.
5. Delineate the logistics of data collection and processing.
6. Determine the appropriate plan of analysis, including hypotheses to be tested and
   power to detect differences; assess the epidemiological and policy implications of
   alternative results.
7. Assess the current social and political ambiance, with consideration of the impact of
   decisions and outcomes.
8. Assess the resource implications and requirements of both the study and alternative
   findings.

Outcome

1. If the feasibility study suggests that there is merit in pursuing an aetiological investigation, the health agency should proceed to Stage 4. This may entail extensive resource commitment, however, and the decision to conduct a study will be tied to the process of resource allocation.
2. If the feasibility study suggests that little will be gained from an aetiological investigation, the results of this process (by now rather extensive) should be summarized in a report to the caller and all concerned parties. In some circumstances, the public or media may continue to demand further investigation regardless of cost or biological merit. The effort devoted to community relationships, media contacts, and Advisory Committee interaction will be critical for an appropriate public health outcome.

Stage 4   Aetiological investigation

Purpose: to perform an aetiological investigation of a potential disease- (or injury-) exposure relationship.

It is important to reiterate that the major purpose of the study is to pursue the epidemiological and public health issues that the cluster generated. In that context, this step is simply a standard epidemiological study, for which all the preceding effort was preparatory.

Procedures

Using the major feasibility study as a guide, a specific protocol for the study should be developed and the study implemented. The circumstances of most epidemiological studies tend to be unique, and specific guidance is not appropriate.

Outcome

The results of this study are expected to be a contribution to epidemiological and public health knowledge. This contribution may take a number of forms, including the demonstration of either an association or non-association between exposure and disease, or the confirmation of previous findings.

Reporting of results

At whatever stage an investigation terminates, administrative closure is critical. Health authorities must remain aware that even internal reports are, in many circumstances, public documents, and can become part of legal proceedings. Even a brief memorandum to the record or a handwritten note summarizing a telephone call are subject to use in court and should be handled accordingly.

It is self-evident that a report should be appropriate to the level of work performed, the seriousness of the problem, and the extent of the readership.

Although a brief note may suffice for a telephone conversation which reassures a concerned citizen that cancer is a common illness, a major monograph may be necessary for an investigation that has proceeded through Stage 4. There is no special formula or format for reporting results. Again, it is self-evident that the report should summarize work performed, should include a compilation of results, should include a summary of community contacts and reaction (together with a record of media coverage, if available), and should contain a summary of findings and recommendations. The standard IMRD format (introduction, methods, results, discussion) is often useful to follow, with the addition of a final section on recommendation and (if necessary) an executive summary.

The use of such a format also facilitates the conversion of an investigation report into a potential publication. Public health workers should undertake these investigations, however, with the foreknowledge that few of their efforts will ultimately be suitable for publication. The reported experience in the United States confirms one of the underlying assumptions of the CDC guidelines: that major associations between exposures and outcomes are rarely demonstrated. The state of Minnesota, for example, has reported results from over 500 investigations of clusters (Bender 1990), only six of which were full-scale investigations; only one of these, in an occupational setting, was published in a peer-reviewed journal (Bender et al. 1989). The states of Missouri (Devier et al. 1990) and Wisconsin (Fiore 1990) have reported similar experiences: large numbers of requests for investigations, only a few of which warrant in-depth evaluation. The Centers for Disease Control itself has been consulted in over 100 such investigations, and major associations between exposures and outcomes, warranting separate publications, have been rare (Caldwell 1990).

Perhaps a more optimistic way of viewing the process of cluster investigation, however, is to recognize that constant vigilance is required to recognize the occasional event with dramatic public health impact. In the following chapters a number of episodes are described in which important observations have resulted from a thorough investigation of a purported association.

References

Bender, A. P. (1990). Appropriate public health response to clusters: the art of being responsibly responsive. American Journal of Epidemiology, 132, S48–S52.
Bender, A. P., et al. (1988). Usefulness of comprehensive feasibility studies in environmental epidemiologic investigations: a case study in Minnesota. American Journal of Public Health, 78, 287–90.
Bender, A. P., et al. (1989). Minnesota highway maintenance worker study: cancer mortality. American Journal of Industrial Medicine, 15, S45–S56.
Black, B. (1990). Matching evidence about clustered health events with tort law requirements. American Journal of Epidemiology, 132, S79–S86.

Caldwell, G. C. (1990). Twenty-two years of cancer cluster investigations at the Centers for Disease Control. *American Journal of Epidemiology*, **132**, S43–S47.

CDC (1987). Thallium poisoning: an epidemic of false positives—Georgetown, Guyana. *Morbidity and Mortality Weekly Report*, **36**, 481–2, 487–8.

CDC (1990). Guidelines for investigating clusters of health events. *Morbidity and Mortality Weekly Report*, **39** (No. RR-11), 1–23.

Devier, J. R., Brownson, R. C., Bagby, J. R., Jr, Carlson, G. M., and Crellin, J. R. (1990). A public health response to cancer clusters in Missouri. *American Journal of Epidemiology*, **132**, S23–S31.

Fiore, B. J. (1990). State Health Department response to disease cluster reports: a protocol for investigation. *American Journal of Epidemiology*, **132**, S14–S22.

Greenberg, M. R. and Wartenberg, D. (1990). Understanding mass media coverage of disease clusters. *American Journal of Epidemiology*, **132**, S192–S195.

Rothenberg, R. B., Steinberg, K. K., and Thacker, S. B. (1990). The public health importance of clusters: a note from the Centers for Disease Control. *American Journal of Epidemiology*, **132**, S3–S5.

Slovik, P. (1987). Perception of risk. *Science*, **236**, 280–5.

Thacker, S. B. and Berkleman, R. L. (1988). Public health surveillance in the United States. *Epidemiologic Reviews*, **10**, 164–90.

24. Studies of disease clustering: problems of interpretation

J. Urquhart

In previous chapters, a distinction has been made between the investigation of specific clusters of disease around a putative point source, and geographical surveillance, which involves the identification of areas of high disease incidence or mortality. Both approaches present difficulties for interpretation, although the chance of spurious results from geographical surveillance is probably higher. In this chapter we discuss the issues related to interpretation in some detail.

Point sources

Ideally, studies carried out to determine the incidence of disease around a point source will have a hypothesis for test which is specified before any data relating to the area are examined. In practice, this is often not possible because the investigator will have prior knowledge of the incidence of the disease in the area of interest which may have come from an earlier *ad hoc* observation or from previous inconclusive studies.

Although it is important to acknowledge the difficulties that are created by prior knowledge of the data, such knowledge does not necessarily invalidate a study. Thus, for example, the studies carried out by Gardner (1989) on the incidence of childhood leukaemia in the area around Sellafield nuclear installation in England (see also Chapter 25) were prompted by the disclosures of a television programme (Yorkshire TV 1983). The programme makers had not set out to investigate the incidence of childhood cancer in the area around Sellafield and observed the apparent excess incidence during the course of a quite different investigation. The chain of prior knowledge was subsequently extended when the government committee (Black 1984) set up to investigate the apparent excess incidence commissioned further studies (Craft *et al.* 1985). Despite the prior knowledge available to Gardner and the subsequent investigators, their studies did provide insights into a possible association between the operation of a nuclear installation and the incidence of childhood leukaemia. These insights were important, not least because they suggested further hypotheses for test in areas around other nuclear installations.

In studies of the incidence of disease around a point source, there will be a prior hypothesis for test if there are existing claims of raised incidence of disease around a similar installation or location. A prior hypothesis may also exist if the investigator is directed to examine a particular location because of a biologically plausible hypothesis.

The first priority before carrying out studies of incidence around the point source must be to establish the underlying incidence of disease. If this is not done, it is not possible to evaluate the results for a particular location.

The studies carried out around the Dounreay nuclear installation in Scotland provide examples of analyses in which there was a prior hypothesis for test. These studies were requested by the Highland Regional Council as part of the evidence to be provided to an enquiry which was considering a planning application for expansion of the Dounreay plant. They were not, therefore, initiated by an observation of raised incidence in the area concerned. The results of the studies of disease incidence around Sellafield provided a clear hypothesis for test relating to the incidence of childhood leukaemia in the area around Dounreay. No prior information was available, however, to suggest which time period was most appropriate for study. Thus, although a highly significant excess incidence was observed for the 12.5 and 25 km zones around Dounreay for the period 1979–84 by Heasman *et al.* (1987), the result must be viewed in the context of a less improbable, but still statistically significant, result observed for the entire period of study from 1968 to 1984 (COMARE 1988) (Table 24.1).

Assessment of an observed excess incidence of disease requires knowledge of the underlying distribution. Thus, for example, in the Dounreay analysis, the

Table 24.1 Incidence of leukaemia and non-Hodgkin's lymphoma in young persons aged 0–24 years in the area around the Dounreay plant

	Within 12.5 km of plant	Within 25 km of plant
1979–84		
Observed	7	7
Expected	0.65	1.23
Observed/expected ratio	7.65	5.77
p	0.00057	0.00029
1968–84		
Observed	6	8
Expected	2	3.86
Observed/expected ratio	3	2.07
p	0.015	0.039

calculation of the probability of an observed result was based on the assumption that the underlying geographical distribution of disease conforms to the Poisson distribution. The assumption of a Poisson distribution was tested for Scotland, using arbitrarily constructed areas of equal population, by Black *et al.* (1991, 1992) and no evidence was found to suggest extra-Poisson variation (see Table 24.2). Ideally (and, in the case of the Dounreay analyses, with the benefit of hindsight) such analyses should be conducted in advance of examinations of the data for a particular area.

Table 24.2   Leukaemia in young persons aged 0–24 years; Scotland 1979–84. Distribution of 301 cases between 557 areas of approximately equal expectation ($E = 0.54$)

No. of cases in area	Expected No. of areas (Poisson)	Observed No. of areas
0	324.51	320
1	175.26	178
2	47.39	54
3	8.55	5
4+	1.30	0

df $= 3$
$\chi^2 = 3.801$
$p > 0.2$

Searching for areas with excess incidence of disease

In studies where searches are carried out amongst many areas to identify those with raised incidence, there is no prior hypothesis for test. For this reason, the method of analysis that is used must deal adequately with the problems created by multiple testing.

Some of the possible pitfalls associated with studies of this kind can be illustrated by reference to an analysis of meningococcal meningitis data for Scotland. Figure 24.1 shows an analysis of data for the period 1980–85 for meningococcal meningitis incidence for children aged 0–4 years for seven postcode sectors. The incidence of meningococcal meningitis in children is raised in at least one postcode sector, KZ12-9. However, the result for this sector was found after examining the incidence of the disease for 893 postcode

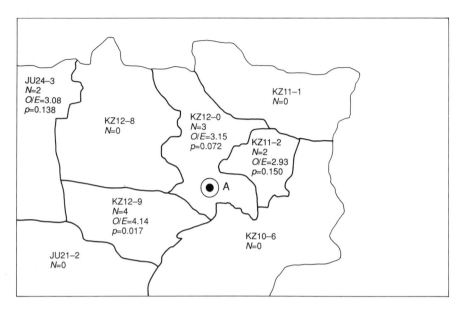

Fig. 24.1 Incidence of meningococcal meningitis in children in the 0–4 years age-group in postcode sectors in the vicinity of a 'point source', 1980–85. The designation of the postcode sectors has been anonymized.

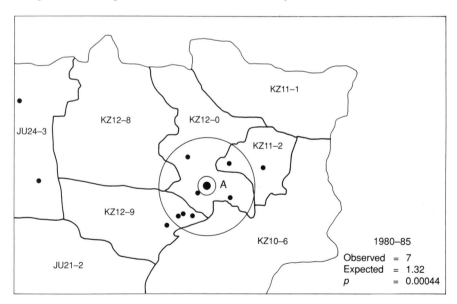

Fig. 24.2 Incidence of meningococcal meningitis in children in the 0–4 years age-group in a defined area around a 'point source', 1980–85. The designation of the postcode sectors has been anonymized.

282 J. Urquhart

sectors and selecting results that looked extreme. The observation that a
nursery school (shown as point source A on the figure) is located in close
proximity to the postcode sector with a raised incidence is a *post hoc* observation, i.e. having located an area with raised incidence, we then looked for a
plausible explanation. The problems associated with this kind of analysis are
further compounded if a more sophisticated analysis is used to 'confirm' the
original analysis. Thus, for example, a precise area approach might be
adopted, in which areas of analysis are constructed from enumeration districts
for which census population data are available. The highly improbable result
shown in Fig. 24.2 might survive sensitivity analysis of variations in boundaries
of space and time; but given the sequence of analysis, it is difficult to escape
the suspicion that the construction of boundaries has been influenced by the
observed result, i.e. that the boundaries used have been constructed to
compress a highly significant result. One further problem with this analysis is
that the calculation of probabilities has been based on unjustified assumptions
of the underlying distribution of disease. Not surprisingly, an analysis on areas
of equal population suggests that the geographical distribution of meningococcal meningitis in children exhibits extra-Poisson variation (Table 24.3) and
the assumption upon which the estimate of probability is based is thus invalid.

Table 24.3 Geographical distribution of
meningococcal meningitis in the 0–4 years
age-group, Scotland 1980–85. Expected
distribution in 234 areas of approximately
equal population assuming Poisson distribution

No. of cases in area	Expected No. of areas	Observed No. of areas
0	86.25	101
1	85.87	69
2	43.02	38
3	14.39	17
4	3.61	7
5+	0.86	2

df = 3
$\chi^2 = 11.49$
$p < 0.01$

The analysis of the meningococcal meningitis incidence data for Scotland
was deliberately conducted in a way that encompasses many of the methodological errors that might arise in studies in which searches are carried out for

areas with raised incidence. It is unlikely that such a proliferation of errors will be present in any one study. However, avoiding such sources of error in studies that are designed to search for clusters is far from easy. The problem is confounded by a variety of other problems that can be experienced in such studies. These relate to the sensitivity of the statistical test, errors in numerator data, errors in denominator data, and the selection of boundaries, all of which have been addressed in previous chapters.

There are several problems of interpretation that can arise when evaluating the results of a study in which searches are made for areas with excess incidence of disease. These problems relate, in particular, to the nature of a possible clustering effect.

The first step in any analysis in which an attempt is made to search for areas of excess incidence is to establish the underlying distribution of disease. However, if the study is restricted to locations within one region alone this may not be possible.

If the underlying distribution appears to have significant departures from a random distribution, the observed effect may either be suggestive of a generalized characteristic of the disease or of clustering at certain locations alone. Clustering at single or multiple locations may be the direct result of the distribution of risk factors.

If the result is suggestive of an excess incidence at a single location, it is necessary to attempt to determine the intensity of the observed effect. If the intensity of clustering appears to be high, consideration should be given to whether there is a local characteristic of the area which could provide a biologically sound explanation. The first priority will be to test such an explanation in another area.

Creating unwarranted concern or false reassurance

Unwarranted public concern may be created if the investigator declares the result for a single area without knowledge of the underlying distribution of the disease. Problems will also arise from the use of inaccurate data, and from failing to test the sensitivity of the result to such errors. If data errors are taken into account after publication of the original observation, it may not be possible subsequently to allay the public concern that has been created.

Particular care must be taken to establish the magnitude of any effect that is found by searching multiple locations. A result which is statistically significant but only marginally raised above some expected value may be a source of undue concern if it is published uncritically. Problems will also arise if the interpretation of results is left to public debate. If such a debate is likely to be initiated, the investigator has a responsibility to at least eliminate explanations of results that would not withstand critical analysis. The assumption is sometimes made that the press and public will interpret caveats correctly. This has often proved not to be the case.

The identification of an area with raised incidence of a disease creates a responsibility for follow-up studies. Particular problems will arise if a study identifies a large number of areas with raised incidence and insufficient resources are available for follow-up. It is entirely unethical to create a demand for follow-up studies in the public arena if such studies are not feasible.

The responsibility of the investigator does not only extend to avoiding unwarranted public concern. Equal responsibilities exist to avoid creating false reassurance. Unjustified reassurance can result from the use of incomplete or inaccurate data or bad experimental design. A particular problem can arise if the study is too insensitive to detect an observed effect. This problem pervades the whole of environmental epidemiology, as discussed in Chapter 22.

Conclusion

Studies that focus attention on the incidence of disease in a particular area may be a source of considerable public anxiety. When such studies are being planned, and when results are to be published, the investigator has a responsibility for appraising ways in which unwarranted anxiety or concern might be created. Investigators have an equally important responsibility to ensure that studies are not conducted which, because of flaws in design or interpretation, provide false reassurance in respect of a legitimate concern.

Studies carried out to examine the incidence of disease at a single location are often technically demanding and create considerable problems of interpretation. These problems are exacerbated in studies in which the aim is to search for locations with an apparent raised incidence.

References

Black, D. (1984). *Investigation of the possible increased incidence of cancer in West Cumbria*. HMSO, London.
Black, R. J., Sharp, L., and Urquhart, J. D. (1991). An analysis of the geographical distribution of childhood leukaemia and non-Hodgkin's lymphoma in Great Britain using areas of approximately equal population size. In *The Geographical Epidemiology of Childhood Leukaemia and non-Hodgkin's Lymphomas in Great Britain 1966–83*, OPCS Studies in Medical and Population Subjects. HMSO, London.
Black, R. J., Sharp, L., and Urquhart, J. D. (1992). Analysing the spatial distribution of disease using a method of constructing geographical areas of approximately equal population size. Contribution to the LRF/IARC monograph on methods of detecting disease clustering, to be published.

COMARE (1988). *Second Report. Investigation of the possible increased incidence of leukaemia in young people near the Dounreay Nuclear Establishment, Caithness, Scotland.* HMSO, London.

Craft, A. W., Openshaw, S., and Birch, J. M. (1985). Childhood cancer in the Northern Region, 1968–82: incidence in small geographic areas. *Journal of Epidemiology and Community Health*, **39**, 53–7.

Gardner, M. J. (1989). Review of reported increases of childhood cancer rates in the vicinity of nuclear installations in the UK. *Journal of the Royal Statistical Society, Series A*, **152**, 307–25.

Heasman, M. A., *et al.* (1987). Leukaemia in young persons in Scotland: a study of its geographical distribution and relationship to nuclear installations. *Health Bulletin*, **45**, 147–51.

Yorkshire TV (1983). *Windscale: the nuclear laundry.* Documentary programme, 1 November.

V Case studies

Introduction

The final section of this book includes six case studies. Five of these are examples of studies conducted in small areas; the remaining study is an example of a geographical correlation study from China.

The first three examples of small-area studies have several features in common. First, an apparent excess of disease was noticed in a particular small area. These excesses were first described anecdotally in the absence of pre-existing hypotheses. In the first example, the excess was first reported by the media following residents' suspicions, in the second case by residents, and in the third by observant clinicians. Thus, the investigations that followed were necessarily *post hoc* and reactive in nature. Secondly, the apparent excess was confirmed without doubt by further, more rigorous investigation—descriptive epidemiological studies. In this phase, the collection of complete and accurate data on the occurrence of illness was an important component. Data obtained during this phase were used to define more precisely the nature of the cluster with respect to the type of disease and the place and time of occurrence as well as other factors such as age and sex. Finally, detailed epidemiological and environmental investigations were able to suggest or identify hitherto unsuspected causes of disease. These investigations included cohort and case-control studies.

The first chapter in the section describes the investigations into childhood leukaemia around the Sellafield nuclear installation in England. As is discussed in the chapter, the original report of an excess mortality spurred a number of enquiries, and led to a series of complex epidemiological investigations. The most recent investigation, a case-control study, produced results which may provide new clues to the aetiology of leukaemia in childhood. This is an excellent example of a cluster occurring around a putative point source but for which there was no hypothesis specified in advance. In addition, the event that was initially suspected to be the 'cause' of the cluster, emission of ionizing radiation into the environment, may not be related at all. (This process is often referred to as search for the guilty and punishment of the innocent.) This highlights the problems of *post hoc* hypotheses relating to point sources.

The second example concerns an epidemic of malignant mesothelioma and lung cancer in a few small villages in central Turkey. Mesothelioma is an extremely rare disease, which is invariably fatal. In populations without occupational exposure to asbestos, the incidence is usually less than 2 cases per million person-years, although in some groups who are occupationally exposed to asbestos, the incidence is up to about 10 000 per million person-years (de Klerk and Armstrong 1991). The rate observed in one of the Turkish villages under study, Karain, may be up to three times higher than the highest rate described in occupationally exposed cohorts. Given the usual rarity of mesothelioma, confirming the epidemic was relatively straightforward. The results of subsequent detailed clinical, epidemiological, and environmental studies identified a mineral fibre, not previously associated with mesothelioma, as the cause of the epidemic.

Studies of cancer are difficult because of the multifactorial nature of the disease and the long periods between exposure to a causative agent and onset of disease. In contrast, asthma, which is the subject of the third example, has immediate precipitating factors. Nevertheless, it took several years of intense investigation before the cause of intermittent asthma epidemics in Barcelona became apparent.

These investigations can all be considered successes to some extent. Indeed, they were chosen for this very reason. In Barcelona, the investigations had direct public health benefit because the source of exposure was removed from the environment. The major benefit from the Sellafield story is the potential for new insights into leukaemogenesis. In Turkey, the epidemic continues, largely because of economic factors. Elsewhere in this book it has been stressed that direct benefits from investigations of clusters are relatively rare. Many 'clusters' are not substantiated and, of those that are substantiated, many have no ready explanation. In the examples given here, as in most such investigations, a great deal of effort, time, and money is expended. The question that public health authorities must always bear in mind is whether the expenditure is justified.

The fourth example is rather different in nature. It describes the studies conducted in a population exposed to dioxin following an explosion at a chemical plant in Seveso. Thus, hypotheses were specified in advance of observing the data, so that the studies were proactive rather than reactive. Since the major investigation was a cohort study, few of the methods for small-area studies discussed in previous sections were used. However, the problems of data quality are as important in this study as in any geographical study. It is included because the cohorts under study were defined geographically on the basis of environmental measurements of dioxin contamination. Furthermore, the design is an efficient method to identify potential adverse effects of acute accidents, many of which will be restricted to small areas.

The final example of a small-area study concerns the incidence of cancer of the larynx and lung around incinerators of waste solvents and oils in Great Britain. It is an example of a study conducted to test a particular hypothesis which was specified in advance of observing the data, although the original hypothesis came about because of concern around one particular incinerator site. A particular strength of the study is the replication at several sites. The example also illustrates the use of many of the techniques given in previous chapters.

The last example is not a study conducted in a small area. It is, rather, an example of a geographical correlation (ecological) study, conducted in various counties of China. The study was designed to exploit the large regional differences in risk of cancers and dietary practices within China. To overcome the problems associated with difficulty in measuring diet and other risk factors in individuals, measurements on all individuals in a sampling unit were combined. Thus, the measurements represent an average over a number of individuals. A major aim of the study, as in most correlation studies, is to generate hypotheses about the cause of disease. The methods employed could be used equally in studies conducted in small areas. Problems common to geographical studies, regardless of the size of the geographical unit, are discussed in this chapter.

Reference

de Klerk, N. H. and Armstrong, B. K. (1991). The epidemiology of asbestos and mesothelioma. In *Malignant mesothelioma*, (ed. D. W. Henderson, K. B. Shilkin, D. Whitaker, and S. L. P. Langlois). Hemisphere, New York.

25. Childhood leukaemia around the Sellafield nuclear plant

M. J. Gardner

The Sellafield nuclear site is located in the north-west of England on the coast of West Cumbria. The site was acquired in 1947 for the production of plutonium for defence purposes, with two nuclear reactors and a spent fuel reprocessing plant being in operation by 1952. These reactors and the reprocessing plant were subsequently closed and replaced between 1956 and 1963 by five further nuclear reactors (one of which was closed in 1981) and, in 1964, by another reprocessing plant. The Sellafield plant reprocesses spent fuel from nuclear power stations in Britain and abroad, and has both stored and discharged to sea low-level radioactive waste—solid and liquid waste, respectively.

Towards the end of 1983 a Yorkshire Television programme called *Windscale: the nuclear laundry* was screened. The television producer had previously made a documentary on the ill-health effects of asbestos on workers, which had successfully influenced the introduction in Britain of stricter control limits on occupational exposure to these fibres. He decided to produce another similarly focused programme and approached the management of Sellafield with a request for their co-operation in making a documentary on the health of the radiation workforce at Sellafield. He was told that there were no definite indications of any major long-term ill-health effects of radiation exposure on their workers—which was largely justified and in accord with studies that had been carried out both by the company itself (Clough 1983) and independently (Smith and Douglas 1986).

Anecdotal suggestion of childhood leukaemia excess

However, while in the area negotiating for the programme, the producer heard incidentally of a number of cases of childhood leukaemia near the nuclear installation, which the local people thought may be too high, and decided to switch the thrust of his programme to discussing these childhood leukaemia cases. He finally presented a programme which suggested that there had been an excess of childhood leukaemia cases in the area near Sellafield—particularly in the village of Seascale some 3 km to the south—and the programme alleged that these cases were linked to the discharges of radioactive liquids from the plant to the Irish Sea, which subsequently polluted the beaches, fish, and seafood. The British government immediately set up an independent inquiry under the chairmanship of Sir Douglas Black to investigate the suggestion and allegation. A major question is 'how should such an allegation be tackled?'

Confirmation of cases

One of the first things that needs to be done is to investigate the cases that are alleged to have occurred. In this instance, because the television production team were not bona fide research workers they did not have access to full confidential clinical details. It was thus necessary to confirm that the cases and their diagnoses existed in medical records—either hospital or cancer registration records, or on death certificates. If the cases are not genuine and not known to the medical profession, then an allegation can effectively be discounted at this stage. On the other hand, if the cases are shown to be genuine, as in this example, then the investigation needs to go further (Black 1984). At the same time as the confirmation of the suggested cases, it was established that there were no further relevant cases of childhood leukaemia that had been unknown to the television producer. One of the next queries needs to be whether there is an excess, given that the cases have been confirmed.

The Black report: geographical studies

Confirmation of excess

The suggestion that the number of cancers, and particularly leukaemia, was in excess among children resident in the neighbourhood of Sellafield was examined by two subsequent geographical analyses. First, it was shown that in Millom Rural District (the local authority administrative area containing Seascale) there had been a raised leukaemia mortality rate among persons aged 0–24 years during 1968–78 (six deaths compared with 1.4 expected at national rates for England and Wales) but not during 1959–67, and not in adjacent Ennerdale Rural District (the local authority administrative area containing Sellafield) during either period of time (Table 25.1). These particular calendar years were used to correspond to the seventh and eighth revisions of the International Classification of Diseases. Rates for other cancers at these ages were not raised, nor were either leukaemia or total cancer rates in the adult populations (Gardner and Winter 1984). The total cancer rates might also have been expected to be raised if radiation, as suggested, was the cause, unless some special argument relating to increased child susceptibility, possibly involving a particular route of exposure, is invoked. Secondly, Craft et al. (1984) reported four cases of lymphoid malignancy among 0–14-year-olds in Seascale during 1968–82, compared with 0.25 expected at registration rates for the overall Northern region of England. Cancer registration started in this region in 1968.

Table 25.1 Mortality from leukaemia under 25 years of age during 1959–78 in Millom and Ennerdale rural districts

Rural district*	Calendar period	Number of deaths		Standardized mortality ratio (SMR)	95% confidence interval for SMR
		Observed (O)	Expected† (E)		
Ennerdale	1959–67	3	3.3	91	19 to 266
	1968–78	4	3.3	121	33 to 310
Millom	1959–67	1	1.6	63	16 to 348
	1968–78	6	1.4	435	160 to 946

* Ennerdale contains the Sellafield nuclear site and Millom contains the village of Seascale.
† At age, sex, and calendar period specific rates for England and Wales.

Statistical aspects

One difficult problem is how to interpret this excess. If we start out on an investigation and find, not what we are expecting (in this case a health risk to the workforce), but something different, unintentionally, how should we react? Is it a chance event that we have stumbled across? Or is it an exposure-related observation waiting to be discovered? Standard statistical hypothesis testing applied to this situation is unhelpful, because it is primarily designed for a priori hypotheses rather than a posteriori hypotheses, where the interpretation of the p value becomes complex. The particular excess discussed in the television programme and the linking of it to Windscale was certainly a *post hoc* argument.

An a priori hypothesis could have been set up given the knowledge that Windscale had discharged vastly more radioactive waste materials into the environment than any other nuclear site in the UK (Black 1984) and given its known record of accidental releases, of which the Windscale fire in 1957 was the worst. However, although there was known to have been some previous concern, for example, by the local District Medical Officer, no detailed study had been launched except that later published by Baron (1984).

'Boundary' definitions

The difficulty of interpretation is increased by the possible selection for analysis of boundaries for geographical areas, calendar years, age-groups, and diagnostic categories that maximize the numerical size of the excess—rather than specification of these defining characteristics in advance of data examination. The potential difficulties raised by this possibly data-guided selection of boundaries are indicated, for example, by the choice of the age-group 0–9 years for a hypothesis test by the television programme collaborators (Urquhart *et al.* 1984) when traditionally the age-group 0–14 years had been used. The exclusion of the ages 10–14 years was clearly not for lack of information, but was possibly influenced by the knowledge that only one case was known at these older ages.

This particular problem was expanded on in the Black report (1984). By variations of the definition of boundaries it is possible to manipulate, if desired, the numerical size of any reported 'excess' and also the associated *p* value from a test of statistical significance. If this procedure is followed, bias is introduced and the *p* value will not be a valid measure of its purpose, i.e. to measure the role of chance in producing the observations. The problem is succinctly described as 'moving the goal posts'.

Putting the figures into context

Another difficulty associated with the interpretation of such an isolated excess is that alone it cannot be seen in the context of other similar geographical areas. With a rare disease like leukaemia in children it can be anticipated that during a limited time period some individually unpredictable areas with small populations will have high observed rates, and others low rates, by the play of chance alone. An examination of areas other than those around Sellafield can help to take the argument further, and some such data were provided (Black 1984; Craft *et al.* 1984). These studies have shown that the immediate areas around Sellafield do have high rates compared to those elsewhere, but not uniquely so.

This is an appropriate and helpful approach, because rates in other localities, regionally and nationally, can be contrasted without any further redefinition of the area basis, calendar years, age, and diagnostic groups. Thus, was the raised rate in Millom extreme or, even though statistically significant at $p < 0.05$, was it in the main part of the distribution? In fact, Millom Rural District, with a standardized mortality ratio (SMR) of 435 (see Table 25.1), had the second highest rate of leukaemia mortality at ages 0–24 years during 1968–78 among 152 similar-sized rural districts around England and Wales (Table 25.2). The area with the highest rate (an SMR of 440) was not geographically close to Millom or near a nuclear installation.

Table 25.2 shows, alongside the observed distribution, the predicted distribution of leukaemia mortality in the 152 rural districts if cases had occurred at random among their combined populations, i.e. assuming uniform risk. It can be seen that, by and large, the observed and predicted distributions are reasonably similar, although there is a suggestion of more areas with SMRs over 100 than would be expected. This comparison, however, is of only limited value as a test of spatial randomness since rates in contiguous rural districts were not examined. It is also of limited value as a test of whether the Sellafield

Table 25.2 Mortality from leukaemia under 25 years of age during 1968–78 in 152 similar-sized rural districts (including Millom) of England and Wales

Standardized mortality ratio	Number of rural districts	
	Observed	Predicted*
0–	78	86
100–	52	48
200–	19	15
300–	1	2.7
400 +	2	0.4

* On the basis of the Poisson distribution.

area has a raised risk from some specific local factor whereas a uniformly lower rate operates in the other rural districts.

Seascale had the third highest registration rate of lymphoid malignancy at ages 0–14 years during 1968–82 among the 675 electoral wards in the Northern Region children's malignant disease registry. If the associated Poisson probabilities are considered, rather than rates, that for Seascale was the lowest of the 675 wards (i.e. Seascale had the lowest one-sided *p* value of 0.0001).

Suggested cause of excess

These two investigations thus tended to support the allegations of the television programme in terms of a raised childhood leukaemia rate near the Sellafield nuclear plant, although making no contribution to an examination of the effects, if any, of radioactive discharges. The plausibility of the suggested cause being radiation followed from the incontrovertible evidence that leukaemia has resulted from high exposure in the past. However, analyses using models of the average radiation dose to the bone marrow received as a consequence of the radioactive discharges from Sellafield did not support the view that an environmental pathway was involved (Black 1984).

Limitations of geographical studies

Geographical analyses of this nature have a number of limitations. For example, the arbitrary nature from an epidemiological viewpoint of the administrative areas used; the potential inclusion of cases after only a short local residential period when the initiating cause of their disease had occurred in another area; the exclusion of cases diagnosed soon after moving away but where the initiating cause had been in the study area; and the use of census-enumerated populations as denominators when high levels of population migration are possible. The effect of such emigration and immigration will tend to dilute disease clusters with a specific localized cause and diminish their detection by geographical studies.

Recommendations for further investigations

The Black inquiry recognized the limitations in the available data, but acknowledged that they pointed to an apparent excess of childhood leukaemia near Sellafield, particularly in Seascale. This was seen as a cause for concern. As a consequence, it was recommended that other epidemiological methods—cohort and case-control studies as described later—should be used to elucidate further the nature of the observed area excess.

In addition, the Black inquiry commented on the reasonable resource and speed, within 2 months, with which two research centres were able to analyse routinely available information, both on mortality and cancer registration, to respond to the Yorkshire Television programme. The first was aided by data partially worked up during the preparation of a cancer atlas for England and Wales (Gardner *et al.* 1983) and the second by the detailed coding and analysis of records in the Northern Region children's malignant disease registry. However, it was thought that the initiation of a research group with the expertise to analyse and interpret such data would be appropriate, both for reactive analyses of the type discussed here and also for prudent proactive examinations. This would include the development of appropriate computerized data-bases—for example, moving away from administrative area to residential address coding using national grid coordinates—and analytical techniques. This particular recommendation led to the formation of the Small Area Health Statistics Unit at the London School of Hygiene and Tropical Medicine (see Chapter 10).

Seascale birth and schools cohort studies

Seascale birth cohort

One of the further epidemiological studies that was recommended by the Black report and which has now been completed was a cohort study (Gardner *et al.* 1987*b*). This was essentially a follow-up study of all children who were born in Seascale during 1950–83, which at the time of starting the study covered most of the period of operation of the Sellafield plant. Using local birth registers for these years, the Office of Population Censuses and Surveys identified 1068 children whose mother's residential address had been in the village. This required an extensive clerical search through microfilm records of births over several registration districts to the end of 1983, which was the latest possible date at the time of searching. In an attempt to ensure the inclusion of all hospital as well as home births, the search included other areas in addition to the main local registration district of Whitehaven. The home addresses given in the birth entries were examined against maps and lists of addresses inside Seascale Civil Parish (the same as the electoral ward area used in the geographical analysis described earlier). Only births where the mother's residential address was inside the civil parish boundary, as opposed to having Seascale as a descriptive postal address, were included.

To try to ensure completeness, a search was also made in the register of births held locally by the West Cumbria Health Authority for immunization and child welfare purposes. This register contained less identifying information on each child so that, for example, forenames were not always recorded, but details on any possible Seascale births found in this way were abstracted. The two differently obtained sets of births were then checked by computer against each other using the recorded information on surname and date of birth. For children in the West Cumbria set who were not in the Office of Population Censuses and Surveys set a further search was made in the Office of Population Censuses and Surveys microfilm records at the appropriate date, and, where found, information on appropriate birth entries was abstracted.

Seascale school cohort

We were made aware of four schools in Seascale which had taken pupils for all or some of the period from 1950. With the co-operation of the local Cumbria Education Department, as well as the headmasters and headmistresses of the schools, we examined the school registers to find out whether the information in them was sufficiently detailed to identify uniquely the children who had attended. For three of the schools the recorded details were of suitable quality for follow-up. The fourth school was a preparatory boarding school for boys which closed during 1972 but had taken some 150 pupils since 1950, of whom about half came from outside Cumbria. Although for each boy the year of birth was recorded, the full date of birth was not and hence follow-up was not feasible. This school had, therefore, to be omitted.

A total of 1546 children who had attended one of the other three schools, and who were born on or after 1 January 1950 as in the Seascale birth cohort, were included. However, any school children who were also born to mothers resident in Seascale Civil Parish at the time of birth, and so were already members of the birth cohort, were left out of this part of the study (Gardner *et al.* 1987*a*).

The allocation of children to birth and schools cohorts in the way described was carried out to avoid duplication in counting children and events such as cancer registration and death. The birth and schools cohorts will not have included all children who were born after 1950 and who lived in Seascale for some period of time. In addition to boys who were pupils only at the excluded

M. J. Gardner

preparatory school, any child who, for example, moved to the village after birth but left before school age, or went to boarding school elsewhere, cannot be identified by the means we have used. The studies, however, will have included most of the Seascale children.

Follow-up of Seascale cohorts

For all eligible children thus identified, details were sent to the National Health Service Central Register with a request for vital status data, including information on deaths, cancer registrations, and emigrations. In addition, we were notified by the Central Register of all areas in which the children had been recorded since birth as registered with general practitioners and the related dates, which allowed estimates to be made of durations of residence in Cumbria. This information was supplemented both by a search for the parents' names in the annual Seascale Electoral Registers and by information from the Seascale Local Authority school register on dates of attendance, to obtain estimates of length of residence in Seascale for each child. The West Cumbria Health Authority register was also searched for recorded information on deaths or cases of cancer among the Seascale children. None of the children or their parents were approached personally for information.

Childhood leukaemia excess limited to Seascale births

Mortality and cancer registration up to 30 June 1986 among the children identified as resident in Seascale were analysed and compared with those values expected at national rates. The person-years method of analysis was used, incorporating calendar period-, cause-, sex-, and age-specific death rates for England and Wales. It was found that cases of leukaemia had occurred only among children born in the village, with an estimated tenfold excess, whereas none occurred in children who had moved in after birth (see Table 25.3). For other cancers there was no suggestion of any excess among the school-children, but a slight suggestion of a possible raised number among those born in the village. The conclusion at this stage was that there was a genuine excess of childhood leukaemia in Seascale and, if there was a genuine local factor causing this excess, then it appeared to operate either very early in life or before birth (Gardner *et al.* 1987*a,b*).

Migration of Seascale children

Table 25.4 gives figures on approximate length of residence in Seascale for the 1068 live births in the birth cohort, by showing the numbers of children who had become pupils at the main school in Seascale by November 1984. If the final four years (1980–83) are excluded, then 556 out of the 978 (57 per cent) children attended the school. The remaining 422 (43 per cent) were not found

Table 25.3 Leukaemia and other cancer cases during 1950–86 in Seascale birth and school cohorts

Diagnosis	Cohort	Number of cases		O/E	95% confidence interval for O/E
		Observed (O)	Expected (E)*		
Leukaemia	Birth	6†	0.6	10.0	3.7–21.8
	Schools	0	0.6	0	0–6.2
Other cancer	Birth	6†	2.2	2.7	1.0–5.9
	Schools	4	3.4	1.2	0.3–3.0

* At age-, sex-, and calendar-period-specific rates for England and Wales.
† Five cases of leukaemia and two cases of non-Hodgkin's lymphoma were diagnosed while resident in Seascale and are included in the case-control study (see Fig. 25.1).

on the school register and can be presumed to have moved out of Seascale between birth and school age, i.e. generally before 5 years of age. This percentage varied little over the 30 years. Forty four (4.5 per cent), however, are known to have attended the school for preschool-age children in Seascale which was open between 1949 and 1968. The general tendency shown in Table 25.4 concurs with the suggestion of a mobile population in Seascale. Some 40 per cent of children born in Seascale did not stay to attend the local school. Additionally, some 75 per cent of children attending the main school in Seascale had migrated in after being born elsewhere. These levels of migration in general are likely to dilute substantially the effect of any local early life

Table 25.4 Children born during 1950–83 to mothers resident in Seascale, according to whether they attended the local authority school up to November 1984

Period of birth	Number of births	Name on school register	
		Yes	Percentage
1950–9	358	202	56
1960–9	391	230	59
1970–9	229	124	54
(1980–3)*	(90)	(9)	(10)
1950–83	1068	565	53

* Children born during these years had mainly not reached school age by November 1984.

factor on the measured incidence of disease in the area among school-age children or older persons.

Organization and resources of study

The time elapsed from the date of the recommendation for the Seascale cohort study in the middle of 1984 to the publication of the results in the scientific papers during the autumn of 1987 was just over 3 years. During this period a project grant proposal had to be written and submitted to the Department of Health for approval of partial funding—the remainder being provided by the Medical Research Council Environmental Epidemiology Unit research budget. Agreement for the basic records required for the study had to be obtained from the Office of Population Censuses and Surveys (for original birth entries of Seascale children from the Registration Division together with follow-up information from the National Health Service Central Register including mortality, cancer registration, and emigration data) and from the Cumbria Education Committee and ex-headmistresses of schools which had previously existed in Seascale (for children's records from school registers). Additionally, ethical committee approval both nationally and locally was obtained.

The study required extensive searching of local hospital and health authority area records—a research assistant was employed locally partly for this purpose —as well as substantial computer data-base preparation and analysis (for example, to link birth and school records to avoid duplicate inclusion of children in both parts of the study), for which a programmer as well as clerical and data-entry staff were also partially employed. A clinical scientist and statistician, as well as others, devoted a substantial period of time to the project. The duration of the project was governed both by the above factors and also the time taken to ensure adequate and correct tracing of the 2614 children included and appropriate elimination of others, for example if their residential address at birth was outside the civil parish boundary.

West Cumbria case-control study

Examining individual factors

The next step, having determined that an excess exists, is to look at individual factors on appropriate cases to determine whether or not any factors can be established that help to explain why the disease occurred (Gardner *et al.* 1990*a,b*). This can be done by a case-control study, in which cases of a disease are compared with healthy children who have not developed the illness. Non-Hodgkin's lymphomas were included, as well as leukaemias, because there is evidence of some relation with ionizing radiation, and also because their diagnoses could have been confused with leukaemia during the early years of this study. Hodgkin's disease was also included, although it is not thought to be related to radiation. Thus it was decided in advance to examine leukaemia and non-Hodgkin's lymphoma separately from Hodgkin's disease in the main analysis and also to look particularly at Seascale.

The West Cumbria Health Authority district was used for the study, although it included a larger area than that (mainly Seascale) in which the excess incidence (mainly of leukaemia) had been reported. Nevertheless, it contains stretches of coastline, including estuaries where concerns had been raised about potential risks from radiation contamination, as well as inland regions away from the coast. In addition, West Cumbria was chosen partly to cover the places of residence of the Sellafield workforce.

Specific objectives

The case-control study that was carried out had very specific objectives. These were to examine whether or not the excess was related to the only generally accepted cause of childhood leukaemia, i.e. prenatal abdominal X-ray of the mother; whether it was related to suggested risk factors for childhood leukaemia, such as viral infections or social class; whether it was related to exposure to radiation as a result of habits which could potentially have enhanced exposure to the radioactive discharges to sea from Sellafield, such as playing on the beach or eating fresh fish or shellfish; or whether exposure to radiation through parental employment at the plant was relevant.

Identification of the cases

As far as possible, a definitive list was compiled of cases of leukaemia and lymphoma diagnosed from 1 January 1950 to 31 December 1985 among persons aged 0–24 years with a residential address in the West Cumbria Health Authority area. Because of lack of cancer registry coverage in the early years of this period, various sources were used to identify the relevant cases, including: *notification* of cases to the Black inquiry; *case records* from a childhood cancer survey in West Cumbria at the time of the Black inquiry; *pathology records* at the West Cumberland Hospital; *death entries*, *death certificates*, and *cancer registrations* for West Cumbria; *circular letters* to general practitioners in West Cumbria; *preschool illness notifications* in the West Cumbria register.

Only cases born and diagnosed in West Cumbria have been included in the analysis. In total, 52 cases of leukaemia, 22 of non-Hodgkin's lymphoma, and 23 of Hodgkin's disease were identified.

Selection of the controls

The selection of controls was from live birth records at the Office of Population Censuses and Surveys. Two groups of eight controls of the same sex as the case were taken from the register into which the case's birth was entered. For one group (area controls) searches were made backwards and forwards from the case's entry in the birth register until the nearest four appropriate controls in each direction were found. Only births to mothers with a West Cumbria address were included. For the second group (local controls) the residence of the control mothers was matched for residence (civil parish, for example, Seascale) of the mothers of the case at the date of birth, although otherwise the procedure was as for the first group.

There was thus, effectively, matching of controls on sex and date of birth. The same individual could have been used as a control in both groups. Thus, if any one of the eight adjacent births of the same sex to a case was also from the same civil parish then this control would have been in each group. Eight controls of each type were taken for each case to increase the statistical efficiency of the study, but it was also envisaged that some case and control parents would either have died or prove impossible to trace. The area controls were taken primarily to repeat the geographical analysis on a case-control basis and the local controls to examine other factors.

For each control a check was made in the National Health Service Central Register and Family Practitioner Committee records to see whether they were still alive, not registered with cancer, and resident in West Cumbria at the date of diagnosis of their associated case, i.e. to check that they had remained in the risk set to that date. After appropriate exclusions, 1001 of 1243 originally selected controls for the 97 cases remained. Of these, 248 served as both area and local controls.

Parents of cases and controls

Identifying particulars, including full name and date of birth, for the parents of each case and control were found where possible from the child's birth certificate and from obstetric and general medical records. The aim was to identify uniquely the parents in the National Health Service Central Register and thus ascertain whether they were still alive. For parents found to be alive, and if they were eligible for the questionnaire part of the study (see below), their current Family Practitioner Committee registration was traced to enable them to be contacted through their own general practitioner.

Use of hospital records

Hospital records were examined for two purposes: first, to obtain detailed information on the case's diagnosis and, secondly, to extract data from the relevant obstetric notes on the pregnancy for both cases and controls. As well as abstracting relevant clinical details, it was ascertained whether or not a histological diagnosis had been made and whether histological material was available. When such material was available the case was the subject of an independent pathological review. We extracted from obstetric records details on exposure to X-rays during the pregnancy, including the parts of the body examined and dates. For abdominal X-ray examinations the number and type of examination were also noted. Recorded information was also obtained on viral infections that the mother suffered during pregnancy, for example chicken pox, influenza, or rubella.

Questionnaire procedure and content

The study included a questionnaire, with information being sought directly from parents of cases and controls. This was carried out through parents' general practitioners. The questionnaire was sent to the case's mother if she was still living and her current residence could be established, and also sent to the mothers of associated controls. For other cases and their controls the questionnaires were forwarded to their fathers. In this way responses from within case-control sets were obtained from parents of the same sex. When both of a case's parents were dead or untraced questionnaires were not sent out for either the case or their controls.

The purposes of the questionnaire were both to obtain information which had been partly collected from hospital records but now directly from the parents and to request data otherwise unavailable. Thus we asked the parent about antenatal care, including X-ray examinations, and infectious illnesses during the relevant pregnancy. Also, we asked for residential and occupational histories of both parents from the time they left school, as well as the residential history of their child. Other data requested included childhood activities on the beach and in the Lake District, family habits in eating fresh fish, seafood, and home-grown vegetables, and the child's birth weight.

Geographical analysis in relation to Sellafield

One aspect of the study was, as indicated, to compare the geographical distributions of the cases and controls in relation to Sellafield. For this purpose residential addresses at birth for cases and controls were identified on Ordnance Survey maps, and national grid references accurate to 100 m squares were obtained for most (87 per cent) addresses. For the remainder the accuracy was less, and in some instances addresses were untraceable, mainly those from the earlier years covered by the study. This method allowed a modified approach to the geography of cases rather than the usual area analysis of mortality and cancer registration statistics. The differences in approach are at least twofold: first, the use of controls rather than census figures to represent the population and, secondly, location at birth rather than at diagnosis. In fact, the cases mainly tended to be diagnosed at the same address or at one close to where they had been born.

Distances of addresses of cases and controls from Sellafield were calculated by taking the national grid reference of the nuclear site to be NY 027 039, as used by the National Radiological Protection Board in its analysis of atmospheric discharges (J. Stather, personal communication). The results given here are for cases and area controls using residential addresses at birth. Table 25.5 shows findings in sectors of increasing 5 km radii moving away from Sellafield, and risks are given relative to the inner circle, which completely contains Seascale and some other smaller villages. All five cases of

Table 25.5 Numbers of cases and controls with relative risks for leukaemia in children by distance from Sellafield of residence at birth for area controls

Distance (km)	Cases ($n = 51$)	Area controls ($n = 350$)	Relative risk	95% confidence interval
≤4	5	14	1	
5–9	5	31	0.35	0.08–1.62
10–14	14	117	0.21	0.05–0.92
15–19	5	35	0.22	0.04–1.22
20–24	9	52	0.22	0.03–1.59
25–29	8	66	0.14	0.02–0.91
≥30	5	35	0.17	0.02–1.88

leukaemia in the inner circle occurred in children born to parents resident in Seascale (see Table 25.3). There was a large fall in relative risk on moving to outside the inner circle, to levels of about one-third and smaller, with some suggestion also of a decreasing risk with further distance. These latter results also applied when analysis was limited to cases born in the birth registration district containing Sellafield rather than throughout West Cumbria.

Paternal employment and radiation exposure at Sellafield

Occupational data on the parents of cases and controls were obtained from three different sources. First, we abstracted parental (mainly fathers') occupations from the birth certificates of their children. Secondly, we obtained occupational histories by questionnaire as described. These two sets of data were coded to both occupation and industry using standard classifications (General Register Office 1966; Central Statistical Office 1968) with some local modifications. Thirdly, we cross-matched our computer file of study subjects with that of the past and present Sellafield workforce to identify people who appeared on both files. This linkage was carried out using surname, initials, and date of birth, with incorporation of forenames, National Health Service numbers, and addresses when available on both files. For those subjects identified as having worked at Sellafield, British Nuclear Fuels plc subsequently supplied us with dates of employment at the site and external whole-body ionizing radiation dosimetry on an annual basis. The radiation dose in each year had been estimated from monitoring with dosemeters worn on the trunk, and our figures come from an information bank on which satisfactory quality checks had been reported (National Radiological Protection Board 1986; Smith and Douglas 1986). The data had been collated prior to our study and hence was 'blind' to the hypothesis being tested and to the particular subgroup of Sellafield workers included. In addition, the personal quantitative measurements were of a high quality for epidemiological study, which is most unusual in occupational investigations.

Analysis showed that for children whose fathers had been employed at Sellafield, and who had had high recorded exposures to ionizing radiation before their child's conception, the relative risk of developing leukaemia was increased (Table 25.6). At the highest levels of paternal exposure given in the Table, i.e. 100 milliSieverts or more in total before their child's conception and 10 milliSieverts or more during the previous 6 months, the relative risks were estimated as about eightfold, not dissimilar to the tenfold excess found in Seascale (see Table 25.3). The numbers are small, but there are suggestions of a gradation in risk with increasing radiation dose, statistically significant using the likelihood ratio test. Three of the four fathers of leukaemia cases in the highest radiation dose groups lived in Seascale.

Table 25.6 Relative risks for childhood leukaemia by father's external ionizing radiation dose during employment at Sellafield before child's conception

Radiation dose (milliSieverts)	Cases	Local controls	Relative risk	95% confidence interval
Total before conception				
0	38	236	1	
>0–49	3	26	0.8	0.2–3.0
50–99	1	11	0.8	0.1–7.7
≥100	4	3	8.4	1.4–52.0
6 months before conception				
0	38	246	1	
>0–4	3	24	1.1	0.3–4.9
5–9	1	3	3.0	0.3–32.6
≥10	4	3	8.2	1.6–41.7

Among the total of five cases of childhood leukaemia in Seascale in this study (see Table 25.3), the four fathers whom we had fully identified and obtained occupational radiation records for had higher overall exposures throughout their Sellafield employment before their child's conception than all the fathers of the matched comparison children who were also born in Seascale (see Fig. 25.1), i.e. the four fathers except case 5 in the figure. These observations led to the suggestion that in some way exposure of a father to radiation during his employment at Sellafield before the conception of his child may be

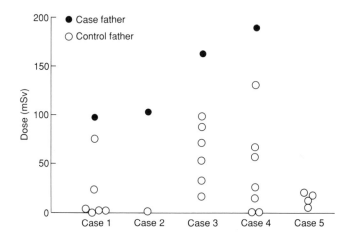

Fig. 25.1 Accumulated external ionizing radiation dose during employment at Sellafield before child's conception in fathers of Seascale leukaemia cases and Seascale controls (the father of case 5 is not yet linked to the radiation dosimetry records).

relevant to the subsequent development of leukaemia in his child, and could explain statistically the excess cases occurring in the village. The results for non-Hodgkin's lymphoma, which were based on fewer cases, were not dissimilar to leukaemia; whereas for Hodgkin's disease, which has not been associated with ionizing radiation in the medical literature, there was no relationship to the father's employment at Sellafield as a radiation worker. Relatively few mothers had been employed at Sellafield and when they had it was mainly in non-radiation jobs.

Other findings

Without going into all the details of the results of this study, it can be said that similar risks were found for prenatal X-rays as had been identified in earlier studies; no important excesses in relation to the suggested risk factors examined were identified; and no apparent risks of leukaemia were indicated in relation to potential exposure to radiation through the Sellafield discharges as assessed.

Organization and resources required

The time taken from the date of the recommendation for the case-control study in the middle of 1984 to the publication of the results in the scientific papers early in 1990 was about 6½ years. This included protocol development, partial funding application, and ethical committee approval, as for the Seascale cohort studies. Major components of this study were searching a variety of sources to identify as far as possible all relevant cases of childhood cancer, including the period before cancer registration commenced in 1968; searching through birth entries at the Office of Population Censuses and Surveys to appropriately select control children for the cases; looking up national grid coordinates for residential addresses at birth of the children; and linking the records of the parents with the Sellafield workforce and radiation dosimetry records. These activities involved many and varied staff working in West Cumbria, at the Central Register and in the Environmental Epidemiology Unit (including a clinical scientist, research assistants, statistician, and programmers) to handle the information retrieval and processing for the more than 3000 individuals (including children and parents) involved in the investigation.

Leukaemogenesis: an occupational risk?

At this stage the perspective has changed from that of a suggested childhood leukaemia excess in Seascale which was possibly related to environmental radiation contamination (as originally reported by the Yorkshire television programme) to a confirmed childhood leukaemia excess in the village which is statistically related to a father's external radiation exposure during work at Sellafield before his child's conception. The evidence has been developed from anecdote by the sequential use of standard epidemiological methods—geographical, cohort, and case-control studies. This finding clearly needs, and is receiving, more attention and detail to try to understand whether it is truly radiation related and, if so, quite how it might operate.

The first point is that there is a well-established excess of childhood leukaemia around Sellafield—while any excesses that have been examined, as part of the logical scientific process, around other nuclear establishments in the UK are of a lower magnitude (Gardner 1989). This excess near Sellafield is strongly associated with fathers having had high exposure to external whole-body penetrating ionizing radiation while working at the installation before their child's conception. But is this association pointing towards a causal mechanism? One possibility is genetic damage, but some geneticists and radio-biologists have considered that the levels of occupational exposure are too low for this to be a plausible pathway according to current knowledge. This conclusion is based, to some extent, on the lack of any similar effect among children born subsequently to Japanese survivors of the atomic bombs. However, the scenarios are somewhat different, contrasting a high short-term exposure with a lower long-term exposure. In addition, some workers at Sella-field will also have been exposed to radionuclides, such as plutonium, which have not yet been analysed for; and there are other exposures in a complex environment that may or may not be relevant. One experimental study in the laboratory using animals supports the idea that a pathway through radiation of the parents is plausible (Nomura 1982), although this one result from Japan needs replication.

Geographical studies have now been carried out in some other countries, such as France (Hill and Laplanche 1990) and the USA (Jablon *et al.* 1990), where the excess seen around nuclear establishments in the UK has not been replicated. It may be that they genuinely do not occur, but it is also possible that the geographical areas used, particularly in the USA, are too large to notice a localized effect. There are two other case-control studies around nuclear installations in the UK. The first of these, around Dounreay, the other nuclear waste reprocessing centre in Britain, failed to replicate the findings near Sellafield, but was based on small numbers (Urquhart *et al.* 1991); the second is around the Aldermaston and Burghfield nuclear sites and has yet to report its findings. Although the results of these studies are of interest, of course, how much they can be considered to be reproductions of the circum-stances at Sellafield is less clear. There are also preliminary plans to do similar case-control studies around a number of the oldest nuclear installations in the USA and France.

References

Baron, J. (1984). Cancer mortality in small areas around nuclear facilities in England and Wales. *British Journal of Cancer*, **50**, 815–24.
Black, D. (1984). *Investigation of the possible increased incidence of cancer in West Cumbria*. HMSO, London.
Central Statistical Office (1968). *Standard industrial classification* (revised 1968). HMSO, London.
Clough, E. A. (1983). The BNFL radiation–mortality study. *Journal of the Society for Radiological Protection*, **3**, (1), 24–7.
Craft, A. W., Openshaw, S., and Birch, J. (1984). Apparent clusters of childhood lymphoid malignancy in Northern England. *Lancet*, **ii**, 96–7.
Gardner, M. J. (1989). Review of reported increases of childhood cancer rates in the vicinity of nuclear installations in the UK. *Journal of the Royal Statistical Society, Series A*, **152**, 307–25.

Gardner, M. J. and Winter, P. D. (1984). Mortality in Cumberland during 1959–78 with reference to cancer in young people around Windscale. *Lancet*, **i**, 216–17.

Gardner, M. J., Winter, P. D., Taylor, C. P., and Acheson, E. D. (1983). *Atlas of cancer mortality for England and Wales, 1968–78*. Wiley, Chichester.

Gardner, M. J., Hall, A. J., Downes, S., and Terrell, J. D. (1987*a*). A follow-up study of children born elsewhere but attending schools in Seascale, West Cumbria (schools cohort). *British Medical Journal*, **295**, 819–22.

Gardner, M. J., Hall, A. J., Downes, S., and Terrell, J. D. (1987*b*). A follow-up study of children born to mothers resident in Seascale, West Cumbria (birth cohort). *British Medical Journal*, **295**, 822–7.

Gardner, M. J., Hall, A. J., Snee, M. P., Downes, S., Powell, C. A., and Terrell, J. D. (1990*a*). Methods and basic data of case-control study of leukaemia and lymphoma among young people near Sellafield nuclear plant in West Cumbria. *British Medical Journal*, **300**, 429–34.

Gardner, M. J., Snee, M. P., Hall, A. J., Powell, C. A., Downes, S., and Terrell, J. D. (1990*b*). Results of case-control study of leukaemia and lymphoma among young people near Sellafield nuclear plant in West Cumbria. *British Medical Journal*, **300**, 423–9.

General Register Office (1966). *Classification of occupations, 1966*. HMSO, London.

Hill, C. and Laplanche, A. (1990). Overall mortality and cancer mortality around French nuclear sites. *Nature*, **347**, 755–7.

Jablon, S., Hrubec, Z., Boice, J. D., and Stone, B. J. (1990). *Cancer in populations living near nuclear facilities*, NIH Publication No. 90–874. National Institutes of Health, Washington.

National Radiological Protection Board (1986). *Radiation dose histories at British Nuclear Fuels plc, Sellafield*, NRPB-M136. NRPB, Chilton.

Nomura, T. (1982). Parental exposure to X-rays and chemicals induces heritable tumours and anomalies in mice. *Nature*, **296**, 575–7.

Smith, P. G. and Douglas, A. J. (1986). Mortality of workers at the Sellafield plant of British Nuclear Fuels. *British Medical Journal*, **293**, 845–54.

Urquhart, J., Palmer, M., and Cutler, J. (1984). Cancer in Cumbria: the Windscale connection. *Lancet*, **i**, 217–18.

Urquhart, J. D., Black, R. J., Muirhead, M. J., Sharp, L., Maxwell, M., Eden, O. B., and Adams Jones, D. (1991). Case-control study of leukaemia and non-Hodgkin's lymphoma in children in Caithness near the Dounreay nuclear installation. *British Medical Journal*, **302**, 687–92.

26. The epidemic of respiratory cancer associated with erionite fibres in the Cappadocian region of Turkey

Y. I. Baris, L. Simonato, R. Saracci, and
R. Winkelmann

In the early 1970s a team from the Department of Chest Diseases of the Hacettepe University of Ankara led by one of us (I.B.) investigated asbestos-related chest diseases in Turkey. The results of several surveys reported parenchymal and pleural diseases in populations living in rural areas, the major source of exposure being mineral fibres, mainly asbestos, originating from the walls of houses whitewashed with asbestos-contaminated soil. Scattered cases of malignant pleural mesothelioma were also found associated with this exposure.

Subsequently, several case-reports of cancers were received and requests were made for the team of the Department of Chest Diseases of the Hacettepe University to visit various areas. In most cases which were assessed, however, no neoplastic disease of the respiratory system was present but, rather, chronic non-malignant lung diseases.

In 1975 a letter from the chief (*muktar*) of the village of Karain, in the province of Nevsehir (Central Turkey), was received at the Department of Chest Diseases in Ankara. The *muktar* claimed that a high number of the inhabitants had cancer, and that for a long time many people in the village had died early from a disease of the chest of unknown cause. Asked to send further information, the chief of the village came to Ankara with a patient, who was diagnosed as having mesothelioma. A quick investigation revealed that other villagers from Karain had also been admitted to hospitals in Ankara or in Kayseri (where the main hospital of the area is located) with a diagnosis of neoplastic or benign disease of the respiratory system.

A medical survey of the population living in Karain was then carried out by the University of Ankara, including information collected on historical cases. Between 1970 and 1976 35 deaths from pleural mesothelioma were reported from a population of less than 600 residents in the village, which corresponds to a crude mortality rate of 8.7 per 1000 person-years (Baris *et al.* 1978). Histological confirmation was obtained for seven cases, corresponding to a crude rate of histologically confirmed mesothelioma of 1.7 per 1000 person-years.

Between 1975 and 1979, a team from the Hacettepe University surveyed other villages in the same area, one of which (Tuzköy) was also found to be affected by the same disease (Artvinli *et al.* 1979, 1982). No industrial activity related to asbestos manufacture and use was present in this area, where agriculture is the predominant activity. Furthermore, according to the Turkish National Institute of Mineralogical Research and Exploitation, there was no deposit of asbestos in the region.

Descriptive investigation

An international collaborative study, jointly conducted by the Hacettepe University of Ankara, the International Agency for Research on Cancer in Lyon, and the UK Medical Research Council's Pneumoconiosis Unit in Penarth, UK, was carried out between 1978 and 1983, in order to:

(1) confirm the high rate of mesothelioma in the area;
(2) to assess the occurrence of other non-neoplastic respiratory diseases; and
(3) to investigate the presence of environmental exposure to mineral fibres, since they are the only known non-occupational cause of mesothelioma.

Four villages in Nevsehir province within 30 km of one another were considered suitable for the study. Two (Karain and Tuzköy) were chosen because of previous reports of mesothelioma cases; one (Sarihidir) because zeolite fibres, suspected as a possible aetiological agent, were reported in the bedrock and road dust samples, but no mesothelioma had at that time been reported; and the fourth (Karlik) was chosen as a control village because no mesothelioma case had been reported since 1970.

The survey consisted of:

(1) an interview of people aged 20 years or older, full-size posterior–anterior chest X-ray, and a brief physical examination in the villages of Karain (327 people), Sarihidir (337 people), and Karlik (228 people)—because of the size of Tuzköy (over 3000 people), the village was excluded from this phase as a recent survey had already been conducted by the Hacettepe University (Artvinli *et al.* 1979, 1982);
(2) recording mortality between 1979 and 1983 in Karain and Karlik, and between 1980 and 1983 in Tuzköy and Sarihidir;
(3) taking measurements of airborne levels of total dust in the four villages, analysis of fibre content of samples, including bulk samples, and analysis by electron microscopy (Pooley 1976) of the fibre content of sheep lung specimens collected in seven villages in the area.

The results have been published in detail previously (Baris *et al.* 1981, 1987). The main findings are summarized here.

During the study period, 141 deaths were recorded, including 29 malignant pleural mesotheliomas, 4 malignant peritoneal mesotheliomas, 17 lung cancers, 1 cancer of the larynx, and 8 cancers of other sites. Twenty-one of the cases of pleural mesothelioma were from Karain, three from Sarihidir, and five from Tuzköy. No person from Karlik died of mesothelioma, either peritoneal or pleural, or from any other respiratory cancer.

The crude death rate from mesothelioma in the affected villages was 8 per 1000 person-years; thus the risk of dying from mesothelioma appears to be higher than recorded anywhere, even among persons exposed occupationally to high levels of asbestos. Mortality from lung cancer was also substantially elevated in the three villages. The population living in the villages affected by high rates of malignant tumours exhibited, particularly for males and for calcified lesions, a moderately higher prevalence of pleural, but not parenchymal lesions than the population of the control village.

Exposure assessment

Rock and dust samples from the villages of Tuzköy and Karain revealed the presence of fine fibres (less than 0.25 μm in diameter and up to 5 μm in length) with an elemental composition close to that of erionite (Pooley 1979). Erionite fibres belong to the family of zeolites, which are crystalline hydrated aluminosilicates of alkali and alkaline earth cations, having a three-dimensional silicate structure (Mumpton 1973).

The most difficult task was to assess the relevant exposure to erionite, the mineral fibre suspected of being responsible for the increased risk of respiratory cancer. Experience in this field is derived from studies on the carcinogenic risk from occupational exposure to high levels of asbestos fibres, and most of the measurements or estimates of exposure to asbestos concern airborne levels of fibres based on short-term (6–8 h) samples taken in conditions of heavy exposure. Whether the same methodology applied to a situation of lifetime exposure to very low levels of airborne fibres is appropriate is, at least in part, questionable.

Because of the long latent period, particularly for mesothelioma, and the lack of historical estimates of exposure, an effort was made to provide supplementary information on exposure based on biological parameters. The data collected are summarized below.

Airborne levels

More than 150 outdoor samples, obtained using the method recommended by the Asbestos International Association (1979), were collected in the affected villages and the control village between 1979 and 1983. The levels of respirable fibres (diameter <3 μm) are shown in Table 26.1. Considering the low values,

Table 26.1 Street samples; concentration (fibres/ml) and identification of fibres ($>5\ \mu$m) (from Baris *et al.* 1987)

	Range (fibres/ml)	Mean (fibres/ml)	Identity
Karain	0.002–0.010	0.006	~80% zeolite, +calcium oxide, sulphate
Karlik	0.002–0.006	0.003	~20% zeolite, +calcium oxide, sulphate
Sarihidir	0.001–0.029	0.009	~60% zeolite, +calcite, quartz, glass, tremolite

the difference in levels between the case villages and the control village (Karlik) is negligible in relation to the magnitude of the risk. The fibre content may be more relevant, though, since there was a higher proportion of zeolitic fibres in the villages with high mesothelioma rates.

The variability of these estimates is shown clearly in Table 26.2. These data were obtained while sweeping walls and floors, both indoors and outdoors, in order to estimate peak levels. Fibre levels up to 1 fibre/ml were recorded from some houses using this method. The main components of these samples were zeolitic fibres.

Table 26.2 Work and recreation areas: concentration (fibres/ml) and identification of fibres ($<5\ \mu$m) (from Baris *et al.* 1987)

	fibres/ml	Identity
Karain		
Fields	0.004	Zeolite, glass, calcium silicates
Schoolyard	0.175	Zeolite
Caves (play)	0.050	Calcium carbonate, sulphate, phosphate
Caves (homes)	0.005–0.31	Zeolite
Karlik		
Fields	0.004	Zeolite, calcium silicates
Schoolyard	0.009	Calcite
Caves	0.005	Calcite
Sarihidir		
Fields	0.007	Zeolite, glass, quartz
Schoolyard	0.015	Zeolite, glass, calcium sulphate
Homes	0.005–1	Zeolite, glass, aluminium silicates

Zeolite content of sputum

In 1979, Sébastien *et al.* analysed 64 sputum samples from volunteers residing in two case villages (Karain and Tuzköy) and two control villages (Karlik and Kizilköy). The samples were analysed blindly for ferruginous bodies using standard techniques (Bignon *et al.* 1974). Although limited by the small numbers involved, and by the possibility of bias due to self-selection, the results indicated that the prevalence of ferruginous bodies was sevenfold higher in the affected villages relative to the controls.

In 1987, a more systematic approach to the collection of sputum samples was used in a survey of all residents in Karain and Karlik aged 20 years or over. Approximately 500 sputum samples were thus collected and coded using randomly generated numbers. They were subsequently sent to Dr P. Sébastien for analysis, which is not yet complete.

Fibre content of lung tissue

The presence of fibres both in humans and in animals have been investigated by Dr F. Pooley at the University College of Cardiff, using standard techniques already applied to asbestos fibres (Pooley 1976).

For religious reasons, it is particularly difficult to get sufficient autopsy or biological material from cases of mesothelioma in the affected villages. The results of the analysis of the fibre content of the lung tissue of two meso-thelioma cases in Tuzköy are shown in Table 26.3. The cumulated dose of zeolite was higher in both cases than for all other fibres, particularly for the case diagnosed at age 42 years.

In an effort to overcome the problem of the lack of human lung samples, we tried an alternative approach using lung tissues from sheep in affected and non-affected villages. A number of sheep aged 5 years or more were killed and the lung tissue analysed using the same methodology as above. The results reported in Table 26.4, although indicating a higher content (one order of magnitude) of zeolites in affected villages, do not show a statistically sig-nificant difference between the two groups of sheep. These data are certainly limited by the relatively shorter life expectancy (on average 8–9 years) of sheep as compared to humans.

Case-control study

After considering the low levels of outdoor airborne fibres, the peak exposure artificially generated indoors, and contamination of the housing blocks with zeolites, particularly erionite, from the quarries used in the past, we hypothesized that indoor fibre pollution of the houses was the main source of exposure. The walls of the old houses are made of blocks of poorly consol-

Table 26.3 Human mesothelioma lung sample (from Baris *et al.* 1987)

D.Y., female aged 42 years: number of fibres ($\times 10^6$/g dried tissue)

zeolite	39.4
chrysotile	14.9
actinolite	0.7
crocidolite	0.35
mullite	0.35
muscovite	0.35
rutile	1.4

S.M., male aged 52 years: number of fibres ($\times 10^6$/g dried tissue)

zeolite	17.1
chrysotile	2.0
actinolite	0.2
mullite	2.9
muscovite	0.4
silica	0.4
rutile	0.8
iron	0.2

Total number of zeolite fibres detected = 197

Table 26.4 Analysis of sheep lung fibre content (from Baris *et al.* 1987)

Type of fibre	Affected villages[1]	Unaffected villages[1]	t	p
Chrysotile	4.27	3.21	0.562	<0.7
Zeolite	0.13	0.01	1.931	<0.3
Crocidolite	0.03	0.13	1.633	<0.4

[1] Average number of fibres ($\times 10^6$/g dried tissue)

idated rocks which easily release dust, not only because of their geological structure, but also because of the dry climate, characterized by a large variation in temperature between day and night, and between cold winters and hot summers.

We therefore carried out a case-control analysis of our data using the presence of fibres in the house blocks as an index of exposure. Cases were inhabitants of Karain diagnosed as having pleural mesothelioma at the 1979 survey, irrespective of their status in 1981 when the study was conducted. Cases with incomplete information on age and house of birth or of residence were excluded, as well as those living in houses previously sampled. For each case, we chose two controls of the same age (±2 years) and sex, randomly selected from the subjects included in the 1979 survey who were still non-cases in 1981.

Houses where subjects were born and, when available, houses where subjects resided were included in the study. Spot specimens from the walls of houses and caves were collected and analysed by optical and electron microscopy. The specimens were randomly allocated in order to assure a reading which was blind of case/control status. A specimen was considered positive when a 'significant number' ($>10^4$ fibres/g) of fibres was found. Out of approximately 100 specimens, 19 were considered positive. No specimen was entirely free of fibres but most of them had a very low content. All fibres identified were zeolites with, in addition, attapulgite in one sample.

Two different statistical analyses were performed: the first using as an index of exposure the presence of fibres in the birth house only; the second using any presence of fibres, irrespective of the type of house. The results of the analysis are reported in Table 26.5. A moderately elevated relative risk was found when any potential exposure to zeolites was included in the analysis, but this disappeared when only exposure to the birth house was considered. In both types of analysis, the case-control study failed to identify a high relative risk for

Table 26.5   Case-control analyses

(a) Using as the index of exposure any presence of zeolite contamination in the house blocks

		Controls	
		E	NE
Cases	E	3	6
	NE	4	4
		RR = 1.5	

(b) Restricted to birth houses

		Controls	
		E	NE
Cases	E	3	1
	NE	1	4
		RR = 1.0	

E, presence of zeolites; NE, little or no presence of zeolites.

pleural mesothelioma associated with zeolite exposure in Karain, possibly due to the difficulties in defining the relevant exposure. The location and number of samples taken from the houses were based on arbitrary decisions. Thus, a high degree of misclassification of exposure was likely.

The prospective study

Individuals from the villages of Karain and Sarihidir (affected) and of Karlik (control) included in the 1979 and 1980 surveys have been followed up for mortality and cancer incidence to 8 October 1987. A combination of various sources was used, including mortality archives in the villages and in the public health centres, archives of the prefecture offices in Urgup, clinical records from Kayseri hospital and from the Department of Chest Diseases of the Hacettepe University in Ankara, and anecdotal information from the *muktars* and other key informants in the villages. No individual follow-up is ongoing in Tuzköy.

These data have been cross-checked at regular intervals (roughly on an annual basis) by the international collaborative group during visits to Turkey between 1979 and 1987, and subsequently computerized at the International Agency for Research on Cancer. We present here the results of the mortality follow-up during the observation period, which started in summer 1979 in Karain and Karlik, and in summer 1980 in Sarihidir, and ended on 8 October 1987 in the three villages.

Causes of death have been coded using the ninth revision of the International Classification of Diseases (WHO 1978). Age-, sex-, and village-specific mortality rates have been computed using a person-year program (Coleman *et al.* 1986) and subsequently directly standardized using the age- and sex-specific distribution of the combined person-years at risk in the three villages as a standard.

Table 26.6 shows the distribution by sex and village of the population under observation, while Table 26.7 presents the vital status as ascertained at the

Table 26.6 Population followed up from 1979 through 1987 by sex and village

	Males	Females	All
Village			
Karain	149	177	326
Karlik	107	122	229
Sarihidir	154	183	337
All	410	482	892

Table 26.7 Vital status at 31 August 1987 by sex and village

	Sex											
	Males status						Females status					
	Alive		Dead		Lost to follow-up		Alive		Dead		Lost to follow-up	
	No.	%	No.	%	No.	%	No.	%	No.	%	No.	%
Village												
Karain	113	75.8	36	24.2	–	–	131	74.0	46	26.0	–	–
Karlik	84	78.5	21	19.6	2	1.9	110	90.2	12	9.8	–	–
Sarihidir	132	85.7	22	14.3	–	–	164	89.6	16	9.3	2	1.1

Table 26.8 Distribution of causes of death by sex and village[1]

Cause of death	Karain Males No.	Males %	Karain Females No.	Females %	Karlik Males No.	Males %	Karlik Females No.	Females %	Sarihidir Males No.	Males %	Sarihidir Females No.	Females %
Lung cancer	–	–	1	2.2	–	–	–	–	6	27.3	1	6.3
Mesothelioma	14	38.9	14	31.1	–	–	–	–	2	9.1	3	18.8
Other cancers	2	5.6	6	13.3	3	14.3	–	–	2	9.1	3	18.8
Other causes	17	47.2	12	26.7	18	85.7	10	83.3	11	50.0	7	43.8
Unknown	3	8.3	12	26.7	–	–	2	16.7	1	4.5	2	12.5
All causes of death	36	100.0	45	100.0	21	100.0	12	100.0	22	100.0	16	100.0

[1] Two deaths with unknown date of birth are excluded from the analysis.

end of the follow-up period. The populations in the villages consist of only a few families, thus facilitating the tracing of the subjects included in the study. Only four subjects were lost to follow-up due to emigration to other areas. Table 26.8 presents the distribution of the deaths recorded by main cause, sex, and village. No cancer of the respiratory tract was recorded in the control village, while both Karain and Sarihidir exhibit an elevated mortality from pleural mesothelioma. Lung cancer appears to be more frequent in Sarihidir, although a certain degree of misclassification is likely because of the diagnostic difficulties, particularly in relation to the incompleteness of histology. Table 26.9 shows the age-standardized rates by sex and village for selected causes of death. Due to the small numbers, and to potential misclassification, all the respiratory cancers, including one death from ill-defined cancer of the respiratory tract, have been analysed together. Except for the females in Sarihidir, the mortality rate from respiratory cancer in the two affected villages exceeded 1000 per 100 000 person-years.

Table 26.9 Mortality rates per 100 000 person-years for selected causes during the follow-up period 1979–87 [1]

	Karain		Karlik		Sarihidir	
	Males	Females	Males	Females	Males	Females
All causes	3349.3	3596.4	1718.7	1007.8	4214.0	1711.1
Respiratory cancers (162, 163, 165.9)	1238.8	1220.0	0.0	0.0	1237.4	551.2
Other cancers	258.3	473.3	277.0	0.0	284.6	233.6
Ill-defined	355.2	951.0	305.8	397.1	1556.7	658.1
Other causes	1497.1	952.0	1135.9	610.7	1135.2	268.2

[1] Age-standardized to the person-years from the three villages combined. Two deaths with unknown date of birth are excluded from the analysis.

Considering the small numbers involved in the analysis, the pattern is very consistent in indicating a rate of respiratory cancer in the populations of Karain and Sarihidir of a magnitude previously unknown in populations exposed to environmental carcinogens.

Conclusion

Detailed clinical, epidemiological, and environmental investigations in Cappadocia have revealed the existence of a new carcinogenic mineral fibre. The epidemic was first reported by the villagers themselves, and confirmed by clinical observation by a team of the Hacettepe University of Ankara. Subsequent multidisciplinary collaboration at international level permitted an efficient approach to defining the nature of the disease, the magnitude of the risk, and the characteristics of exposure. Their task was obviously made easier by the rarity of the disease (mesothelioma) in most populations and the specificity (mineral fibres) of its known aetiological agents.

The carcinogenic risk from exposure to erionite fibres was evaluated by the International Agency for Research in Cancer in 1987, which concluded that there was sufficient evidence both in humans and in animals of carcinogenicity. Fibrous erionite is probably the most striking example of consistency between epidemiological and experimental evidence. It induces mesotheliomas in 100 per cent of rats by inhalation (Wagner *et al.* 1985), while a cumulative lifetime dose of 1 fibre/yr/ml appears capable of inducing, for mesothelioma, a mortality rate of 996 per 100 000 person-years in the exposed population (Simonato *et al.* 1989). Mechanisms of carcinogenesis of mineral fibres are still unknown, but experimental research could make further progress by investigating the physico-chemical properties of erionite fibres.

With respect to the situation in the villages, although the data strongly suggest the role of contaminated houses as the main source of carcinogenic risk, no systematic measures have been taken to control the exposure. The rebuilding of the village of Sarihidir on the other side of the river Kizilirmak after a flood in 1960 did not completely stop the exposure to fibres, as some of the new houses were built partly with blocks of tufa from old houses. The persistence of both exposure to the carcinogenic agent and the risk of respiratory cancer has been documented by the results of the investigations. Some families in Karain have left the village and built new modern houses in the neighbourhood. However, no more than 30 per cent of the population has left the village. Furthermore, the abandoned houses have been occupied subsequently by immigrants from the south-east of Turkey, thus actually increasing the size of the population at risk. A few years ago, the villagers in Tuzköy decided to move their village. A new site has already been chosen, but the funds have not been provided. Thus, the epidemic of respiratory cancer in the small villages of the Cappadocian region of Turkey will continue.

References

Artvinli, M. and Baris, Y. I. (1979). Malignant mesotheliomas in a small village in the Anatolian region of Turkey: an epidemiologic study. *Journal of the National Cancer Institute*, **63**, 17–22.
Artvinli, M. and Baris, Y. I. (1982). Environmental fibre-induced pleuro-pulmonary diseases in an Anatolian village: an epidemiologic study. *Archives of Environmental Health*, **37**, 177–81.
Asbestos International Association (1979). *Recommended technical method No. 1*, AIA Health and Safety Publication. Asbestos International Association, London.

Baris, Y. I., *et al.* (1978). An outbreak of pleural mesothelioma and chronic fibrosing pleurisy in the village of Karain/Ürgup in Anatolia. *Thorax*, **33**, 181–92.

Baris, Y. I., Saracci, R., Simonato, L., Skidmore, J. W., and Artvinli, M. (1981). Malignant mesothelioma and radiological chest abnormalities in two villages in Central Turkey. *Lancet*, **ii**, 984–7.

Baris, Y. I., *et al.* (1987). Epidemiological and environmental evidence of the health effects of exposure to erionite fibres: a four-year study in the Cappadocian region of Turkey. *International Journal of Cancer*, **39**, 10–17.

Bignon, J., Sébastien, P., Jaurand, M. C., and Hem, B. (1974). Microfiltration method for quantitative study of fibrous particles in biological specimens. *Environmental Health Perspectives*, **9**, 155–60.

Coleman, M., Douglas, A., Hermon, C., and Peto, J. (1986). Cohort study analysis with a Fortran computer program. *International Journal of Epidemiology*, **15**, 134–7.

Mumpton, F. A. (1973). Worldwide deposits and utilization of natural zeolites. *Industrial Mineralogy*, **73**, 1–11.

Pooley, F. D. (1976). An examination of the fibrous mineral content of asbestos lung tissue from the Canadian chrysotile mining industry. *Environmental Research*, **12**, 281–98.

Pooley, F. D. (1979). Evaluation of fibre samples taken from the vicinity of two villages in Turkey. In *Dust and diseases*, (ed. R. Lemen and J. H. Dement), pp. 41–4. Pathotox Publishers, Park Forest South.

Sébastien, P., Bignon, J., Baris, Y. I., Awad, L., and Petit, G. (1979). Ferruginous bodies in sputum as an indication of exposure to airborne mineral fibers in the mesothelioma villages of Cappadocia. *Archives of Environmental Health*, **39**, 18–23.

Simonato, L., Baris, Y. I., Saracci, R., Skidmore, J. W., and Winkelmann, R. (1989). Relation of environmental exposure to erionite fibres to risk of respiratory cancer. In (ed. J. Bignon, J. Peto, and R. Saracci), IARC Scientific Publications, No. 90, pp. 398–405. International Agency for Research on Cancer, Lyon.

Wagner, J. C., Skidmore, J. W., Hill, R. C., and Griffiths, D. M. (1985). Erionite exposure and mesotheliomas in rats. *British Journal of Cancer*, **51**, 727–30.

World Health Organisation (1978). *Manual of the international statistical classification of diseases, injuries and causes of death* (9th revision conference). WHO, Geneva.

27. Soya bean as a risk factor for epidemic asthma

J. M. Antó and J. Sunyer

Background to asthma epidemics

Asthma epidemics are rare phenomena sporadically described in the medical literature. Some of the information about asthma epidemics is anecdotal and a general theory to explain both their occurrence and causes has not yet been developed. In this section the most well-known asthma epidemics are described.

Some of the first asthma outbreaks were attributed to ricin dust inhalation. On 11 August 1952 in Bauru, Brazil, a city of 60 000 inhabitants, 150 people suffered sudden asthma crises (Mendes and Ulhoa Cintra 1954). It was soon observed that the affected people suffered the asthma crisis near to a ricin mill, leading investigators to suspect a point-source origin for the outbreak. Skin reactivity was assessed in 30 patients, 28 of whom were positive to a ricin allergen. In four cases a specific bronchoprovocation test was performed: all presented with an immediate asthma crisis. Based on this evidence, the mill was closed for 1 year while several changes that precluded new releases of ricin dust to atmospheric air were introduced. Similar episodes also attributed to ricin dust inhalation have been reported in Toledo, Ohio (Figley and Elrod 1928) and South Africa (Ordman 1955).

The most well-known asthma epidemics were detected at the emergency room of The Charity Hospital in New Orleans, USA. One of the largest asthma outbreaks that occurred in this city took place on 26 August 1955, affecting more than 350 patients, all of whom were treated at the same emergency room in a period of less than 24 hours; two patients died. Lewis *et al.* (1962) advanced the hypothesis that the New Orleans asthma outbreaks were due to the inhalation of particles emanating from a waste dump site where spontaneous underground burning was occurring. However, the fact that the asthma outbreaks persisted years after the waste dump site had been removed led to this possibility being ruled out.

In a series of studies, Salvaggio *et al.* (Salvaggio and Klein 1967; Salvaggio *et al.* 1970, 1971*a,b*; Salvaggio and Seabury 1971) concluded that the New Orleans asthma epidemics had affected a subgroup of atopic asthmatics and were probably not caused by atmospheric pollution or by chemical industrial releases. Although the causes were not clearly identified, the authors pointed out (Salvaggio *et al.* 1971*b*) that there was strong evidence that a group of natural allergens, such as spores of different fungal species, ambrosia pollen, and amorphous particles similar to vegetable detritus, had a causative role in the epidemics. The presence of these allergens in atmospheric air in higher than normal levels would be favoured by appropriate meteorological conditions.

Goldstein and Salvaggio (1984), following an epidemiological approach originally developed to study asthma epidemics in New York, analysed the New Orleans data for the period 1969–77, and concluded that the incidence of asthma epidemics had notably decreased. According to the authors, their findings could not be attributed to an improvement in socio-economic conditions of the susceptible population or to better medical care, rather than to change in exposure to an environmental agent.

Unusual increases in the number of emergency room admissions for asthma in New York on a given day were first observed by Greenburg *et al.* (1964) when assessing the relationships between air pollution, meteorological conditions, and health indicators in a retrospective time-series study. Goldstein and Rausch (1978) analysed the emergency room admissions of three hospitals (Cumberland, Kings County, and Harlem) in New York during the period 1969–71. The series of the daily number of asthma emergency room admissions showed a reasonably good fit to the Poisson distribution. However, a number of unusual asthma days, based on departures from a Poisson distribution, were observed which occurred simultaneously at the three hospitals. These hospital clusters of unusual asthma days led to the hypothesis that an environmental factor present in the city could have been triggering the asthma outbreaks. In a further study, a relationship between the presence of unusual asthma days and the levels of sulphur dioxide and black smoke was excluded (Goldstein and Weinstein 1986).

Other studies carried out in New York have analysed the daily variations in the number of emergency room admissions for asthma (Goldstein and Cuzick 1983), their seasonality (Goldstein and Currie 1984), and the meteorological conditions present on the unusual asthma days (Goldstein 1980). The fact that most of the unusual asthma days coincided with Sundays, Mondays, Thanksgiving days, and the day following them, led the authors to suspect that the cause of these increases of asthma could be related to indoor environmental agents. However, despite such intensive epidemiological investigation, the causes of the unusual asthma days in New York remain to be elucidated.

Another interesting asthma outbreak was detected by Packe and Ayres (1985) at the East Birmingham Hospital, Birmingham, UK, on 6 and 7 July 1983, following a striking increase in the number of asthma emergency room admissions. In a period of 36 hours, 26 asthma cases were treated at the emergency room, compared to the daily mean of 2–3 cases in the days preceding the outbreak. A retrospective analysis of the period 1980–84 by these authors showed that other asthma outbreaks had not occurred. This outbreak coincided with an important increase of several airborne spores, particularly *Sporobolomyces* and *Didymella exitialis* (*D. exitialis*), suggesting a possible aetiological clue. To analyse the influence of the ascospores of *D. exitialis* in the asthma outbreak, Packe and Ayres (1986*a*) compared a group of 18 epidemic asthma patients to non-epidemic asthma controls. Skin reactivity to several allergens including *D. exitialis* was tested but showed no differences between the groups. Although the appropriateness of the controls has been disputed by Morrow-Brown (1986), the results indicate that the rise of *D. exitialis* in the air was not the cause of this asthma outbreak (Packe and Ayres 1986*b*).

Other asthma epidemics have been described in Brisbane, Australia (where more than 90 patients were woken up by sudden nocturnal dyspnoea over a period of a few hours) (Morrison 1960) and Bahia Blanca, Argentina (Piccolo *et al.* 1988), without acceptable explanation of their causes.

From the methodological point of view, the most interesting contribution to the study of asthma outbreaks comes from the work of Goldstein and Rausch (1978) who established a precise analytical strategy. They defined an unusual asthma day as a day in which the number of emergency room visits for asthma was so high that the probability that such a number or a higher one was the result of chance was 0.025 or less. This probability was calculated by assuming a Poisson distribution, with the 15-day moving average representing the number of cases expected. The authors considered that unusual asthma days coinciding on the same day in different hospitals of the city were more likely to reflect the effect of environmental agents acting throughout the city.

A general pattern can be detected from consideration of all these outbreaks: most of them were identified through an abrupt increase in the number of people needing acute care for an asthma crisis, frequently at an emergency room. The term 'abrupt' in these outbreaks denotes that the increase took place in hours. Thus the most relevant finding in terms of outbreak detection was a time cluster. Even in New York, where such increases in emergency room admissions for asthma were identified retrospectively when analysing time-series data for other purposes, the dominant trait was the presence of time clusters. The only exceptions were the outbreaks attributed to ricin dust inhalation, where a geographical cluster was the more prominent feature.

Identification of asthma epidemics in Barcelona

The first information concerning asthma epidemics in Barcelona came in 1983 from a letter published in *Lancet* by Ussetti *et al.* (1983) reporting a retrospective study of six outbreaks. The first outbreak occurred in 1981. The emergency room of the Hospital Clinic of Barcelona had a sudden influx of patients suffering severe asthma crises. All outbreaks showed similar characteristics: most of the cases arrived at the hospital within a period of 4 hours, reporting the onset of symptoms soon before their admission to the emergency room. The asthma attacks were also unusually severe, with many patients needing mechanical ventilation.

Average 24 h levels of sulphur dioxide and black smoke were not unusually high, but short-term peaks in air pollution could not be excluded. During a new outbreak, high levels of nitrogen oxide were recorded during the hours at which most of the patients arrived at the emergency room. This coincidence of time led Ussetti *et al.* (1984) to suspect an aetiological role for this contaminant.

The publication of reports of these outbreaks in a medical journal was widely reported by the local mass media, which emphasized the possible relationship to air pollution. Several meetings were organized between physicians, researchers, and health officers to discuss the available evidence as well as the need for further studies or interventions. Finally, the Barcelona Asthma Collaborative Group was organized to undertake a multicentre study of asthma at the emergency rooms. This study was designed to overcome the main limitations of the preliminary reports: identification of outbreaks had been based on the subjective experience of clinicians, emergency room admissions on epidemic and control days were not available for other respiratory diseases, assessment of epidemics had been restricted to only one hospital in the city, and a population-based description of the outbreaks was not available.

The respiratory emergency room admission register of Barcelona

A respiratory emergency room admissions monitoring system was established during 1984 with the aim of permitting extensive descriptive analysis of asthma outbreaks occurring since that time. The emergency rooms of the four largest hospitals in the city were recruited. They provided a reasonably wide geographical coverage and accounted for more than 90 per cent of all hospital emergency admissions in Barcelona. For each hospital, the total daily number of emergency admissions was registered and a distinction was made between medical and surgical causes for admission. Among medical emergencies, the total daily number of admissions for respiratory causes was also registered.

Patients were identified who were admitted to the emergency rooms for asthma or chronic bronchitis and who were living in Barcelona. Their age, sex, address, day and hour of arrival, and details of their referral were recorded. Specific operational definitions of emergencies for asthma and chronic bronchitis were established by identifying lists of equivalent terms used by emergency room clinicians for the diagnosis of both diseases. A panel of respiratory physicians from all the participant hospitals was convened and the terms to be included in the final list were selected by consensus. Special difficulties were observed in differentiating asthma from other respiratory disorders with wheezing in children. The following terms were included under the category of asthma: asthmatic bronchitis, spastic bronchitis, bronchial hyperreactivity, status asthmaticus, and bronchospasm. Another list was made for chronic bronchitis. Data were collected from the clinical records at the emergency rooms by personnel specially trained to identify admissions for asthma and chronic bronchitis using the list of accepted terms. The validity and other methodological aspects of this register have been discussed elsewhere (Antó and Sunyer 1990).

A point-source asthma outbreak

On 26 November 1984 a marked influx of patients suffering from asthma attacks was detected at the emergency room of the Hospital Clinic. The monitoring system, together with the information provided by the administration of an *ad hoc* questionnaire permitted Antó *et al.* (1986*a*) to produce a complete description of this outbreak. Forty-three emergency admissions for asthma in adults and 22 in children (under 14 years) were registered (Fig. 27.1). Based on the Poisson distribution, the probability that this outbreak had been a random event was very low for adults ($p = 1.5 \times 10^{-17}$) but not statistically significant for children ($p = 0.087$). The number of emergencies for chronic bronchitis and other respiratory diseases was as usual. Hourly clustering was assessed by means of a Knox and Lancashire (1982) approximation to the scanning method (Wallenstein 1980). The greatest number of patients (70 per cent)

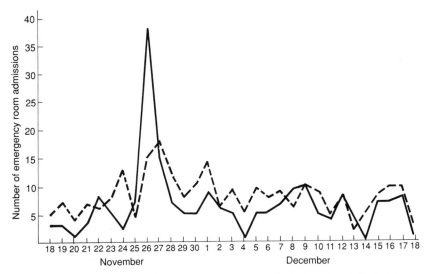

Fig. 27.1 Daily number of asthma emergency room admissions in adults ($\geqslant$14 years; solid line) and in children ($<$14 years; dotted line) from 18 November to 18 December 1984.

arrived at the hospital between noon and 4 p.m., the 4 h cluster being highly significant ($p = 1.4 \times 10^{-27}$).

The geographical distribution of cases was studied, considering both the places where the symptoms started, as reported in the questionnaire, and the patients' addresses. For adults, a striking cluster of cases in the harbour areas of the city was observed (Fig. 27.2). The most affected district showed an age-standardized rate of 21.7 asthma admissions per 100 000 inhabitants (95 per

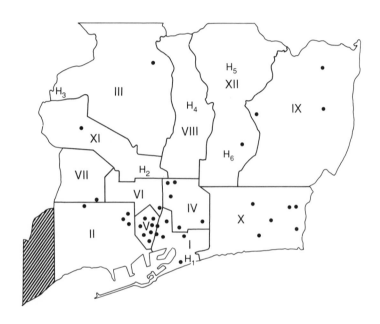

Fig. 27.2 Places at which attacks of asthma started. The map shows standard boundaries of areas I–XII Barcelona. Dots represent the places where attacks started in adults on 26 November 1984. Hatching indicates an industrial area. H represents the hospitals participating in the register.

cent confidence limits for the Poisson distribution, 10.8–38.9) compared to rates ranging from 0.64 to 2.67 per 100 000 inhabitants in the less affected districts (range of the 95 per cent confidence limits, 0.02–8.41). Most of the cases in the epidemic area arrived at the emergency room in a period of a few hours, revealing a simultaneous time and space clustering, this pattern being highly suggestive of a point-source epidemic.

The 24 h average for SO_2 was 54 $\mu g/m^3$ and that of black smoke was 98 $\mu g/m^3$. The highest hourly mean for NO_2 was 10 p.p.b. Meteorological data showed high atmospheric pressure and stagnancy of the air with a very low wind speed. Routinely measured air pollutants, pollen, and fungal spores did not exhibit a sharp increase in their normal levels and were considered an unlikely cause of the asthma outbreak.

The fact that the most affected neighbourhood was next to the harbour and near to an industrial area led us to consider that it could contain the point source of the causative factor. Asthma is often caused by chemical substances at the workplace or other airborne allergens present in indoor or outdoor environments. In those cases when the agent acts through an IgE-mediated mechanism asthma crises may appear only minutes after inhalation of the agent. Other biological mechanisms acting over longer periods of time, as well as other routes of exposure, such as foods or water, could hardly cause such a time–space cluster. Thus we advanced the hypothesis that a biological or chemical agent, spread from a point source contained in the harbour or in an industrial area next to it, was the cause of the asthma outbreak.

Descriptive analysis of 12 outbreaks: the confirmation of the point-source hypothesis

In order to assess the consistency of this temporal and geographical pattern, the 12 outbreaks identified by hospital-based physicians between 1981 and 1986 were studied.

Age-standardized rates of emergency room admissions for asthma for each epidemic day were compared to the corresponding rates for the 15-day moving average. The statistical significance of the difference between these rates was assessed by assuming a Poisson distribution (Goldstein and Rausch 1978). All 12 outbreaks showed a significant increase in the number of admissions for asthma in the population over 14 years of age (Table 27.1). Although asthma attack rates in the child population also increased in 11 of the outbreaks, they were not statistically significant (Table 27.1). The average daily rate of emergency room admissions for asthma over the 12 outbreak days for people under 14 years was 4.26 per 100 000 inhabitants (95 per cent confidence limits, 2.38–7.10) whereas the same rate for the control periods was 2.53 (95 per cent confidence limits, 1.16–4.80). By contrast, the corresponding rates for people aged 14 years old and over were 2.94 (95 per cent confidence limits, 2.12–3.97) for the outbreak days and 0.37 (0.12–0.86) for the control periods. No statistically significant increases in rates of admissions for chronic bronchitis on epidemic days were detected.

The presence of hourly clusters on epidemic days was assessed by means of the moving-window test, a Knox and Lancashire (1982) approximation to the scan statistic. All outbreaks showed statistically significant 4 h clusters and most of them even exhibited 1 h clusters (Fig. 27.3).

The geographical distribution of cases of asthma was determined according to patients' addresses. Mean age-adjusted attack rates by district were obtained for the 12 epidemics (Table 27.2). Emergency room admissions of

Table 27.1 Number of emergency room admissions for asthma and chronic bronchitis in outbreak days compared to the 15-day moving average (control period)

Outbreak day Control period p-value[1]	No. of cases of asthma		No. of cases of chronic bronchitis
	<14 years old	>14 years old	>15 years old
5 Aug. 1981	5	34	9
29 Jul.–12 Aug. 1981	3.4	5.4	4.1
p-value	NS[2]	6.7×10^{-12}	NS
8 Jun. 1982	15	36	6
1–15 Jun. 1982	5.7	5.8	5
p-value	NS	3.7×10^{-14}	NS
11 Aug. 1982	9	30	9
4–18 Aug. 1982	2.1	4.6	4.2
p-value	NS	1.1×10^{-10}	NS
17 Aug. 1982	4	29	6
10–24 Aug. 1982	2.8	4.4	4.8
p-value	NS	1.4×10^{-10}	NS
26 Oct. 1982	17	38	10
19 Oct.–2 Nov. 1982	9.2	4.0	4.9
p-value	NS	6.4×10^{-18}	NS
10 Jan. 1983	7	33	15
3–17 Jan. 1983	3.9	4.6	13
p-value	NS	7.0×10^{-13}	NS
25 Oct. 1983	31	76	9
18 Oct.–1 Nov. 1983	16.4	5.9	5.4
p-value	NS	0.0×10^{-50}	NS
26 Nov. 1984	22	43	16
19 Nov.–2 Dec. 1984	9	5.7	9.2
p-value	0.05	2.4×10^{-17}	NS
21 Jan. 1986	17	81	16
14–28 Jan. 1986	12.3	6.9	21.2
p-value	NS	0.0×10^{-50}	NS
6 May 1986	18	28	24
29 Apr.–13 May	9.6	5.9	12.3
p-value	NS	1.5×10^{-7}	NS
17 Sept. 1986	8	25	17
10–24 Sept. 1986	12.4	5.2	9.3
p-value	NS	1.0×10^{-6}	NS

11 Nov. 1986	26	53	22
4–18 Nov. 1986	19	6	12
p-value	NS	3.5×10^{-24}	NS
All outbreaks	14.9	43.1	13.2
Control periods	8.8	5.4	8.7

[1] *p*-value was assessed by Poisson distribution (see Goldstein and Weinstein 1986).
[2] NS, non-significant (*p* > 0.05).

asthma during outbreaks were distributed over most districts, although over the 12 asthma episodes districts, I, V, and VI had the highest mean rates. Similarly, the ratio of the rate of emergency asthma admissions on epidemic days to the rate on control days was highest in these same districts, with an average rate ratio higher than 17. Inspection of the maps in which cases were plotted according to the reported place of onset of symptoms, instead of place of residence, showed that, in most outbreaks, cases reporting the onset of symptoms within 4 h clusters occurred primarily in the coastal districts (especially districts I, V, and VI). Since these districts also experienced the highest attack rates, the two observations together were suggestive of a close relationship between time and space clustering. The comparison between maps

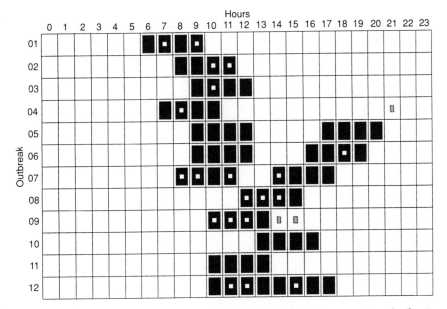

Fig. 27.3 The hourly distribution of asthma cases in Barcelona outbreaks (by time of admittance to the emergency room). ◻ 1 h cluster and 4 h cluster; ■, 4 h cluster; ▨, 1 h cluster.

Table 27.2 Geographical distribution of age-standardized rates by municipal districts for 12 outbreaks (1981–86) per 100 000 people

Outbreak day	I	II	III	IV	V	VI	VII	VIII	IX	X	XI	XII
5 Aug. 1981	4.14	2.87	–	1.60	3.66	8.56	5.24	4.50	–	0.71	4.45	0.98
8 Jun. 1982	4.14	1.80	1.65	2.42	12.41	2.42	2.56	1.37	0.77	4.30	4.25	0.95
11 Aug. 1982	2.07	2.04	0.78	1.49	6.59	7.10	1.73	2.34	1.19	3.58	2.14	–
17 Aug. 1982	8.34	5.74	–	4.95	–	5.64	0.91	1.98	0.30	2.85	2.14	–
26 Oct. 1982	7.00	2.63	0.78	6.08	1.47	2.93	1.78	1.55	0.66	3.59	1.97	3.78
10 Jan. 1983	9.10	2.81	0.88	3.14	14.36	4.45	1.84	1.44	1.01	2.15	–	1.99
25 Oct. 1983	8.97	5.26	1.64	7.1	9.12	10.98	2.63	8.22	2.37	6.35	3.29	5.79
26 Nov. 1984	11.06	5.89	1.49	2.33	21.75	2.15	1.48	0.64	2.48	4.84	2.67	1.43
21 Jan. 1986	11.60	4.60	2.20	9.20	9.80	11.60	7.30	2.30	3.20	6.50	6.30	4.00
6 May 1986	9.82	1.09	–	3.14	5.56	6.13	–	0.78	1.18	5.98	–	0.47
17 Sep. 1986	11.20	1.09	0.88	3.32	–	1.48	–	0.36	1.1	0.71	2.15	1.49
11 Nov. 1986	8.59	5.97	1.68	2.65	12.04	6.56	4.5	0.78	3.02	4.54	4.31	1.49

Municipal districts

based on the place of residence with maps based on place of symptoms showed that rates calculated from the former tended to underestimate the degree of spatial clustering in the inner districts, leading, in consequence, to an over-estimation in the peripheral districts.

In conclusion, the time and space distribution of emergency room admissions for asthma in all 12 outbreaks provided strong additional evidence in favour of the point-source hypothesis. The confirmation of the point-source nature of the epidemics was important in terms of aetiology since it led us to consider it very unlikely that ordinary atmospheric chemical pollution or habitual aeroallergens had been responsible for the asthma epidemics in Barcelona.

The meteorological characteristics common to all outbreaks (lack of wind, high barometric pressures, low relative humidity, and lack of rainfall) were considered likely to have contributed to the stagnation and rise in concentra-tion of an airborne agent. The data on wind direction, predominantly from the south-east and south-west in the hours of the outbreaks, and the distribution of cases of asthma in the city were consistent with the possibility that the origin of the outbreaks was localized in the south-western part of the city, close to the coast. As had been suggested previously, two main areas where possible point-source industrial emissions of the casual agent might be taking place were considered:the harbour area, where different industrial processes regularly take place and the Zona Franca, an important industrial area nearby. As we will see later, this hypothesis was established prior to having any clue as to the true aetiology of the asthma outbreaks.

Aetiological hypothesis generation and testing: the soya bean hypothesis

Most of the patients affected in the epidemics were interviewed by administer-ing a standardized questionnaire in the emergency room, or at home during the hours or days following the episodes. No plausible aetiological hypothesis was forthcoming on the basis of the questionnaires.

During an air pollution episode, a group of epidemic asthma patients were followed by means of a morbidity diary administered by telephone, which showed that they were not affected, despite a large increase in the usual air pollution levels (Antó *et al.* 1986*b*). In addition, on the occasion of each outbreak since 1984 several local agencies, such as the harbour administration, fire department, or local police, were approached to identify any unusual environmental event potentially related to the appearance of asthma out-breaks. Again, no evidence was obtained on possible asthma triggers until the first months of 1987, when the harbour administration reported that at least two asthma epidemics occurred on days when soya beans were unloaded in the harbour. Data on ship unloadings were not available at that time for all known outbreaks. Nevertheless, the observation excited our interest, since grain handling has frequently been related to asthma.

To assess a possible relationship between soya bean unloading and asthma outbreaks, the presence of specific IgE antibodies against 22 different commercial antigens, including both Barcelona's airborne common antigens and soya bean antigens, was determined in a group of 18 serum samples of epidemic asthma patients. IgE reactivity was assessed blindly by radioallergosorben test (RAST) by the same technician. Results showed that 13 out of 18 showed specific IgE antibodies to soya bean antigen, whereas only four positive responses were observed to the rest of the antigens. These results were considered strongly suggestive of a possible relationship between the unloading of soya bean in the Barcelona harbour and asthma outbreaks.

In September 1987, two months after the RAST-screening data became available, another outbreak occurred, affecting more than 100 people and causing two deaths. For the first time since the organization of the Barcelona Asthma Collaborative Group, the occurrence of the outbreak was widely covered by the mass media in a climate of acute social concern. Although at that time it was believed that data pointing to soya bean unloading as the cause were only preliminary and needed further confirmation, it was decided to recommend to the local and regional health authorities the interruption of soya bean unloading activities in the harbour.

Aetiological studies

In order to test the soya bean hypothesis, two epidemiological studies were designed. The relationship between soya bean unloadings in the harbour and the occurrence of asthma outbreaks was investigated in a time–ecological study. The relation between epidemic asthma and serum IgE antibodies reactive with soya bean antigen was tested in a case-control study. As will be shown, both epidemic asthma day and epidemic patient definitions used for subject selection were based on the respiratory emergency room monitoring system.

The relationship between asthma outbreaks and soya bean unloading: a time–ecological study

During the period 1985–86, 13 asthma epidemic days had been identified by means of epidemiological analysis. All products identified as having been loaded or unloaded at the docks during at least one asthma outbreak were also studied (Antó *et al.* 1989*a*). The days on which each product was loaded or unloaded was recorded during the same 2 yr period. In the case of soya beans, the use of two harbour silos (A and B) for soya bean unloading was also examined.

All 13 asthma-epidemic days in these 2 years coincided with soya bean unloading (lower 95 per cent confidence interval of the risk ratio 7.2). Of the remaining 25 products studied, only wheat was related to the epidemics of asthma, although when adjusted for the unloading of soya bean the relation was not statistically significant (risk ratio 5.03; 95 per cent confidence interval, 0.95–26.46). The unloading of soya bean also occurred on 27 May 1985 and 21 October 1985, two days which could be considered potential epidemic days but which were not identified by our method (false negative epidemics). When the site of soya bean unloading (silo A or B) was taken into account, the association was too high to be determined for silo A ($p < 0.001$), but not statistically significant for silo B ($p = 0.22$). This latter observation was consistent with the characteristics of the silos, as silo A did not have bag filters installed in the cyclone dust-collection system, thereby allowing the release of soya bean dust into the air.

A case-control study of serum IgE reactivity to soya bean allergen

On 4 and 7 September, 1987, two large asthma epidemics occurred, causing 157 emergency room admissions for asthma. Serum samples were taken from 86 of these patients at the emergency room, who were considered as cases in this study (Sunyer *et al.* 1989). Controls were selected from emergency room admissions for asthma seen during the period October 1987 to January 1988, when no epidemic days occurred and when soya bean was unloaded under controlled conditions. Potential controls previously seen for asthma on an epidemic day were excluded. Eighty-six controls were individually matched to cases by age, sex, and area of residence. In 64 of 86 cases (74.4 per cent) there was a reaction with commercial soya bean antigen extracts, compared with only 4 of 86 controls (4.6 per cent) (odds ratio 61; lower 95 per cent confidence limit 8.1). For the antigen prepared with a soya bean dust extract collected from the ship whose unloading coincided with one epidemic the association was stronger (odds ratio unquantifiably high; lower 95 per cent confidence limit 11.7). No other serological covariates included in the study confounded the association between serum anti-soya-bean IgE antibodies and epidemic asthma. These results strongly supported a causal relation between the releases of dust during the unloading of soya bean and the occurrence of asthma outbreaks. The results also suggested that the asthma outbreaks had an underlying allergic mechanism.

Immunological evidence of the presence of the antigen in the air on epidemic days

Soya bean allergens on urban aerosols collected with glass-fibre filters were studied in a sample of 24 h average filters corresponding to epidemic and non-epidemic days (Antó *et al.* 1989*b*; Rodrigo *et al.* 1990). The antigens were assayed by a RAST inhibition technique that used antiserum from epidemic asthma patients. The reference antigen preparation was an extract of soya bean hull from beans collected in the harbour. The results showed highly statistically significant differences between soya bean antigen concentrations on epidemic days compared to those on non-epidemic days (the average soya bean antigen concentrations were 2583.1 and 29.2 units, respectively). These findings provided evidence that an airborne soya bean particulate antigen, reactive with serum from epidemic asthma patients, reached the city on epidemic days.

Evaluation of the environmental measures established at the point source (silo)

Preliminary analysis of environmental control measures introduced in silo A in September 1987 has demonstrated that during 838 consecutive days after the installation of bag filters in the silo, epidemic asthma days did not occur. Twenty asthma epidemic days were identified during a period of 973 days before the intervention ($p > 0.0001$). Specific IgE antibodies against soya bean have been assayed in 38 epidemic asthma patients 2 yr after the intervention. Although the mean average levels of IgE to soya bean showed a 50 per cent reduction, the proportion of epidemic patients with specific IgE antibodies against soya bean antigens has not changed (79 per cent v. 72 per cent). Two main conclusions can be established at this time: first, the intervention in the harbour that took place in September 1987 was effective and prevented the occurrence of new outbreaks; secondly, although, overall, the serum levels of specific IgE against soya bean have fallen by half, most epidemic patients are sensitized to soya bean (Antó 1990).

Organization and development of the research process

The formal research has extended over a period of 7 years. At least three different steps can be distinguished: 1982–84, hospital-based physicians identified asthma outbreaks and initiated a more intensive effort to elucidate the causes of these phenomena; 1984–87, several epidemiological initiatives were carried out under the auspices of the Barcelona Asthma Collaborative Group, mainly the establishment of the respiratory emergency room admissions register, the establishment of the point-source hypothesis, and the preliminary observation that asthma outbreaks could be related to soya bean unloading in one silo at the city harbour (this step ended with the environmental intervention at the harbour's silo); 1988–89, specific studies to formally assess the suspected causal relationship were carried out, particularly a time–

ecological and a case-control study. Throughout this period a large number of persons and institutions have been involved in the project. From 1984 the research was directed and co-ordinated by the Health Department of the Barcelona Local Council, where two epidemiologists from the staff (part-time) and one research fellow (full-time) were dedicated to the project. In addition, during the second step (1984–87) the Barcelona Collaborative Asthma Group set up two committees, one clinical–epidemiological, the other toxicological, which involved some 20 researchers.

From the organizational point of view there are several aspects that deserve comment. A great deal of collaboration among the different health administrations took place. This collaboration was crucial at least in two aspects: first, data collection from different hospitals, as well as from different environmental data-bases, was facilitated by this high degree of collaboration; secondly, the decision to suspend all soya bean operations at the city harbour, which had important economic and logistic consequences, was again largely facilitated by the concerted action. No less important were the contributions of outside experts and institutions in the form of scientific advice. A complete list of these contributions is given in the acknowledgements section of the reports, but the collaboration with the Division of Environmental Hazards and Health Effects at the Centers For Disease Control (CDC), Atlanta, USA deserves specific mention. In August 1987 a workshop was held at CDC to fully discuss the available data and the soya bean hypothesis. Both CDC staff and other outstanding American researchers participated, together with members of the Barcelona Asthma Collaborative Group, in reviewing the available evidence and suggesting further studies and methodological guidelines. In addition, a formal collaboration with the Allergy Unit of the Mayo Clinic has led to preliminary characterization of the soya bean allergen as well as to its measurement in the Barcelona atmospheric air in different studies (Rodrigo *et al.* 1990).

Conclusion

Asthma outbreaks in Barcelona can be considered as an example of clusters which frequently challenge public health departments. In a recent scientific conference on clustering, Rothman (1990) cogently argued why the study of individual clusters of disease—single clusters defined by space–time coordinates—do not offer hopeful prospects for scientific advance.

Although most of the methodological difficulties enumerated by Rothman usually are present in the study of clusters of cancer, asthma epidemics constitute a very different problem. In this final section we comment on several aspects that could be of general interest for the study of similar problems.

First, time and place are the axes which express the local occurrence of diseases. Both dimensions are closely interrelated: both spatial clusters and temporal clusters are subsets of space–time clusters (Knox 1989). Although some problems are frequently seen as geographical clusters, whereas others are more frequently identified as temporal clusters, this choice may depend upon the investigator's wishes and upon the model in mind. Rothman (1990) has pointed out that the relative magnitude of space–time clustering is influenced by the length of the induction period and, in the case of transmissible diseases, by the pathogenicity of the causative agent. A long induction period allows the cases to appear scattered both in time and space, thus attenuating the clustering pattern. By contrast, if the induction period is short, space–time clustering will be easily identifiable. Asthma outbreaks in Barcelona were caused through an immediate allergic mechanism (IgE) which prompted the appearance of cases in minutes or hours following the exposure and led to a striking space–time cluster. This is consistent with other reported asthma outbreaks since most of them were easily identified by hospital-based physicians. Asthma outbreaks related to castor bean dust inhalation were also likely to have been caused through an IgE mechanism. Also, in other outbreaks in which aetiology has not been elucidated, similar mechanisms have been proposed (Salvaggio *et al.* 1971*b*; Packe and Ayres 1985).

In addition to these factors, the local conditions under which the risk factors are distributed, both in time and space, are also relevant to describe the occurrence of the disease. In our case the most relevant conditions were the factors related to the point source, such as their periodic emissions of dust, the large doses of antigen contained in these emissions, and probably the meteorological conditions which on some days allowed soya bean dust to reach the city. These factors probably explain why the asthma clustering in Barcelona occurred in the form of repeated space–time clusters following a geographical point-source distribution. Indeed, respiratory episodes due to air pollution such as the ones that occurred in Tokyo–Yokohama (Phelps and Koike 1962) or Philadelphia (Rchenk *et al.* 1949), followed a broader (area-source) geographical distribution. Conversely, outbreaks attributed to dust coming from a castor bean mill in South Africa (Ordman 1955) or to sulphuric acid coming from a titanium oxide factory in Japan (Kitawa 1984) clearly followed a point-source pattern. In the case of Barcelona a point-source general hypothesis was established early, leading us to focus the search for a hypothesis in a more concrete direction, although the identification of the causative agent took several years of continuous research. On the other hand, the periodic emissions of soya bean dust to the atmospheric air determined a large series of outbreaks, allowing the inclusion of a reasonable number of observations in the ecological study of the harbour activities.

For some diseases for which causes are largely unknown, and where the application of classical epidemiological methods is difficult, the study of clusters could result in important scientific advances. As a result of the study of Barcelona asthma epidemics, a new cause of asthma has been identified (Anonymous 1989) and other asthma outbreaks caused by the same agent have been reported in other cities (Hernando *et al.* 1989). Even 2 years after the cessation of the outbreaks a case-control study demonstrated other factors interrelated to soya bean dust inhalation in causing asthma epidemics. In this study, an interaction between soya bean dust exposure, allergy to common aeroallergens, and smoking determined a higher risk of suffering the epidemics, pointing out that the interaction among these factors could be relevant in causing asthma among the general population as has been demonstrated in the occupational workforce (Sunyer *et al.* 1992). Finally, and probably more important, the investigation of the Barcelona asthma epidemics led to an environmental intervention to modify the causative point source which has prevented the occurrence of new outbreaks (Antó 1990) and the associated morbidity and mortality.

In conclusion, we suggest that in some circumstances the investigation of health event clusters could be of local, general and scientific interest. Several factors should be considered when deciding whether or not to carry out an epidemiological investigation, including possible biological mechanisms and available knowledge about the nature of the health event. In the case of clusters of asthma, we advocate an intensive multidisciplinary investigation whenever possible.

Acknowledgements

We acknowledge Dr Antoni Plasència for his contribution in the temporo-spatial study of the 12 outbreaks. We also acknowledge all members of the Barcelona Asthma Collaborative Group for their participation in the study of Barcelona asthma outbreaks. This work was supported in part by the following grants from the Fondo de Investigacion Sanitaria (FIS) 84/1851; 86/1847; 88/2029; 90/649.

References

Anonymous (1989). Asthma and the bean. *Lancet*, **ii**, 538–40.

Antó, J. M. (1990). Barcelona asthma epidemics: new evidence two years after their control. *European Respiratory Journal*, **3**, (Suppl. 10), 61s.

Antó, J. M. and Sunyer, J. (1990). Epidemiologic studies of asthma epidemics in Barcelona. *Chest*, **98**, (5), 185S–190S.

Antó, J. M., Sunyer, J., and the Barcelona Asthma Collaborative Group (1986*a*). A point-source asthma outbreak. *Lancet*, **i**, 900–3.

Antó, J. M., Sunyer, J., and Plasencia, A. (1986*b*). Nitrogen dioxide and asthma outbreaks. *Lancet*, **ii**, 1096–7.

Antó, J. M., Sunyer, J., Rodriguez-Roisin, R., Suarez-Cervera, M., Vazquez, L., and the Toxicoepidemiological Committee (1989*a*). Community outbreaks of asthma associated with inhalation of soybean dust. *New England Journal of Medicine*, **320**, 1097–102.

Antó, J., Sunyer, J., Grimalt, J., Aceves, M., and Reed, C. E. (1989b). Outbreaks of asthma associated with soybean dust. *New England Journal of Medicine*, **321**, 1128.

Figley, K. D. and Elrod, R. H. (1928). Endemic asthma due to castor bean dust. *Journal of the American Medical Association*, **90**, 79–82.

Goldstein, I. F. (1980). Weather patterns and asthma epidemics in New York City and New Orleans, USA. *International Journal of Biometeorology*, **24**, 329–39.

Goldstein, I. F. and Currie, B. (1984). Seasonal Patterns of asthma: a clue to etiology. *Environmental Research*, **33**, 201–15.

Goldstein, I. F. and Cuzick, J. (1983). Daily patterns of asthma in New York and New Orleans: an epidemiologic investigation. *Environmental Research*, **30**, 211–23.

Goldstein, I. F. and Rausch, L. E. (1978). Time series analysis of morbidity data for assessment of acute environmental health effects. *Environmental Research*, **17**, 266–75.

Goldstein, I. F. and Salvaggio, J. (1984). The decline of New Orleans asthma epidemics. *Reviews of Environmental Health*, **4**, 133–46.

Goldstein, I. F. and Weinstein, A. I. (1986). Air pollution and asthma: effects of exposures to short-term sulfur dioxide peaks. *Environmental Research*, **40**, 332–45.

Greenburg, L., Field, F., Reed, J. I., and Erhardt, C. L. (1964). Asthma and temperature change. *Archives of Environmental Health*, **8**, 642–7.

Hernando, L., Navarro, C., Marquez, M., Zapatero, L., and Galvan, F. (1989). Asthma epidemics and soybean in Cartagena (Spain). *Lancet*, **i**, 502.

Kitawa, T. (1984). Cause analysis of the Yokkaichi asthma episode in Japan. *Journal of the Air Pollution Control Association*, **34**, 743–6.

Knox, E. G. (1989). Detection of clusters. In *Methodology of enquiries into disease clustering*, (ed. P. Elliott), pp. 17–22. Small Area Health Statistics Unit, London.

Knox, E. G. and Lancashire, R. (1982). Detection of minimal epidemics. *Statistics in Medicine*, **1**, 183–9.

Lewis, R., Gilkeson, M. M., and McCaldin, R. O. (1962). Air pollution and New Orleans asthma. *Public Health Reports*, **77**, 947–54.

Mendes, E. and Ulhoa Cintra, A. (1954). Collective asthma, simulating an epidemic provoked by castor-bean dust. *Journal of Allergy and Clinical Immunology*, **25**, 253–9.

Morrison, I. (1960). It happened one night. *Medical Journal of Australia*, **i**, 850–1.

Morrow-Brown, H. (1986). Skin sensitivity to aero-allergens. *Lancet*, **i**, 980.

Ordman, D. (1955). An outbreak of bronchial asthma in South Africa, affecting more than 200 persons, caused by castor bean dust from an oil-processing factory. *International Archives of Allergy and Applied Immunology*, **7**, 10–24.

Packe, G. E. and Ayres, J. G. (1985). Asthma outbreak during a thunderstorm. *Lancet*, **ii**, 199–204.

Packe, G. E. and Ayres, J. G. (1986a). Aeroallergen skin sensitivity in patients with severe asthma during a thunderstorm. *Lancet*, **i**, 850–1.

Packe, G. E. and Ayres, J. G. (1986b). Aeroallergens in an asthma outbreak. *Lancet*, **i**, 980.

Phelps, H. W. and Koike, S. (1962). Tokio-Yojohama asthma. *American Review of Respiratory Disease*, **86**, 55–63.

Piccolo, M. C., Perillo, G., Ramón, C., and Didio, V. (1988). Outbreaks of asthma attacks and meteorological parameters in Bahia Blanca, Argentina. *Annals of Allergy*, **60**, 107–10.

Rchenk, H. N., Heimann, H., Clayton, G. D., Gafafer, W. M., and Westler (1949). Air pollution in Donora, Pennsylvania. Epidemiology of the unusual smoke episode of October 1948. *Public Health Bulletin*, **306**, 1–171.

Rodrigo, M. J., *et al.* (1990). Identification and partial characterization of the soybean dust allergens involved in the Barcelona asthma epidemic. *Journal of Allergy and Clinical Immunology*, **85**, 778–84.

Rothman, K. J. (1990). A sobering start for the cluster busters' conference. *American Journal of Epidemiology*, **132**, S6–S13.

Salvaggio, J. E. and Klein, R. C. (1967). New Orleans asthma. I. Characterization of individuals involved in epidemics. *Journal of Allergy*, **39**, 227–34.

Salvaggio, J. and Seabury, J. (1971). New Orleans asthma IV. Semi-quantitative airborne spore sampling, 1967–1968. *Journal of Allergy*, **48**, 82–95.

Salvaggio, J., *et al.* (1970). New Orleans asthma II. Relationship of climatologic and seasonal factors to outbreaks. *Journal of Allergy*, **45**, 257–65.

Salvaggio, J., Zaslow, L., Greer, J., and Seabury, J. (1971a). New Orleans asthma III. Semi-quantitative aerometric pollen sampling, 1967–1968. *Annals of Allergy*, **29**, 305–11.

Salvaggio, J., Seabury, J., and Schoenhardt, E. A. (1971b). New Orleans asthma V. Relationship between asthma admission rates, semiquantitative pollen and fungal spore counts, and total particulate aerometric sampling data. *Journal of Allergy*, **48**, 96–114.

Sunyer, J., *et al.* (1992). Risk factors of soybean epidemic asthma: the role of smoking and atopy. *American Review Respiratory Disease*, (in press).

Ussetti, P., Roca, J., Agusti, A. G. N., Montserrat, J. M., Rodriguez-Roisin, R., and Agusti-Vidal, A. (1983). Asthma outbreaks in Barcelona. *Lancet*, **ii**, 280–1.

Usetti, P., Roca, J., Agusti, A. G. N., Montserrat, J. M., Rodriguez-Roisin, R., and Agusti-Vidal, A. (1984). Another asthma outbreak in Barcelona. *Lancet*, **i**, 156.

Wallenstein, S. (1980). A test for detection of clustering over time. *American Journal of Epidemiology*, **111**, 367–72.

28. The Seveso accident

P. A. Bertazzi, A. C. Pesatori, and C. Zocchetti

Seveso, an industrious, quiet, and prosperous town in the province of Milan in northern Italy, has become synonymous with environmental pollution and associated problems. The accident at Seveso was actually only the most recent in a series of accidents arising during the industrial preparation of 2,4,5-trichlorophenol (IPCS 1989), yet its characteristics were somehow unique, and made it the prototypic example of the environmental and health hazards associated with the manufacture and use of toxic chemicals. The ingredients for a real but incompletely understood major industrial hazard were all there: a chemical plant located in the immediate vicinity of an inhabited area; an extremely toxic, unintentional by-product formed during the preparation of a compound employed for pesticide manufacturing; an accidental explosion caused by an uncontrolled development during the synthesis process; and finally, foreseeable health effects, the nature of which was only partially known but certainly included late and subtle appearance and, possibly, damage to future generations.

The mode of occurrence of the accident and its immediate aftermath have been reported in detail by Hay (1982) and Silano (1981). On Saturday 10 July 1976, at the Icmesa chemical plant, shortly before closing down for the weekend, the reactor in department B was left in unusual conditions. A few hours later, a 'parasitic' reaction took place which raised the temperature and caused a pressure surge that blew safety devices. The fluid mixture of chemicals contained in the reactor was discharged through a vent pipe directly into the atmosphere and formed a toxic cloud containing trichlorophenol, sodium trichlorophenate, ethylene glycol, sodium hydroxide, and, as ascertained a few days later, substantial quantities of 2,3,7,8-tetrachlorodibenzo-p-dioxin (TCDD).

In the following few days, unequivocal signs of serious environmental contamination were noted. They included damage to vegetation, casualties of birds and courtyard animals, and especially among children, burns, caustic lesions, and swelling in uncovered parts of the body. These signs provided an early and most worrisome picture of the extent and seriousness of the toxic hazard present in the area.

In the immediate aftermath of the accident, the main concern shared by the population, family physicians, and health officials was the identification and treatment of any persons exhibiting signs and symptoms of exposure to the toxic chemicals (Carreri 1978). For this reason, and because of the social and political pressure under which health activities had to be planned and conducted, little attention was devoted to the planning of formal epidemiological investigations (Bruzzi 1983a). When, on the tenth day, the presence of TCDD in the reactor discharge was confirmed, it became clear that primarily the population affected by the accident had to be defined in terms of potential for exposure, and not only for the presence of acute effects. Like many other toxic chemicals, dioxin was considered capable of causing delayed health sequelae, possibly manifesting themselves even after decades. This concern suggested the need to design *ad hoc* studies and surveillance systems, aimed at discovering mid- and long-term effects attributable to accident exposure.

Extent of contamination and exposure level

The amount of TCDD released has been the subject of numerous and quite contrasting estimates, but recent re-evaluations by Di Domenico *et al.* (1990) led to estimates of the order of tens of kilograms. TCDD is a poorly water-soluble compound with high affinity for soil and water sediment, and with a significant potential for bioaccumulation. The soil was thus the first and main environmental medium available to define the extent and level of contamination. Measurements in the surface soil provided evidence of decreasing levels with increasing distance from the point source of release and suggested that the cloud had been moving in a definite direction, with gradual dispersion on the edges of the main pathway. Measurements in the deeper soil layers suggested that the vertical gradients varied only slightly with time, with over 90 per cent of the detectable TCDD still found in the upper 15 cm after several months. Measurements were also made in other environmental/ecological systems. In vegetation (leaves, grass, vegetables), TCDD levels decreased rapidly with distance from the factory; both pre-existing tissues and new growth were found to be contaminated, and the ability of plants to absorb and translocate TCDD was shown, with a progressive increase in TCDD level with plant maturation. In farm animals TCDD was detected in the liver, and several wild mammals showed positive levels of TCDD in both skin and liver. Measurements in cow's milk showed the highest levels in samples from the farms closest to the trichlorophenol plant (Silano 1981; Cerquiglini Monteriolo *et al.* 1982; Pocchiari *et al.* 1983).

The environmental analyses, mainly those performed on soil samples, led to the delimitation of zones with different mean levels of contamination (Fig. 28.1). In the area most heavily contaminated (zone A), mean soil levels of TCDD ranged from 15.5 μg/m^2 to 580 μg/m^2. The zone covered nearly 90 hectares and extended south–southeast up to a distance of 2200 m from the plant, in the direction of the dominant wind at the time of the accident. There

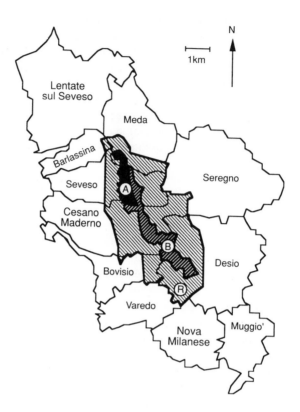

Fig. 28.1 Sketch of the Seveso accident scenario. The three contaminated zones (A, B, and R) and the surrounding area adopted as reference are shown.

were 181 families with more than 700 individuals living within zone A's boundaries; they were evacuated in three steps by the beginning of August 1976. A second contaminated area (zone B) was delimited, extending in the same direction for 270 hectares, with 1721 families (more than 5000 individuals). The levels of TCDD soil contamination did not exceed, on average, 50 μg/m^2. People in this area were requested to comply with strict regulations regarding personal and home hygiene, and consumption of water and local food. Children between the ages of 1 and 12 years and women in their first trimester of pregnancy were ordered to leave the area during the daytime. Animals (cattle, poultry, rabbits, etc.) were sacrificed. Surrounding the two zones was an area with low-level and patchy contamination, referred to as the 'zone of respect' (zone R), in which TCDD levels were generally below 5 μg/m^2. More than 30 000 persons had their residence within the boundaries of this 1430 hectare zone, where consumption of local crops and animal raising was also prohibited.

Another major and obvious indicator of exposure was represented by early signs and symptoms of contact with the chemical cloud (irritative symptoms and dermal chemical lesions). Specific signs of exposure to TCDD (chloracne) began to appear on the fourth day. It is easy to appreciate how relevant these early signs were for establishing individual exposure.

Attempts were made to integrate the various pieces of information in order to obtain comprehensive estimates of exposure. Frequency of chloracne turned out to be fairly, if not completely, related to the estimated levels of ground contamination (Caramaschi *et al.* 1981). Other data by Merlo *et al.* (1986) included animal deaths in addition to TCDD in soil and skin changes, which raised some questions about the accuracy of the established boundaries of the contaminated areas.

Thousands of blood samples were collected after the accident for blood chemistry testing. At that time, no methods existed which were sufficiently sensitive to measure low dioxin concentrations in small blood samples, but such methods have been developed recently. Fortunately, the blood samples had been stored in a proper way. Results of the first few measurements have been reported by Mocarelli *et al.* (1990) concerning 19 zone A residents (10 children with chloracne and nine other persons), and 10 subjects from outside the contaminated zones. The TCDD levels found among zone A children who developed chloracne were the highest ever reported in humans and ranged between 828 part per trillion (p.p.t.) and 56 000 p.p.t. Seven of those children had serum levels higher than 12 000 p.p.t. Zone A residents without chloracne had TCDD levels ranging between 1770 and 10 400 p.p.t. Only one of the residents outside the contaminated areas had detectable levels of TCDD. The programme of serum TCDD testing is continuing and the increase in the number of samples examined will, it is hoped, yield better quantitative estimates of exposure potential in the different locations.

Thus, exposure classification of subjects in the area was essentially based on environmental contamination data. Individual exposure was specified by zone, and period of residence was used as a surrogate indicator of level and duration of exposure. Limited biological data documented the potentially high exposure in the area closest to the source. Other groups of people could be classified as exposed on other grounds. This was the case, for example, with the nearly 200 chloracne cases (Caramaschi *et al.* 1981), with workers in the plant (Zedda *et al.* 1976), and with people involved in reclamation works (Ghezzi *et al.* 1982).

Epidemiological methods

Study base

The identification and enumeration of the study population greatly benefited from the delimitation of the extent of contamination; yet, it was by no means a straightforward process. In the early phase, it was obvious to focus on persons evacuated from zone A, on persons with dermal signs of contact with the chemical cloud (especially those with chloracne), and on individuals who were considered a priori as highly susceptible (e.g. pregnant women, children). Numerous investigations by Homberger *et al.* (1979) and Bisanti *et al.* (1980) on health outcomes possibly associated with dioxin exposure (e.g. neuro-logical, immunological, hepatic impairment; birth defects and abortion rate) were carried out among these subgroups.

In a second phase, a few years after the accident, the establishment of a registry covering the resident population of the municipalities concerned was initiated. Investigations on mortality, cancer morbidity, and birth defects were conducted by Abate *et al.* (1982), Bruzzi (1983*b*) and Puntoni *et al.* (1986) which provided interim results describing the mid-term health experience of residents in the contaminated zones.

In a third, more recent, phase, a further refined definition of the study base was achieved. The population of any geographical area is subject to change with time. Moreover, since in our case the area happened to be hit by the disruptive event of a 'chemical disaster', the population changes did not occur according to the usual, 'natural' patterns. One can easily anticipate a migration away from the area by those people who suffered physically, emotionally, or economically because of the accident. Unfortunately, people who leave the area may well be the most relevant to the ascertainment of late health effects of accident exposure. Thus, this selective migration may cause a serious bias in the study results. As time passes, in addition, a dilution phenomenon related to the moving out of exposed and moving in of non-exposed subjects should be expected, causing a shifting towards the null of the effect estimates provided by epidemiological studies. In order to avoid these probable sources of bias, Bertazzi *et al.* (1989) adopted a cohort approach. Two prerequisites had to be met, i.e. the identification and complete enumeration of eligible subjects, and the availability of reliable information systems to trace people who left the area. The only comparable and comprehensive identification and enumeration source turned out to be the official residence registrations at the vital statistics offices of the 11 towns within the accident scenario (Fig. 28.1). The decision was thus made to rely on administrative boundaries and official record files so as to ensure reliability of the population data. There were, none the less, people living in the area at the time of the accident who did not have their official residence there, as well as people having their residence but not living in the area. Their exact number was unknown, but was certainly not large, so that the effect of this misclassification was deemed negligible. Priority was given to the need for getting uniform, basic information for each individual in order to identify and follow up the cohort. The available information included: full name, gender, place and date of birth, town and full address of residence at the date of the accident or first entry into the area, vital status inclusive of date, place, and cause in case of death, and date and new town of residence for those who moved.

The study population thus comprised all persons of any age and both sexes ever resident in one of the 11 towns, at any time from the date of the accident onwards (including new-borns and immigrants), irrespective of their current residence. The information about towns and street addresses allowed subjects to be attributed to one of the three exposure zones or to the surrounding non-contaminated area. Admission into the study cohort was discontinued as of 31 December 1986; after that date no potential for exposure was deemed to exist any more for newcomers into the area.

Follow-up procedures

The follow-up of the Seveso cohort was based on individual information recorded on vital statistics registries which are maintained by every municipality in Italy. This population statistics system covers the whole national territory. Individual changes (residence, status, etc.) are continuously updated. Even for people who migrate abroad but maintain Italian citizenship, a special vital status registry exists in their hometown. When a person moved outside the study area to any municipality in Italy, the towns were contacted in turn, until the person was located and vital status ascertained. Indeed, every year, about 3500 cohort members moved outside the study area. Updating the information for the entire population as of 31 December 1986 for the purposes of the 10-year mortality analysis involved contacting some 4300 municipalities over the entire country. Even so, the tracing was successful in over 99 per cent of cases (Bertazzi *et al.* 1989).

Because there is no national registration system of cancer cases, the cancer incidence study had to be limited to people residing in the study area and those who had moved within the Lombardy region (nearly 9 000 000 inhabitants). For every hospital in the region, the information on each hospitalization, from admission to discharge (except name and surname of the patient), is centrally recorded and stored. The linkage of the information on admission date, birth date, gender, and residence of the subject at the time of hospitalization with the records of our cohort members, allows the identification of the study subjects discharged by any hospital within the region with a diagnosis mentioning cancer. The examination of the original medical records leads to the ascertainment of the true diagnosis and date of occurrence. The cancer incidence study covers malignant tumours at any site plus benign tumours of the liver, bladder, and central nervous system, first diagnosed after the date of the accident (10 July 1976).

Reference data

Another crucial element in designing the study was the selection of reference data. Different sets of data, both national and local, were available as reference standards. The national rates available for mortality were discarded because of marked interregional differences; local rates were not deemed completely satisfactory either. For mortality, local rates had the drawback of including the large metropolitan area of Milan, hence influenced by a set of variables affecting mortality which were not shared by our study population; and, for cancer incidence, even though a tumour registry was in operation in a nearby province, the calendar years covered were not the same, and the quality of data for the registry population and our cohort, and the social and cultural backgrounds were not fully comparable.

It appeared that the most suitable source of reference data was the population of the accident area not affected by TCDD contamination (Fig. 28.1). People living in this territory surrounding zone R shared with the index population the main characteristics related to life-style and occupational environment, personal habits, and social and educational background. They were traced concurrently and with the same methods as people from the contaminated zones. All tracing procedures were implemented without knowledge of cohort members' exposure status.

Statistical methods

Standard techniques were applied for the analysis of mortality data (Breslow and Day 1987). In the treatment of cancer data, special care has been devoted to the problem of multiple cancers using ideas in Lynge and Thygesen (1990). Each cancer site has been analysed separately. Each person has been considered 'at risk' from the date of the accident or first entry into the area to the date of incidence of that specific cancer, the date of death, or the end of the follow-up period, whichever came first. This approach allows genuine multiple cancers of different sites to be enumerated correctly (and person-years computed accordingly) taking into account the problem of prevalent cases. When grouping of sites has been analysed (e.g. all cancers, digestive cancers) the first occurrence in that 'group' of sites has been considered, discarding subsequent occurrences of cancers of the same 'group' (for 'all cancers' this is equivalent to considering only the first occurrence of cancer).

Comparisons of rates have been performed using standard Poisson regression techniques (Frome 1983), separately by sex, and controlling for age (five-year strata) and calendar period (before and after 1981). Relative risks and 'large sample' 95 per cent confidence intervals were estimated, as well as the number of 'expected' deaths (or cancer cases). More than 100 mortality causes and more than 70 cancer sites have been analysed.

Advantages and problems of the approach

The cohort approach had the ability to overcome the most severe of the limitations inherent in any geographical epidemiological study. In particular, migration could be taken into consideration, which allowed the investigation to focus on the group of people actually exposed because of their place and time period of residence. Another useful feature was the availability of dates of residence at each address held in any municipality. This enabled length of residence to be used as a surrogate for duration of exposure, and the time period since first residence in the contaminated area as a surrogate for induction/latency time.

The completeness of the population coverage was highly satisfactory. The reason such high rates of completeness were achieved in the follow-up was almost entirely because 'hard' records were used (official population registries, death certificate and hospital discharge forms). The validity of such an approach also played a major role in deciding which studies to consider feasible in the long run, since previous investigations by Mocarelli *et al.* (1986) and Assennato *et al.* (1989) had experienced major problems in maintaining completeness of follow-up.

Systematic errors in estimating the denominator could be excluded confidently. Subjects lost in follow-up were those not registered in any of the 11 towns embracing the area of TCDD contamination. The use of the nationwide vital statistics system ensured successful tracing of more than 99 per cent of the subjects. As for the numerator, completeness of case ascertainment was different for causes of death and cancer diagnoses. For deaths, only chance losses occurred and the ascertainment can be considered virtually complete. However, incomplete ascertainment of cancer cases came about for several reasons. The system of data collection precluded the detection of cancer cases admitted to hospitals outside Lombardy and cases treated as out-patients only. Additional losses were due to errors in recording or coding data on place of birth and place of residence on the hospital discharge form, or to incorrect coding of discharge diagnoses.

In the feasibility phase of the study, estimates had already been made of the completeness of ascertainment of cancer cases. The proportion of non-detected cases in the Lombardy hospitals was first estimated with an *ad hoc* investigation in the two main hospitals of the study area. For a 1.5 year period all hospital records (20 000 in Desio hospital and 7500 in Seregno) were checked, and all those reporting a diagnosis of cancer (International Classification of Disease codes 140-239) in subjects with residence in one of the 11 municipalities of the study area were extracted and compared with records obtained from the regional files of discharge diagnoses. Considering benign and malignant tumours together, the proportion of cases not detected by our system was about 12 per cent, while the proportion of malignant tumours undetected was smaller, and ranged from 2.6 per cent to 6.8 per cent. Erroneous coding of the discharge diagnosis was the major reason for non-detection, although the erroneous coding was not related to specific types or sites of tumour.

We also tried to estimate the proportion of cases lost because they were diagnosed as out-patients. We checked all cytohistological referrals positive for any neoplasm at the Pathology Service of San Gerardo Hospital in Monza, the largest hospital next to the study area. For the period 1979–82, 280 in-patient and 220 out-patient cancer cases were identified among residents in the study area. Among the hospitalized cancer cases, 93 per cent had been correctly identified by our data collection system, yielding a 7 per cent proportion of loss which was consistent with the previous evaluation. The proportion of undetected cases among out-patient diagnoses rose, however, to 20 per cent. Some 50 per cent of missing cases were skin cancers.

Every year, 0.6 per cent of the study population moves outside Lombardy, a proportion which might be considered reassuring given the possibility of major biases due to losses to follow-up. None the less, we decided to investigate whether it would be possible to get information on cases outside Lombardy by sending an *ad hoc* questionnaire to family physicians once the subject had been located. A sample of about 500 people who had moved to three different regions, Veneto (north), Abruzzo (center), and Calabria (south) were chosen. We obtained from the local health service the names and addresses of all relevant family physicians in Abruzzo and Veneto, and 83 per cent of them in Calabria. After that, a questionnaire was sent to each physician in which information about possible cancer occurrence in the subjects was sought. Although the quality of responses was good, the number was quite low (55 per cent from Abruzzo, 61 per cent from Veneto, and 65 per cent from Calabria) and the procedure proved to be too cumbersome, expensive, and time-consuming. Consequently, we decided to search for cancer cases outside Lombardy only for particular groups at highest risk; for example, all chloracne cases are followed up for cancer occurrence even after leaving the Lombardy region.

The use of the surrounding population as the source of reference mortality and morbidity data had numerous advantages. All available economic, social, cultural, environmental, and occupational macro-indicators supported a close comparability between the index and reference populations. Also, availability and access to medical and diagnostic facilities was similar between the two areas. Even so, there were problems, including the size of the population in the referent area. Stability of rates was checked by comparing findings in the area with those of the entire Lombardy region. A few discrepancies emerged, which have been taken into consideration (Bertazzi *et al.* 1989). Another problem was related to the temporal trend of occurrence of certain causes of death. Data for the period prior to the accident were available only for mortality, and Bertazzi (1989) showed that for one cause at least, brain cancer, mortality in the TCDD-contaminated area was higher *before* the accident. Problems of accuracy of death certificate diagnosis had also to be addressed, so that interpretation of the mortality findings for certain causes (e.g. cancer of peritoneum) was substantially influenced by arguments about accuracy (Bertazzi *et al.* 1989).

With regard to exposure, in addition to the absence of individual data on exposure, two further problems emerged when using environmental data on

TCDD contamination for epidemiological purposes. One was the evolution of analytical methods which, when used years after the accident, were found by Cerlesi *et al.* (1989) to give new and different estimates of the TCDD levels in the soil. The second problem was linked to the soil sampling scheme originally employed, which was based on discrete measurements taken with a low resolution and varying sampling grid. Spatial modelling of the data was thus needed to get quantitative estimates for the whole contaminated area. A theoretical model of fall-out, based on the physico-chemical characteristics of the cloud and properties of the materials therein, was used by Ratti *et al.* (1987) and suggested a log-normal local distribution of TCDD along the release path. Each point of the area has been characterized in terms of polar coordinates (distance from the point source, and angle). The analytical form of the model was derived from available data. Points with the same estimated TCDD value were connected so as to generate contours delimiting areas to be used as iso-concentration zones in future analyses.

Results and interpretation

The majority of the health investigations on early and mid-term effects of TCDD exposure yielded inconclusive results, due to flaws in the study design, or difficulties in conducting the study in the complex crisis situation determined by the accident. Problems included lack of appropriate reference groups, poor standardization of methods and procedures, and low and/or biased compliance of subjects to be examined.

Between 1976 and 1982 more than 4500 laboratory tests were performed, to investigate, in particular, liver enzyme induction and lipid metabolism on a group of children aged 6–10 years at the date of the accident. Boys from the highly polluted zone A showed increased γ-glutamyl transpeptidase (GGT) and alanine aminotransferase (ALT) levels in comparison with a group of control children. These differences were restricted to values within the reference limits and disappeared over a period of time (Mocarelli *et al.* 1986).

The group of 193 cases of chloracne was followed up to 1985 by Assennato *et al.* (1989) and the health findings were compared with a reference group of the same sex and similar size and age. Chloracne dermal lesions disappeared in all subjects but one. The only statistically significant change in laboratory tests was a decrease in mean values of serum cholesterol and triglycerides in the chloracne group between 1976 and 1982.

Urinary D-glucaric acid (an indirect, but valid and reliable, indicator of liver enzyme induction) was measured at different times between 1976 and 1981. In 1976, Ideo *et al.* (1985) found that children from zone A with chloracne exhibited significantly increased levels of urinary D-glucaric acid excretion compared to children from the same area without chloracne.

An increased frequency of peripheral neuropathy, although of mild and non-acute type, was found in 1978 by Filippini *et al.* (1981) among subjects with probably heavy exposure to TCDD. A later investigation on 152 children with chloracne by Barbieri *et al.* (1988) indicated signs of involvement of the peripheral nervous system at higher rate than in a comparison group, even though a definite peripheral neuropathy was not evident in any of the chloracne subjects.

Cytogenetic findings after induced abortion in women involved in the accident and non-exposed women were studied by Tenchini *et al.* (1983) and failed to show obvious effects related to TCDD exposure. In an embryological and histomorphological study of 30 interrupted pregnancies and four spontaneous abortions, Rehder *et al.* (1978) found no indications of mutagenic, teratogenic, or fetotoxic effects of TCDD.

Infants born between 1977 and 1982 were examined for the presence of any congenital malformation. Analysis was performed according to the type of birth defect, and mother's residence on 10 July 1976, with special attention devoted to those born in the first quarter of 1977 (Mastroiacovo *et al.* 1988). The results failed to demonstrate an increased risk of birth defects associated with the accident experience of this population.

An International Steering Committee (Regione Lombardia 1984) guided the early phase of scientific work on the consequences of the Seveso accident. The Committee concluded that 'it is obvious that no clear-cut adverse health effects attributable to TCDD, besides chloracne, have been observed'. At that time, post-accident surveillance programmes were discontinued, while long-term investigations (mortality and cancer incidence) were re-designed to ascertain, in the long run, possible unusual health experiences in the exposed population and their relation to the accident, and to contribute in clarifying the role of TCDD in causing cancer in humans.

Results of the mortality study for the 10.5 year period following the accident have been published (Bertazzi *et al.* 1989). The male population of the contaminated zones experienced a statistically significant increase in mortality from chronic ischaemic heart disease (relative risk (RR) = 1.56). The increase was highest (RR = 3.2) in zone A, where the impact of the chemical contamination and of the psycho-social stress caused by the accident was strongest. In this zone, mortality from cerebrovascular disease was found to be significantly elevated as well (RR = 3.3). Among female subjects, a similarly increased pattern of cardiovascular mortality was noted (RR in zone A = 1.9). Two mechanisms have been hypothesized to explain the increased pattern of cardiovascular mortality, i.e. TCDD toxicity and post-disaster stress which might have precipitated pre-existing conditions. Both may have contributed. Confounding could reasonably be ruled out (Bertazzi 1989; Bertazzi *et al.* 1989) because of the close similarity of the index and referent populations in terms of major risk factors.

Tables 28.1 and 28.2 show selected cancer mortality findings for males and females, respectively. Overall, the relative risk for cancer deaths tended to be slightly below 1.00. Among males, suggestive increases were seen for several cancer causes, in particular for soft tissue sarcomas (RR = 5.4, two cases), melanoma (RR = 3.3, three cases), and myeloid leukaemia (RR = 2.5, five cases). As expected, very few events were observed in the small population of zone A. The population of zone B exhibited the clearest suggestions of a possibly increased cancer occurrence, a finding that might be consistent with their post-accident experience (they remained in the polluted area, and compliance to restrictive regulations was never evaluated). Mortality from cancer of the liver (one of the target organs of TCDD toxicity) failed to show any increase. Two soft tissue sarcomas were observed in the largest sub-cohort which comprised persons living in the least polluted area (zone R), and resulted in a noteworthy increase of the relative risk. Leukaemia, and specifically myeloid leukaemia, also showed a noteworthy increase, particularly when considered together with the probably associated cause, 'blood disease'. Noteworthy findings among females were the consistent and seemingly zone-related increase of mortality from biliary cancer (based, however, on only a few deaths), and a deficit of breast cancer of borderline significance. The suggestive increase of brain cancer deaths was similar to the finding among males. Hodgkin's disease, but not leukaemias, exhibited a near significant increase.

The mortality study was descriptive in nature, hence results do not permit the conclusive association of any of the unusual cancer mortality findings with accidental exposure to TCDD in 1976. Other factors that limit a causal interpretation are the short time period elapsed since first exposure, the small number of deaths from certain causes, and exposure definition based on ecological rather than individual indicators.

Mortality of the young members of the cohort (1–20 years of age) was analysed separately. Leukaemia deaths showed an increase above expectations, although statistically non-significant, in both males and females. A suggestive increase of congenital anomalies was also noted by Pesatori *et al.* (1990); however, five out of the seven observed anomalies in the contaminated area turned out to have occurred in children born before the accident.

Interim results of the cancer incidence investigation (Pesatori *et al.* 1991) confirmed the increased risk of biliary cancer, particularly among females. Myeloid leukaemia was clearly elevated in both males and females. In addition, a statistically significant increase of lymphoreticulosarcomas was noted among males (RR = 5.5, three cases).

The incident cancer cases will constitute the basis for initiating case-control studies on specific cancer types for which an association with TCDD is suggested as possible, not only by these but also by the previous findings of Boyle *et al.* (1989), Wiklund *et al.* (1989), Hoar Zahm *et al.* (1990), Suskind (1990), and Fingerhut *et al.* (1991). Case-control studies will allow closer

Table 28.1 Mortality from selected causes, 1976–86, in the male population of the three contaminated zones of the Seveso area

Cause of death (ICD 9)[1]	Zone A		Zone B		Zone R		Total	
	Observed deaths	RR[2] 95 CI[3]	Observed deaths	RR 95 CI	Observed deaths	RR 95 CI	Observed deaths	RR 95 CI
All cancers (140–209)	3	0.46 0.1–1.4	52	1.19 0.9–1.6	270	0.86 0.8–1.0	322	0.97 0.9–1.0
Liver cancer (155)	–	–	3	1.20 0.4–3.8	7	0.40 0.2–0.8	10	0.48 0.2–0.9
Lung cancer (162)	2	0.95 0.2–3.8	20	1.45 0.9–2.3	77	0.78 0.6–1.0	99	0.87 0.7–1.1
Soft tissue sarcoma (171)	–	–	–	–	2	6.33 0.9–45.0	2	5.43 0.8–38.6
Melanoma (172)	–	–	1	9.06 1.1–77.6	2	2.58 0.5–13.3	3	3.33 0.8–13.9
Bladder cancer (188)	–	–	3	2.17 0.7–6.9	7	0.70 0.3–1.5	10	0.87 0.4–1.7
Brain cancer (191)	–	–	–	–	5	1.37 0.5–3.6	5	1.17 0.4–3.1
Leukaemia (204–208)	–	–	3	2.44 0.8–7.8	4	0.47 0.2–1.3	7	0.70 0.3–1.5
Myeloid leukaemia (205)	–	–	1	4.14 0.5–32.1	4	2.36 0.8–7.4	5	2.53 0.9–7.3
Blood disease (280–289)	–	–	–	–	6	4.28 1.5–12.0	6	3.70 1.3–10.4

[1] ICD 9, code of the International Classification of Diseases, ninth revision.
[2] RR, relative risk.
[3] 95 CI, 95 per cent confidence interval of RR estimate.

Table 28.2 Mortality from selected cancer causes, 1976–86, in the female population of the three contaminated zones of the Seveso area

Cause of death (ICD 9)[1]	Zone A		Zone B		Zone R		Total	
	Observed deaths	RR[2] 95 CI[3]	Observed deaths	RR 95 CI	Observed deaths	RR 95 CI	Observed deaths	RR 95 CI
All cancers (140–209)	3	0.80 0.3–2.5	14	0.60 0.4–1.0	159	0.87 0.7–1.0	176	0.84 0.7–1.0
Liver cancer (155)	–	–	–	–	3	0.43 0.1–1.4	3	0.38 0.1–1.2
Cancer of the gallbladder and biliary tract (156)	1	12.07 1.6–88.7	2	3.86 0.9–16.2	5	1.18 0.5–3.1	8	1.66 0.8–3.6
Soft tissue sarcoma (171)	–	–	1	16.99 1.8–163.6	–	–	1	1.98 0.2–1.9
Breast cancer (174)	1	1.06 0.1–7.5	5	0.87 0.4–2.1	28	0.64 0.4–0.9	34	0.67 0.5–1.0
Brain cancer (191)	–	–	–	–	5	2.42 0.9–6.7	5	2.11 0.8–5.9
Hodgkin's disease (201)	–	–	1	5.87 0.7–47.7	3	2.65 0.7–10.2	4	3.01 0.9–10.3
Leukaemia (204–208)	–	–	1	1.08 0.1–7.9	3	0.43 0.1–1.4	4	0.50 0.2–1.4

[1] ICD 9, code of the International Classification of Diseases, ninth revision.
[2] RR, relative risk.
[3] 95 CI, 95 per cent confidence interval of RR estimate.

control of possible confounding factors such as life-style, occupation, personal accident experience, etc. In addition, the use of biological indicators will be pursued, to characterize individual exposure better as well as to reveal possible signs of susceptibility in certain subjects.

Overall, the available results do not provide either fully comprehensive documentation of the effects of the accident on the exposed subjects, or conclusive evidence of the effects of TCDD on humans. As already mentioned, the reasons range from a latency period still too brief, to problems of study design and conduct encountered in the post-disaster setting. The extension of the follow-up, along with the new studies being initiated, will certainly contribute to bridging the existing gap in knowledge about human toxicity of TCDD and long-term health sequelae of the Seveso accident.

References

Abate, L., *et al.* (1982). Mortality and birth defects from 1976 to 1979 in the population living in the TCDD populated area of Seveso. In *Chlorinated dioxins and related compounds*, (ed. O. Hutzinger, R. W. Frei, E. Merian, and F. Pocchiari), pp. 571–87. Pergamon Press, Oxford.

Assennato, G., Cervino, D., Emmett, E. A., Longo, G., and Merlo, F. (1989). Follow-up of subjects who developed chloracne following TCDD exposure at Seveso. *American Journal of Industrial Medicine*, **16**, 119–25.

Barbieri, S., Pirovano, C., Scarlato, G., Tarchini, P., Zappa, A., and Maranzana, M. (1988). Long-term effects of 2,3,7,8-tetrachlorodibenzo-*p*-dioxin on the peripheral nervous system. *Neuroepidemiology*, **7**, 29–37.

Bertazzi, P. A. (1989). Industrial disasters and epidemiology. A review of recent experiences. *Scandinavian Journal of Work Environment and Health*, **15**, 85–100.

Bertazzi, P. A., Zocchetti, C., Pesatori, A. C., Guercilena, S., Sanarico, M., and Radice, L. (1989). Ten-year mortality study of the population involved in the Seveso incident in 1976. *American Journal of Epidemiology*, **129**, 1187–200.

Bisanti, L., *et al.* (1980). Experiences from the accident of Seveso. *Acta Morphologica Hungarica*, **28**, 139–57.

Boyle, C. A., Decouflé, P., and O'Brien, T. R. (1989). Long-term health consequences of military service in Vietnam. *Epidemiologic Reviews*, **11**, 1–27.

Breslow, N. E. and Day, N. E. (1987). *Statistical methods in cancer research*, Vol. II, *The design and analysis of cohort studies*. International Agency for Research on Cancer, Lyon.

Bruzzi, P. (1983*a*). Health impact of the accidental release of TCDD at Seveso. In *Accidental exposure to dioxins. Human health aspects*, (ed. F. Coulston and F. Pocchiari), pp. 215–25. Academic Press, London.

Bruzzi, P. (1983*b*). Birth defects in the TCDD polluted area of Seveso: results of a four-year follow-up. In *Accidental exposure to dioxin. Human health aspects*, (ed. F. Coulston and F. Pocchiari), pp. 271–80. Academic Press, New York.

Caramaschi, R., Del Corno, G., Favaretti, C., Giambelluca, S. E. , Montesarchio, E., and Fara, G. M. (1981). Chloracne following environmental contamination by TCDD in Seveso, Italy. *International Journal of Epidemiology*, **10**, 135–43.

Carreri, V. (1978). Review of the events which occurred in Seveso. In *Dioxin, toxicological and chemical aspects*, (ed. F. Cattabeni, A. Cavallaro, and G. Galli), pp. 1–5. Spectrum Publications, New York.

Cerlesi, S., Di Domenico, A., and Ratti, S. (1989). 2,3,7,8-tetrachlorodibenzo-*p*-dioxin (TCDD) persistence in the Seveso (Milan, Italy) soil. *Ecotoxicology and Environmental Safety*, **18**, 149–64.

Cerquiglini Monteriolo, S., Di Domenico, A., Silano, V., Viviano, G., and Zapponi, G. (1982). 2,3,7,8-TCDD levels and distribution in the environment at Seveso after the ICMESA accident on July 10, 1976. In *Chlorinated dioxins and related compounds*, (ed. O. Hutzinger, R. W. Frei, E. Merian, and F. Pocchiari), pp. 126–7. Pergamon Press, Oxford.

Di Domenico, A., Cerlesi, S., and Ratti, S. (1990). A two-exponential model to describe the vanishing trend of 2,3,7,8-tetrachlorodibenzodioxin (TCDD) in the soil at Seveso, Northern Italy. *Chemosphere*, **20**, 1559–66.

Filippini, G., Bordo, B., Crenna, P., Massetto, N., Musicco, M., and Boeri, R. (1981). Relationship between clinical and electrophysiological findings and indicators of heavy exposure to 2,3,7,8-tetrachlorodibenzo-dioxin. *Scandinavian Journal of Work Environment and Health*, **7**, 257–62.

Fingerhut, M. A., *et al.* (1991). Cancer mortality in workers exposed to 2,3,7,8-tetrachlorodibenzo-*p*-dioxin. *New England Journal of Medicine*, **324**, 212–18.

Frome, E. L. (1983). The analysis of rates using Poisson regression models. *Biometrics*, **39**, 655–74.

Ghezzi, I., *et al.* (1982). Potential 2,3,7,8-tetrachlorodibenzo-*p*-dioxin exposure of Seveso decontamination workers. *Scandinavian Journal of Work Environment and Health*, **176**, (Suppl. 1), 9–17.

Hay, A. (1982). *The chemical scythe. Lessons of 2,4,5-T and dioxin*, pp. 197–227. Plenum Press, New York.

Hoar Zahm, S., *et al.* (1990). A case-control study of non-Hodgkin's lymphoma and the herbicide 2,4-dichlorophenoxyacetic acid (2,4-D) in eastern Nebraska. *Epidemiology*, **1**, 349–56.

Homberger, E., Reggiani, G., Sambeth, J., and Wipf, H. K. (1979). The Seveso accident: its nature, extent and consequences. *Annals of Occupational Hygiene*, **22**, 327–70.

Ideo, G., Bellati, G., Bellobuono, A., and Bisanti, L. (1985). Urinary D-glucaric acid excretion in the Seveso area, polluted by tetrachlorodibenzo-*p*-dioxin (TCDD): five years of experience. *Environmental Health Perspectives*, **60**, 151–7.

IPCS International Program on Chemical Safety (1989). *Polychlorinated dibenzo-para-dioxins and dibenzofurans*, Environmental Health Criteria 88. World Health Organization, Geneva.

Lynge, E. and Thygesen, L. (1990). Occupational cancer in Denmark. Cancer incidence in the 1970 census population. *Scandinavian Journal of Work Environment and Health*, **16**, (Suppl. 2), 1–35.

Mastroiacovo, P., Spagnolo, A., Marni, E., Meazza, L., Bertollini, R., and Segni, G. (1988). Birth defects in the Seveso area after TCDD contamination. *Journal of the American Medical Association*, 1668–72.

Merlo, F., Puntoni, R., and Santi, L. (1986). The Seveso episode: the validity of epidemiological inquiries in relation with the definition of population at risk. *Chemosphere*, **15**, 1777–86.

Mocarelli, P., Marocchi, A., Brambilla, P., Gerthoux, P. M., Young, D., and Mantel, N. (1986). Clinical laboratory manifestations of exposure to dioxin in children: a six-year study of the effects of an environmental disaster near Seveso, Italy. *Journal of the American Medical Association*, **256**, 2687–95.

Mocarelli, P., Patterson, O. G., Jr, Marocchi, A., and Needham, L. L. (1990). Pilot study (phase II) for determining polychlorinated dibenzo-*p*-dioxin (PCDD) and polychlorinated dibenzofuran (PCDF) levels in serum of Seveso, Italy resident collected at the time of exposure: future plans. *Chemosphere*, **20**, 967–74.

Pesatori, A. C., Zocchetti, C., Tironi, A., Landi, M. T., and Bertazzi, P. A. (1990). Mortality among persons aged 1–20 years after accidental exposure to dioxin (TCDD). *23rd International Congress on Occupational Health, 22–28 September, Montreal.*

Pesatori, A. C., *et al.* (1991). Cancer incidence and dioxin exposure: the Seveso experience. *Eighth International Symposium on Epidemiology in Occupational Health, Paris, 10–12 September.*

Pocchiari, F., Di Domenico, A., Silano, V., and Zapponi, G. (1983). Environmental impact of the accidental release of tetrachlorodibenzo-*p*-dioxin (TCDD) at Seveso (Italy). In *Accidental exposure to dioxins. Human health aspects*, (ed. F. Coulston and F. Pocchiari), pp. 5–35. Academic Press, London.

Puntoni, R., Merlo, F., Fini, A., Meazza, L., and Santi, L. (1986). Soft tissue sarcomas in Seveso. *Lancet*, **ii**, 525 (letter).

Ratti, S. P., Belli, G., Bertazzi, P. A., Bressi, G., Cerlesi, S., and Panetsos, F. (1987). TCDD distribution on all the territory around Seveso; its use in epidemiology and a hint into dynamical models. *Chemosphere*, **16**, 1765–73.

Regione Lombardia (1984). *Final report and recommendations of the 6th International Steering Committee Meeting*. Regione Lombardia, Milan.

Rehder, H., Sanchioni, L., Cefis, F., and Gropp, A. (1978). Pathologischembryologische Untersuchungen an Abortusfällen im Zusammenhang mit dem Seveso-Unglück. *Schweizerische Medizinische Wochenschrift*, **108**, 1617–25.

Silano, V. (1981). Case study: accidental release of 2,3,7,8-tetrachlorodibenzo-*p*-dioxin (TCDD) at Seveso, Italy. In *Planning emergency response systems for chemical accidents*, pp. 167–203. World Health Organization, Regional Office for Europe, Copenhagen.

Suskind, R. (1990). The association of selected cancers with service in the US military in Vietnam. *Archives of Internal Medicine*, **150**, 2449–50.

Tenchini, M. L., Grimaudo, C., Pacchetti, G., Mottura, A., Agosti, S., and De Carli, L. (1983). A comparative cytogenetic study on cases of induced abortions in TCDD-exposed and nonexposed women. *Environmental Mutagenesis*, **5**, 73–85.

Wiklund, E., Dich, J., and Holm, L. E. (1989). Risk of soft tissue sarcoma, Hodgkin's disease and non-Hodgkin lymphoma among Swedish licensed pesticide applicators. *Chemosphere*, **18**, 395–400.

Zedda, S., Cirla, A. M., and Sala, C. (1976). Contaminazione accidentale da tetraclorodibenzoparadiossina. Considerazioni sull'episodio ICMESA. *La Medicina del Lavoro*, **67**, 372–8.

29. Cancer of the larynx and lung near incinerators of waste solvents and oils in Britain

P. Elliott, J. A. Beresford, D. J. Jolley, S. H. Pattenden, and M. Hills

The background and methods of the Small Area Health Statistics Unit (SAHSU) are outlined in Chapter 10. Here we give an example of an enquiry carried out on the SAHSU data-base of cancer incidence around incinerators of waste solvents and oils in Britain. This followed reports by Gatrell and Lovett (undated, 1990), Diggle (1990), and Gatrell (1990) of a 'cluster' of cases of cancer of the larynx around an incinerator at Charnock Richard, Coppull, Lancashire. The example illustrates the problems of interpretation that arise when the health statistics around an industrial site are scrutinized without a prior hypothesis (following complaints from the public concerning a possible health hazard related to emissions from the site), and also the steps that can be taken to further investigate the problem. Further details of the study are published (Elliott *et al.* 1992*a*).

Background

The site at Charnock Richard which gave rise to the enquiry was used as an incinerator from 1972 to 1980; the original incinerator was replaced by a new design around 1976. In response to complaints and concern about odours, nuisance, and possible health hazards, the local council commissioned a study to investigate the possible health effects. An analysis (unpublished) of the incidence of leukaemia and selected solid tumours was carried out for electoral wards in the vicinity of the incinerator. Cancer sites studied included bladder, oesophagus, stomach, larynx, and lung. No statistically significant excesses were found (cited by Gatrell and Lovett, undated).

Chorley and South Ribble Health Authority, in which the incinerator was located, near its southern boundary, then commissioned a preliminary investigation into the geographical distribution of selected cancers within the Health Authority. Cases of cancers of the oesophagus, stomach, rectum, liver, larynx, lung, and bladder diagnosed between 1974 and 1983 were mapped, by converting the unit postcode of their address of residence at registration to Ordnance

Survey grid references using the Central Postcode Directory. On visual inspection of the maps, nothing unusual was seen for cancers of the lung, stomach, rectum, bladder, and oesophagus. For cancers of the liver and larynx, however, apparent 'clusters' were detected by eye, although the 'cluster' of cancer of the liver was not in the vicinity of the incinerator and was not considered further. That left a possible 'cluster' of five cases of cancer of the larynx (out of a total of 58 cases registered in the Health Authority from 1974 to 1983), all of whom lived in Coppull, including four cases living within 2 km of the incinerator site. It was concluded that the spatial distribution of cancer of the larynx was sufficiently unusual to warrant further investigation and more rigorous statistical analysis (Gatrell and Lovett undated, 1990).

The statistical method adopted is described by Diggle (1990) and Gatrell (1990). In summary, it uses a Poisson point process model which states that the intensity of disease (that is, the mean number of cases per unit area) in the neighbourhood of a point is proportional to the product of a background intensity (which reflects, for example, the age and sex distribution at the point) and a function of distance from the putative source of pollution. The model provides a statistical test of whether proximity to the source is (significantly) related to the incidence of the disease in question, in this case cancer of the larynx.

The method requires a measure of background intensity against which the intensity of the disease under study is compared. The authors chose not to use population data for this purpose, arguing instead for the use of a surrogate measure of the natural spatial variation in disease. In the analyses described by Diggle (1990), the distribution of the 978 cases of cancer of the lung occurring in the Chorley and Ribble Health District during the period was used. According to Gatrell and Lovett (undated) the map of lung cancer cases reflected the underlying population distribution, and lung cancer was assumed *not* to be associated with the point of interest (the incinerator site). Using this model, the incidence of cancer of the larynx was found to be significantly associated with distance from the incinerator, although 'Most of the evidence for the raised incidence near the incinerator derives from the cluster of four cases . . .' (Diggle 1990).

In summary, following complaints about the incinerator at Charnock Richard, *post hoc* visual inspection of data for a number of cancers in the local Health Authority revealed a possible 'cluster' of cases of cancer of the larynx nearby. This visual impression was supported by formal statistical analysis in which the distribution of cases of cancer of the larynx around the incinerator was compared to an 'expected' distribution based on the distribution of cases of cancer of the lung.

Methods

After SAHSU had conducted an initial examination of the data for Charnock Richard, the enquiry was extended to all 10 licensed incinerators of waste solvents and oils in Great Britain (including Charnock Richard) which began operation before 1979, and which could be identified by the Department of the Environment as having burned a similar type of waste to the incinerator at Charnock Richard.

Cancer of the lung (International Classification of Disease, eighth and ninth revision, 161) was included in the study as well as cancer of the larynx (ICD 162). Not only is cancer of the lung the most common respiratory cancer, but it shares a number of epidemiological features with cancer of the larynx (e.g. strong social class gradient, with higher rates in the lower social classes; strong relationship with cigarette smoking), and has been associated with ambient air pollution secondary to combustion processes (Doll and Peto 1981). As described above, lung cancer was also used in previous analyses of the data for Charnock Richard to give information on the expected spatial distribution of cases of cancer of the larynx.

Only those cases were included for which a complete postcode of address at the time of registration was available. As described in Chapter 10, the postcode allows cases to be located (via a grid reference attached) and linked to population data at the level of census enumeration district (ED). Postcoded cancer registration data for 1974–84 (England and Wales) and 1975–87 (Scotland) were analysed. On preliminary examination of the data, there were over 2000 cases of cancer of the larynx with inadequate postcoding out of a total of more than 22 000 cases (10 per cent), but after a special postcoding exercise there remained only 73 cases with doubtful postcodes possibly near the sites which could not be included in the analyses. For the purposes of this enquiry, no extra postcoding was undertaken for cancer of the lung, although further postcoding of *all* cancers has subsequently been carried out by the Office of Population Censuses and Surveys (OPCS). Confirmation was sought of the registration details of all cases of cancer of the larynx near the sites in Scotland and a 10 per cent random sample of cases near the sites in England (one duplicate registration was discovered).

For solid tumours, a lag period should be assumed between first exposure to a putative agent and development of clinical disease; here, we have allowed lag periods of 5 and 10 years (10 years is likely to be biologically more appropriate). In the analysis using a five-year lag period, the years over which cases were recorded started 5 years after each site was registered or began operation; cases were recorded similarly for the ten-year lag period. Where the exact dates of operation of a site were unknown, it was assumed that operations started from the date of first registration of the site.

Population counts from the small-area statistics for the 1981 census gave data on population at the level of the census ED. Standard national incidence rates (for Great Britain) for cancer of the larynx and lung by sex and five-year age-group were obtained directly from the SAHSU data-base. To take account of regional differences in reporting levels and incidence rates, standardized registration ratios (SRRs) were also calculated for each cancer registry included in the study. The expected values for each site calculated from national rates were then multiplied by the SRR relevant to that site, to give regionally adjusted expected values, which were used in subsequent analyses.

Standard rates for cancer of the larynx were based on the whole period (1975–84) for which data for Great Britain were available, for all 10 incinerator sites. *All* cases (fully postcoded and incompletely postcoded) were used in the calculation of rates because a special attempt had been made to obtain post-codes on all cases near the sites. For cancer of the lung, standard rates were based only on postcoded cases; to allow for secular trends in completeness of postcoding and in incidence, the expected values for each site were obtained using standard rates based on the same years as those for which the site was under study.

To allow for possible socio-economic confounding, the national age–sex-specific rates were also calculated separately within strata based on Carstairs' index, an areal measure of socio-economic status, values of which were calculated for all EDs in Great Britain. These strata were made up of EDs which were in the same quintile of the national (i.e. Great Britain) distribution of values of Carstairs' index as described in Chapter 11. A further (sixth) stratum comprised EDs for which the index could not be measured (approximately 5 per cent of the EDs and 0.7 per cent of persons).

To find the expected number of cases adjusted for Carstairs' index, the component EDs (and hence the underlying population) of each area of analysis were classified according to strata of Carstairs' index. Expected numbers of cases within these strata were then found in the usual way by standardization for age and sex, and summed over strata to give the stratified expected value for that area.

Statistical methods

Two sets of circles were selected a priori for analysis around each site. First, circles of 3 and 10 km were chosen to examine observed/expected (*O/E*) ratios close to and further away from the sites. The larger circle (10 km) was considered to enclose the area of any hypothesized effect. The smaller circle was selected to represent an area close to the sites for which sufficient data for meaningful inference (across all sites) could be expected. Secondly, circles of radius 0.5, 1.0, 2.0. 3.0, 4.9, 6.3, 7.4, 8.3, 9.2, and 10.0 km were chosen, again a priori. The first four circle sizes were selected to investigate effects close to the sites, and the latter six to give successive bands between circles of approximately equal areas.

The numbers of cases observed, the numbers expected (based on regionally adjusted standard rates with and without stratification by Carstairs' index) and the *O/E* ratios were found for the bands between the various circles around each site. Observed and expected numbers were also summed over all sites to give an overall estimate of *O/E* for each band. The analysis proceeded in two phases, based first on the choice of two circles, made a priori, and second on all 10 circles. For the 3 km circle and outer band (between 3 and 10 km), *O/E* ratios were calculated together with their 95 per cent confidence intervals using the Poisson distribution, to give independent measures of disease frequency near and more distant from the source. An analysis based on Stone (1988) using all 10 circles was then carried out (see Chapter 20) to give likelihood ratio tests (and *p*-values) for *overall* departure from *O/E* = 1 around the site, and also *trend* in *O/E* with distance from the site.

Results

Charnock Richard

Observed and expected numbers of cases of cancer of the larynx and lung, *O/E* ratios and 95 per cent confidence intervals for the bands from 0 to 3 km and 3–10 km, for five- and ten-year lag periods, are shown in Table 29.1. For cancer of the larynx with the ten-year lag, there was only one case within 3 km. With the five-year lag, there were six cases within 3 km (*O/E* 1.43 unstratified and 1.57 stratified by Carstairs' index). From 3 to 10 km, there were 76 cases observed (*O/E* 0.95 unstratified and 0.96 stratified). None of these results approached statistical significance at the 5 per cent level. When data for all 10 bands were examined with a five-year lag, no cases of cancer of the larynx were observed until five were seen in band 3 (i.e. from 1 to 2 km from the site) with an expected number (Carstairs' stratified) of 1.5, giving an *O/E* ratio for that band of 3.34. However, when *O/E*s for all 10 bands were tested using Stone's method, there was no evidence of overall departure from unity (*p* = 0.22) nor for trend of decreasing risk with distance (*p* = 0.13). For cancer of the lung, *O/E* ratios were non-significantly less than 1 near the sites (Table 29.1).

Pooled analysis

Table 29.2 shows observed and expected numbers of cases, aggregated over all 10 sites, for the bands from 0 to 3 km and 3–10 km and for five- and ten-year lag periods. For cancer of the larynx, the largest *O/E* ratio was 1.08 and all 95 per cent confidence intervals (CIs) included unity. For cancer of the lung with a five-year lag period and without stratification, there was a 3 per cent excess from 3 to 10 km of the sites which (because of the large numbers) was nominally significant at the 5 per cent level, but which disappeared after stratification by Carstairs' index. With a ten-year lag period without stratification, there was a significant 8 per cent deficit from 3 to 10 km, which all but disappeared after stratification. The confidence intervals of all the other *O/E* ratios for lung cancer shown in Table 29.2 include unity. When all 10 bands were examined, none of the tests overall (testing for *O/E* different from 1) or tests for trend (of decreasing risk with distance from site) approached statistical significance at the 5 per cent level.

Table 29.1 Charnock Richard: observed (O) and expected (E) numbers of cases, O/E ratios and 95% confidence intervals within bands 3 km and 3–10 km of the site, without and with stratification by Carstairs' index. Five- and ten-year lag periods, males and females combined, cancer of the larynx and lung

Site of cancer	Lag period (yr)	Carstairs' stratified	Band (km)	No. of cases		O/E ratio	95% confidence interval	
				Observed	Expected		Lower	Upper
Larynx	5	No	0–3	6	4.2	1.43	0.52	3.12
	5	No	3–10	76	80.0	0.95	0.75	1.19
	10	No	0–3	1	1.6	0.64	0.01	3.55
	10	No	3–10	27	30.0	0.90	0.59	1.31
	5	Yes	0–3	6	3.8	1.57	0.58	3.42
	5	Yes	3–10	76	78.8	0.96	0.76	1.21
	10	Yes	0–3	1	1.4	0.70	0.02	3.89
	10	Yes	3–10	27	29.5	0.91	0.60	1.33
Lung	5	No	0–3	58	75.3	0.77	0.58	1.00
	5	No	3–10	1418	1433.7	0.99	0.94	1.04
	10	No	0–3	24	31.8	0.75	0.48	1.12
	10	No	3–10	607	605.6	1.00	0.92	1.09
	5	Yes	0–3	58	69.3	0.84	0.64	1.08
	5	Yes	3–10	1418	1419.3	1.00	0.95	1.05
	10	Yes	0–3	24	29.2	0.82	0.53	1.22
	10	Yes	3–10	607	599.7	1.01	0.93	1.10

Table 29.2 Pooled analysis: observed (*O*) and expected (*E*) numbers of cases, *O/E* ratios and 95% confidence intervals within bands 3 km and 3–10 km of the sites, without and with stratification by Carstairs' index. Five- and ten-year lag periods, males and females combined, cancer of the larynx and lung

Site of cancer	Lag period (yr)	Carstairs' stratified	Band (km)	No. of cases Observed	No. of cases Expected	O/E ratio	95% confidence interval Lower	95% confidence interval Upper
Larynx	5	No	0–3	48	44.5	1.08	0.79	1.43
	5	No	3–10	342	321.0	1.07	0.96	1.19
	10	No	0–3	20	19.0	1.05	0.64	1.63
	10	No	3–10	50	57.3	0.87	0.65	1.15
	5	Yes	0–3	48	46.0	1.04	0.77	1.38
	5	Yes	3–10	342	330.3	1.04	0.93	1.15
	10	Yes	0–3	20	18.5	1.08	0.66	1.67
	10	Yes	3–10	50	53.2	0.94	0.70	1.24
Lung	5	No	0–3	914	907.8	1.01	0.94	1.07
	5	No	3–10	6659	6437.5	1.03	1.01	1.06
	10	No	0–3	361	393.5	0.92	0.83	1.02
	10	No	3–10	1054	1149.4	0.92	0.86	0.97
	5	Yes	0–3	914	943.7	0.97	0.91	1.03
	5	Yes	3–10	6659	6660.5	1.00	0.98	1.02
	10	Yes	0–3	361	385.7	0.94	0.84	1.04
	10	Yes	3–10	1054	1072.4	0.98	0.92	1.04

Data reproduced from the *Lancet*, with permission.

Discussion

We found no evidence of association between cancer of the larynx or lung and incinerators of waste solvents and oils of the type found at Charnock Richard. The 'cluster' of cases of cancer of the larynx originally described near Charnock Richard was found following visual inspection of the data for a number of cancers. A statistically significant association with cancer of the larynx near Charnock Richard, in comparison with the geographical distribution of cancer of the lung, was found by Diggle (1990) but not confirmed here using Stone's method. It may be that the (non-significant) deficit of cancer of the lung shown here within 3 km of the incinerator exaggerated the findings for cancer of the larynx in Diggle's analysis. (Also the point process model is less generalisable than Stone's method; see Chapter 19.) In addition, as discussed by Diggle (1990), his analysis could take no account of the *post hoc* nature of the original finding.

The analyses set out here are a good illustration of the approach adopted by SAHSU in response to reports of a suspected cluster of disease around an industrial site. After examination of the data for Charnock Richard, the enquiry was widened to include all incinerators in Great Britain that could be identified as having burned similar waste. From an initial *post hoc* observation at Charnock Richard, a formal null hypothesis (of no excess risk of cancer of the larynx) could be set up for the analyses around all sites, taking into account the age–sex structure of the population and the socio-economic profile of the study areas. In the event, there was no evidence to reject that null hypothesis; if such evidence *had* been found, then further investigation would have been indicated, for example, review of case notes, collection of environmental data, or the setting up of formal case-control studies. These points are discussed more fully by Elliott et al. (1992a,b) and in Chapters 2 and 23.

References

Diggle, P. J. (1990). A point process modelling approach to raised incidence of a rare phenomenon in the vicinity of a prespecified point. *Journal of the Royal Statistical Society, Series A*, **153**, 349–62.

Doll, R. and Peto, R. (1981). The causes of cancer. Quantitative estimates of avoidable risks of cancer in the United States today. Oxford University Press, Oxford.

Elliott, P., et al. (1992a). Incidence of cancer of the larynx and lung near incinerators of waste solvents and oils in Great Britain. *Lancet*, **339**, 854–8.

Elliott, P., et al. (1992b). The Small Area Health Statistics Unit: a national facility for investigating health around point sources of environmental pollution in the United Kingdom. *Journal of Epidemiology and Community Health*, in press.

Gatrell, A. C. (1990). *On modelling spatial point patterns in epidemiology: cancer of the larynx in Lancashire*. Research Report No. 9, North West Regional Research Laboratory, Lancaster University.

Gatrell, A. C. and Lovett, A. A. (undated). *Cancers in Chorley and South Ribble Health Authority: Preliminary results of a study on geographical distributions*. Report to the Chorley and South Ribble Health Authority, Department of Geography, University of Lancaster.

Gatrell, A. C. and Lovett, A. A. (1990). *Burning questions: incineration of wastes and implications for human health*. Research report No. 8, North West Regional Research Laboratory, Lancaster University.

Stone, R. A. (1988). Investigations of excess environmental risks around putative sources: statistical problems and a proposed test. *Statistics in Medicine*, 7, 649–60.

30. A study of geographical correlations in China

R. Peto, J. Chen, T. C. Campbell, J. Li, J. Boreham, Z. Feng, and L. Youngman

After some years of analysis, we have at last reported on one of the most diverse geographical correlational studies in the world, involving age-standardized death rates from almost 100 separate causes or groups of causes in each of 65 rural Chinese counties, plus a representative survey of almost 300 characteristics of the populations in each of those counties (Chen *et al*. 1990). The characteristics, most of which were assessed by survey of a random sample of 50 adults from each of two randomly chosen villages in each county, included blood biochemistry, urine biochemistry, diet, smoking, drinking, and much else besides.

A study such as this, which describes the geographical variation of some hundreds of factors in a country as heterogeneous as China, may be used either directly or indirectly for medical research. Its direct value is as a source of correlations between diseases, between diseases and factors that might affect those diseases, or between one factor and another. Its indirect value is simply as a source of statistical information that can be exploited in many different ways. Parts of it may be used to help develop an overall description of some recent large developments in preventive medicine in China, while other parts may be used to help design more specific studies of particular questions.

Both a particular strength and, paradoxically, a particular weakness of the study is the vast heterogeneity between different counties of many of the death rates, and of many of the other characteristics. The reason why such hetero-geneity is a strength is obvious: for example, the massively significant correla-tions between age-standardized mortality from schistosomiasis (chiefly, in China, *Schistosoma japonicum*, which chronically affects the large intestine) and colorectal cancer ($r = 0.89$, $2p < 0.001$) is unusual in that this geographical correlation provides of itself very strong evidence of an important causal relationship (Fig. 30.1). The reason why wide variation in real disease rates is a weakness, however, is that failure to find a strong correlation between a particular disease and a particular factor that has been reliably measured is not good evidence that the factor is unimportant. Instead, it merely indicates that geographical variation in that particular factor does not determine the main

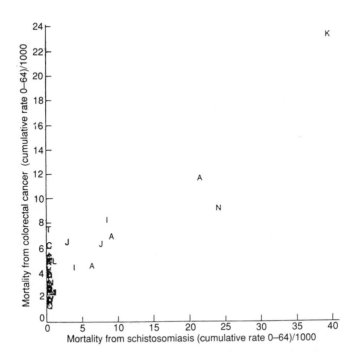

Fig. 30.1 Relationship between mortality from schistosomiasis and colorectal cancer in China.

geographical variation in that particular disease. For example, there are in China a few patches of particularly high mortality from cancer of the oesophagus—indeed, in the worst affected counties the disease is about 100 times more common than in some of the low-incidence areas, and some of these differences are known to have persisted for centuries. Smoking is a more recent habit, and the variation in tobacco use from one part of China to another happens not to correlate with the main variations in cancer of the oesophagus ($r = -0.18$, for total current tobacco consumption), even though, in each area, tobacco may multiply up the local risk factors and thereby account for more than half the male deaths from cancer of the oesophagus (specific studies to this particular hypothesis are now in progress).

Furthermore, a review (Doll and Peto 1981) of what was known about the causes of cancer in developed countries, such as the USA stated:

'Trustworthy epidemiological evidence, it should be noted, always requires demonstration that a relationship holds for individuals (or perhaps small groups) within a large population as well as between large population groups. Correlation between the incidence of cancer in whole towns or whole countries and, for example, the consumption of particular items of food can, at most, provide hypotheses for investigation by other means. Attempts to separate the roles of causative and of confounding factors by the statistical techniques of multiple regression analysis have been made often, but evidence obtained in this way is, at best, of only marginal value.

It is commonly, but mistakenly, supposed that multiple regression, logistic regression or various forms of standardization can routinely be used to answer the question of whether the correlation of exposure (E) with disease (D) is due merely to a common correlation of both with some confounding factors (C). The trouble is that unless the confounding factors are something such as age or sex that can be estimated with negligible measurement error, adjustment by any standard statistical techniques of the correlation of E with D for the measured values of C will reduce but will not extinguish the correlations of E with D even if, given the error-free (but unknown) values of C, no correlation between E and D would remain. Moreover, it is obvious that multiple regression cannot correct for important variables that have not been recorded at all.'

That was written chiefly about geographical studies that are far less thorough and reliable than our study in China. However, consideration of the evidence provided by the geographical correlations in our study on a few previously established causal relationships (e.g. tobacco/lung cancer, cholesterol/ coronary heart disease, selenium/Keshan disease, hepatitis B/hepatoma) suggests that the statement above may well remain valid even in our study.

Plasma cotinine, for example, is a nicotine metabolite that is a highly specific marker of tobacco use, yet cotinine levels are negatively correlated with lung cancer (simply because the chief cause of lung cancer is prolonged cigarette smoking, and in many parts of China other types of tobacco still yield more nicotine than cigarettes do). Perhaps the most important observation, therefore, is not the geographical correlation of 1983 tobacco with 1973–5 disease, but the very high levels of cigarette smoking in many areas, which experience in other countries (and in Shanghai) shows will eventually result in massive mortality rates in middle age.

Likewise, plasma apolipoprotein B is a marker of the type of blood cholesterol that causes most coronary heart disease (CHD) in countries such as the US, where meat and dairy products are now used widely and in which CHD has now become the most common cause of death. In our study, however, it is apparent that dairy and animal produce is used very little, and CHD rates are low and are only weakly correlated with apolipoprotein B ($r = 0.38$, $2p < 0.01$), suggesting that variation in that type of blood cholesterol is not at present the chief reason for any variation in CHD within China. Again, perhaps the most useful observation is not the geographical correlation but the absolute mean fat intake level (15 per cent of dietary energy, as opposed to 40–45 per cent in some Western countries), the absolute mean cholesterol level (mean = 127 mg/dl, which is only just over half what is commonly seen in the UK or US), and the absolute mortality rate attributed to CHD (which is less than one-tenth of that in the UK or US).

If other specific case-control studies are to be undertaken, then, as for studies of smoking, this geographical study may help to choose counties where studies have a particularly good chance of being fruitful. For example, there is one county that has a moderately high oesophageal cancer rate, a low ascorbate intake, and a high level of endogenous nitrosation. These characteristics may or may not be connected, but they would make that county a promising place to try to discover whether endogenous nitrosation is of much relevance to human cancer. In another county, the population drinks on average a few litres of wine a week; one uses water-pipes extensively; one has an unusually high proportion of female smokers; one has massive stroke death rates; one has even more massive death rates from chronic lung disease; in one, the population consumes milk regularly; a few have mean cholesterol levels of less than 100 mg/dl (and might repay an autopsy study of coronary arteries); some still have really low plasma selenium levels; and so on. (Research into the causes of chronic lung disease is particularly indicated, for the rates are already extraordinarily high for reasons that may at present have little to do with tobacco, especially among females.)

A further difficulty with geographical correlation studies is that they may be of little scientific value (particularly if the correlations are not particularly strong) unless the sources of variation of the putatively causative factors can be characterized reliably. There are several sources of variations to be assessed —variation within one village, variation between different villages in the same county, variation between the same county in different years, and variation between the same county in different decades. The first is dealt with by studying several people per village. (For many factors, the biochemical assay costs can be greatly reduced by making a physical pool of parts of the blood samples, e.g. from all the males in one village, and then assaying the pool instead of assaying each male separately, and averaging the answers.) The second is dealt with by examining the correlation between the values in the two different villages. Only if (as, for example, for plasma selenium) it is strong have the real differences between counties (in plasma selenium) been sufficiently well characterized for between-county correlations to be straightforwardly interpretable. Variation from one year to another has been dealt with by undertaking a complete resurvey in 1989–90; only factors whose measured values in the early 1980s correlate with their measured values in the late 1980s can usefully be correlated with chronic disease patterns. Finally, of course, even if the patterns of exposure in the 1980s have been measured in a way that is statistically reliable, they may not correlate with the disease patterns now but a few decades hence. Failure to appreciate this has led to much misinterpretation of 'positive' correlations between air pollution and lung cancer in countries where cigarette smoking became widespread first among urban males. Conversely, it has also led to much misinterpretation of 'null' correlations of national lung cancer rates with current smoking habits (Doll and Peto 1981). In Chinese males, as in many European female populations, the large recent increases in cigarette consumption will have their chief effects on lung cancer only after a delay of several decades.

References

Chen, J., Campbell, T. C., Li, J., and Peto, R. (1990). *Diet, mortality and lifestyle in China.* Oxford University Press, UK; Cornell University Press, US; and People's Medical Publishing House, People's Republic of China.

Doll, R. and Peto, R. (1981). *The causes of cancer.* Oxford University Press.

Index